Constructing the Viennese Modern Body

This book takes a new, interdisciplinary approach to analyzing modern Viennese visual culture, one informed by Austro-German theater, contemporary medical treatises centered on hysteria, and an original examination of dramatic gestures in expressionist artworks. It centers on the following question: How and to what end was the human body discussed, portrayed, and utilized as an aesthetic metaphor in turn-of-the-century Vienna? By scrutinizing theatrically "hysterical" performances, avant-garde puppet plays, and images created by Oskar Kokoschka, Koloman Moser, Egon Schiele and others, Nathan J. Timpano discusses how Viennese artists favored the pathological or puppet-like body as their contribution to European modernism.

Nathan J. Timpano is Assistant Professor of Art History at the University of Miami.

Studies in Art Historiography
Series Editor: Richard Woodfield
University of Birmingham

The aim of this series is to support and promote the study of the history and practice of art historical writing focusing on its institutional and conceptual foundations, from the past to the present day in all areas and all periods. Besides addressing the major innovators of the past it also encourages the re-thinking of ways in which the subject may be written in the future. It ignores the disciplinary boundaries imposed by the Anglophone expression "art history" and allows and encourages the full range of enquiry that encompasses the visual arts in its broadest sense as well as topics falling within archaeology, anthropology, ethnography, and other specialist disciplines and approaches.

5 **The Expressionist Turn in Art History**
A Critical Anthology
Edited by Kimberly A. Smith

6 **Mariette and the Science of the Connoisseur in Eighteenth-Century Europe**
Kristel Smentek

7 **Vladimir Markov and Russian Primitivism**
A Charter for the Avant-Garde
Jeremy Howard, Irēna Bužinska, and Z. S. Strother

8 **Architecture and the Late Ottoman Historical Imaginary**
Reconfiguring the Architectural Past in a Modernizing Empire
Ahmet A. Ersoy

9 **Michael Baxandall, Vision and the Work of Words**
Edited by Pater Mack and Robert Williams

10 **Circulations in the Global History of Art**
*Edited by Thomas DaCosta Kaufmann, Catherine Dossin,
and Béatrice Joyeux-Prunel*

11 **Video Art Historicized**
Traditions and Negotiations
Malin Hedlin Hayden

Constructing the Viennese Modern Body

Art, Hysteria, and the Puppet

Nathan J. Timpano

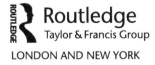

Routledge
Taylor & Francis Group

LONDON AND NEW YORK

First published 2017
by Routledge
2 Park Square, Milton Park, Abingdon, Oxon OX14 4RN

605 Third Avenue, New York, NY 10017

First issued in paperback 2020

Routledge is an imprint of the Taylor & Francis Group, an informa business

Library of Congress Cataloging-in-Publication Data
A catalog record for this book has been requested

ISBN 13: 978-0-367-73618-7 (pbk)
ISBN 13: 978-1-138-22018-8 (hbk)

Typeset in Sabon
by codeMantra

Contents

List of Illustrations   vi
List of Plates   ix
Acknowledgments   x

Introduction: A Conundrum of the Viennese Modern Body   1

1   "The Semblance of Things": Re-Visioning Viennese Expressionism   17

2   "The Woman Emerges": Medical Vision and the Spectacle of Hysteria   43

3   Performing Hysteria: A Vogue for Hystero-Theatrical Gestures   66

4   A Tale of Three Hysterics: Elektra, Isolde, and Salome   91

5   The Inanimate Body Speaks: The Language of the Marionette Theater   121

6   Pathological Puppets: The Body and the Marionette in Viennese Expressionism   153

Bibliography   189
Index   203

List of Illustrations

I.1   Gustav Klimt, *Adele Bloch-Bauer I*, 1907, oil, silver and gold leaf on canvas. Acquired through the generosity of Ronald S. Lauder, the heirs of the Estates of Ferdinand and Adele Bloch-Bauer, and the Estée Lauder Fund, Neue Galerie, New York.   1

I.2   Pablo Picasso, *Les Demoiselles d'Avignon*, 1907, oil on canvas. Acquired through the Lille P. Bliss Bequest, The Museum of Modern Art, New York.   2

I.3   Wassily Kandinsky, *Untitled*, 1910, watercolor and Indian ink and graphite on paper. Musée National d'Art Moderne, Centre Georges Pompidou, Paris.   3

I.4   Gustav Klimt, *Philosophy*, 1900–07, oil on canvas. Destroyed by fire in 1945 at Schloss Immendorf.   7

I.5   Gustav Klimt, *Medicine*, 1900–07, oil on canvas. Destroyed by fire in 1945 at Schloss Immendorf.   8

I.6   Paul Régnard, *Tétanisme*, image of Augustine, hysterical patient of Jean-Martin Charcot, published in *Iconographie photographique de la Salpêtrière*, vol. II, c. 1878, photograph.   10

I.7   Egon Schiele, *Nude Pregnant Woman Reclining*, 1910, gouache and black chalk on paper. Leopold Museum, Private Collection, Vienna.   10

1.1   Gustav Klimt, *Judith II (Salome)*, 1909, oil on canvas. Galleria d'Arte Moderna di Ca'Pesaro, Venice.   29

1.2   Oskar Kokoschka, *The Awakening*, from *The Dreaming Youths*, 1907, printed 1908, color lithograph. Wien Museum Karlsplatz, Vienna, Austria.   30

1.3   Egon Schiele, *The Hermits*, 1912, oil on canvas. Leopold Museum, Vienna.   35

2.1   French School, *L'arche de pont*, in *Iconographie photographique de la Salpêtrière*, c. 1884, print. Bibliothèque de la Faculté de Médecine, Paris, France.   53

2.2   Pierre Aristide André Brouillet, *A Clinical Lesson at the Salpêtrière*, 1887, oil on canvas. Paris Descartes University, Paris.   54

2.3   Jean-François Badoureau, *Hystero-epileptic attack: period of contortions*, in *Iconographie photographique de la Salpêtrière*, after a drawing by M. Richer, 1876, pen and ink on paper. Private Collection.   60

3.1   W. & D. Downey, Sarah Bernhardt as Adrienne Lecouvreur,
      19th century, sepia photograph on paper. Bequeathed by Guy Little.
      Victoria and Albert Museum, London.   70

3.2   Henri de Toulouse-Lautrec, *Jane Avril Dancing*, c. 1892, oil on
      cardboard. Musée d'Orsay, Paris.   71

4.1   Anna Bahr-Mildenburg as Klytaemnestra in Richard Strauss'
      Elektra, 1909, photograph. Theatermuseum, Vienna.   94

4.2   Anna Bahr-Mildenburg as Klytaemnestra in Richard Strauss'
      Elektra, 1910, photograph. Theatermuseum, Vienna.   95

4.3   Annie Krull as Elektra and Johannes Sembach as Aegisth in
      Richard Strauss' *Elektra*, 1909, photograph.   96

4.4   Maria Gärtner as Elektra in Richard Strauss' *Elektra*, 1909,
      photograph. Theatermuseum, Vienna.   97

4.5   Anna Bahr-Mildenburg as Isolde in Richard Wagner's *Tristan
      and Isolde*, c. 1900, photograph. Theatermuseum, Vienna.   100

4.6   Alfred Roller, costume design for Anna Bahr-Mildenburg as
      Isolde in Richard Wagner's *Tristan and Isolde* (1903), dated 1904,
      mixed media on paper. Theatermuseum, Vienna.   101

4.7   Alexander Moissi as King Oedipus in Hugo von Hofmannsthal's
      and Max Reinhardt's *Oedipus Rex*, c. 1910, photograph.   102

4.8   Anna Bahr-Mildenburg, c. 1928/30, photograph. Theatermuseum,
      Vienna.   104

4.9   Egon Schiele, *Woman with Blue Hair*, 1908, gouache, watercolor
      and pencil on paper. Private Collection.   105

4.10 Gustave Moreau, *The Apparition*, 1874–76, oil on canvas. Musée
      Gustave Moreau, Paris, France.   106

4.11 Franz von Stuck, *Salome*, 1906, distemper on canvas. Städtische
      Galerie im Lenbachhaus, Munich.   109

4.12 Franz von Stuck, *Dancing Salome*, 1906, oil on wood panel.
      Private Collection.   109

4.13 Maud Allan as Salome in *The Vision of Salomé*, c. 1908,
      photograph. Private Collection.   110

4.14 Josef von Divéky, *Poster for the Cabaret Fledermaus*, 1907,
      color lithograph. Sammlungen der Universität für angewandte
      Kunst Wien, Vienna.   113

5.1   Lotte Pritzel, *Puppets for the Cabinet*, c. 1910, photograph
      reproduced on page 333 in *Deutsche Kunst und Dekoration*
      (October 1910–March 1911).   134

5.2   Wayang golek, 19th–20th century, fabric and painted wood.   135

5.3   Wayang kulit shadow puppets from Java, Indonesia, late 18th–early
      19th century, leather, wood and paint. Private Collection.   136

5.4   Richard Teschner, The Golden Shrine with rod-puppets,
      c. 1912, photograph. Theatermuseum, Vienna.   137

5.5   Richard Teschner in front of the Figure Mirror, 1941,
      photograph. Theatermuseum, Vienna.   137

5.6   Richard Teschner, Scene from *Nawang Wulan*, as performed in the
      Golden Shrine, 1912, photograph. Theatermuseum, Vienna.   138

5.7   Richard Teschner, Princess and prince rod-puppets from *Princess and Water Elf*, 1913, photograph reproduced on page 171 in *Deutsche Kunst und Dekoration* (October 1913–March 1914).   140

5.8   Richard Teschner, Scene from *Princess and Water Elf*, with the naked magician levitating above the chained prince, 1913, photograph. Theatermuseum, Vienna.   141

6.1   Unknown, *Oskar Kokoschka's Alma-Puppe as Venus*, circa 1918–19, photograph. Private Collection.   163

6.2   Oskar Kokoschka, *Woman in Blue*, circa 1920, oil on canvas. Staatsgalerie, Stuttgart.   164

6.3   Oskar Kokoschka, *Man with Doll*, circa 1922, oil on canvas. Staatliche Museen zu Berlin, Nationalgalerie, Berlin.   165

6.4   Oskar Kokoschka, *Seated "Woman" with Exposed Breasts*, circa 1920, ink on paper. Musée Jenisch, Stiftung Oskar Kokoschka, Vevey.   166

6.5   Arthur Roessler's study at Billrothstrasse 6 in Vienna, showing his Javanese puppets and Egon Schiele's *Setting Sun* on the back wall, circa 1920, photograph. Wien Museum Karlsplatz, Vienna.   169

6.6   Egon Schiele, *Self-Portrait as Saint Sebastian*, 1914/15, watercolor and Indian ink on paper. Wien Museum Karlsplatz, Vienna.   172

6.7   Anton J. Trčka, Egon Schiele, 1914, photograph. Neue Galerie, New York.   173

6.8   Egon Schiele, *Erwin Dominik Osen*, 1910, gouache, watercolor and black chalk on paper. Leopold Museum, Private Collection, Vienna.   174

6.9   Egon Schiele, *Mime van Osen*, 1910, gouache and black chalk on paper. Leopold Museum, Private Collection, Vienna.   174

6.10   Unknown, Erwin Osen and the dancer Moa, c. 1910, photograph. Egon Schiele Archive, Albertina Museum, Vienna.   175

6.11   Egon Schiele, *Self-Portrait with Black Vase and Spread Fingers*, 1911, oil on wood panel. Wien Museum Karlsplatz, Vienna, Austria.   177

6.12   Egon Schiele, *Levitation (The Blind II)*, 1915, oil on canvas. Leopold Collection, Vienna.   177

6.13   Egon Schiele, *Preacher (Nude Self-Portrait with Blue-green Shirt)*, 1913, gouache and pencil on paper. Leopold Museum, Vienna.   179

6.14   Egon Schiele, *Self-Portrait with Striped Armlets*, 1915, gouache and pencil on paper. Leopold Museum, Vienna.   180

6.15   Egon Schiele, *Self-Portrait in Jerkin with Right Elbow Raised*, 1914, gouache, black chalk and pencil on paper. Private Collection.   181

6.16   Egon Schiele, *Two Women Embracing (Two Friends)*, 1915, watercolor, gouache and pencil on paper. Museum of Fine Arts (Szépművészeti) Budapest, Hungary.   182

List of Plates

Plate 1 Oskar Kokoschka, *Hans Tietze and Erica Tietze-Conrat*, 1909, oil on canvas. Abby Aldrich Rockefeller Fund, The Museum of Modern Art, New York.   87

Plate 2 Egon Schiele, *Nude Self-Portrait*, 1910, gouache, watercolor and white heightening. Graphische Sammlung Albertina, Vienna, Austria.   87

Plate 3 Koloman Moser, *The Love Potion—Tristan and Isolde*, 1915, oil on canvas. Leopold Museum, Private Collection, Vienna.   88

Plate 4 Oskar Kokoschka, *Portrait of Lotte Franzos*, 1909, oil on canvas. The Phillips Collection, Washington, D.C., USA. Acquired 1941.   88

Plate 5 Egon Schiele, *Seated Female Nude with Tilted Head and Raised Arms*, 1910, gouache, watercolor and black ink on paper. Private Collection.   89

Plate 6 Gustav Klimt, *Judith I*, 1901, oil on canvas. Österreichische Galerie im Belvedere, Vienna.   89

Plate 7 Egon Schiele, *Portrait of Albert Paris von Gütersloh*, 1918, oil on canvas. Minneapolis Institute of Art, Minneapolis, USA. Gift of the P. D. McMillan Land Company.   90

Plate 8 Egon Schiele, *Two Girls, Lying in an Entwined Position*, 1915, gouache and pencil on paper. Graphische Sammlung Albertina, Vienna, Austria.   90

Acknowledgments

I wish to acknowledge and thank the many individuals that contributed in significant ways to the realization of this book. My gratitude goes to Adam Jolles, Roald Nasgaard, Robert Neuman, and Natalya Baldyga for their many insightful comments on an early version of this project. I am indebted to Perri Lee Roberts, Mihoko Suzuki, and my colleagues at the University of Miami who offered thought-provoking feedback on my manuscript during my year as a faculty fellow at the Center for the Humanities. I am grateful for Matthew Armistead, who provided an adept eye as my proofreader; to my initial editor at Ashgate, Margaret Michniewicz, for her enthusiasm of this project; and to Isabella Vitti and the wonderful editors at Routledge, for their patience and professional expertise throughout this process. I am equally indebted to the outside reviewers of my manuscript, whose astute comments greatly enhanced and clarified my overall arguments, and to Richard Woodfield, who generously included my book in his *Studies in Art Historiography* series. I likewise offer much thanks to Christoph Brenner, Christina Stubenrauch, and Chris Vorstius, who aided me with particularly difficult German translations.

The writing of this book was made possible through the support of a number of national and international grants, including a Fulbright fellowship to Austria, a DAAD grant to Germany, and a Scholar-in-Residence grant from the Robert Gore Rifkind Center for German Expressionist Studies at LACMA. At the Rifkind Center, a number of stimulating conversations with Tim Benson and Erika Esau aided in the analyses presented in this book. I want to recognize, moreover, the following institutions that helped to facilitate research for this project: the Department of Art and Art History at the University of Miami, the Department of Art History at Florida State University, the Federal Republic of Germany's Deutscher Akademischer Austauch Dienst, the Austrian-American Fulbright Commission in Vienna, and the Harvard Art Museums at Harvard University. Thanks are especially owed to Laura Muir, curator at the Harvard Art Museums, for her guidance and support of this project during my tenure at the Busch-Reisinger Museum. Research for this book would not have been possible without access to a number of special collections and archives housed within the city of Vienna, including the collections of the Österreichische Nationalbibliothek, the Kunsthistorisches Museum Wien, the Theatermuseum, the Egon Schiele-Archiv at the Albertina Museum, and the library at the Institut für Kunstgeschichte at the University of Vienna. I am indebted to these institutions for opening their doors and sharing their wealth of information with me.

Earlier versions of portions of Chapter One appear in "The dialectics of vision: Oskar Kokoschka and the historiography of expressionistic sight," *Journal of Art*

Historiography 1, no. 5 (December 2011): 1–13; and portions of Chapters Five and Six in "Body Doubles: The *Puppe* as *Doppelgänger* in Fin-de-Siècle Viennese Visual Culture," in *The Doppelgänger*, ed. Deborah Ascher Barnstone, vol. 3, *German Visual Culture* (Oxford and New York: Peter Lang, 2016), 119–46.

Finally, my deepest gratitude goes to my wife, Kiara Timpano, for her unwavering support, continual encouragement, and wise observations, all of which contributed significantly to the fruition of this book.

Introduction

A Conundrum of the Viennese Modern Body

> Until a few years ago, the artist [Gustav Klimt] ranked as a second-tier modern master both at auction and in the estimation of most art critics and historians. Unlike another painting that was made in 1907, Picasso's "Demoiselles d'Avignon," [Klimt's] "Adele" was the climax, rather than the big-bang launch, of an era.[1]
>
> —Peter Schjeldahl, 2006

According to Peter Schjeldahl, art critic for *The New Yorker*, some scholars of European modernism have only given a passing thought to Gustav Klimt's place in the history of early twentieth-century art. Schjeldahl's appraisal of Klimt's beguiling, gold-covered painting *Adele Bloch-Bauer I* (1907, Figure I.1) thus raises a recurring issue facing *fin-de-siècle* Viennese painters, namely that of their inevitable comparison to more dominant European modernists. The critic's analysis also serves as a

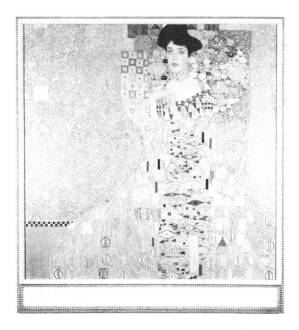

Figure I.1 Gustav Klimt, *Adele Bloch-Bauer I*, 1907, oil, silver and gold leaf on canvas. Acquired through the generosity of Ronald S. Lauder, the heirs of the Estates of Ferdinand and Adele Bloch-Bauer, and the Estée Lauder Fund, Neue Galerie, New York.

Source: Photo: Neue Galerie New York / Art Resource, NY.

reminder that the whole of European modernism, not simply Austrian symbolism, has historically been bound to a narrative that privileges the movement away from figurative painting toward abstraction. In this particular story of modern art, Pablo Picasso's "big-bang launch," with his proto-cubist canvas *Les Demoiselles d'Avignon* (1907, Figure I.2), or Wassily Kandinsky's slightly later exploration of non-objective painting in Munich in 1910 (see Figure I.3), invariably outshine Klimt's shimmering *Adele*. One explanation for this is that Klimt and his fellow Viennese artists continued to pursue an avant-garde exploration of the human body rather than anticipating or embracing abstract compositions.

So what makes a first-tier modern master, and who exactly is qualified to confer this status? And, if a non-figurative aesthetic became synonymous with such prestige, how does one account for the continued interest in the non-abstracted human body in Viennese visual culture at a time when Paris and Munich-based artists were turning away from figuration? In contrast to French and German modernism, the literature on Austrian modernism, and particularly expressionism, is marked by the noticeable absence of such critical enquiries. Indeed, the current scholarship on European modernism on the whole tends to confer a high standing—based purely on chronology—to the "first" non-figurative compositions, suggesting that abstractions from the recognizable world were invariably more modern than representations of the human body. Artists who initially explored cubism or non-objective painting were thus the (seemingly) clear winners in the race to discover new modes of pictorial expression in the early twentieth century, a period often referred to as Vienna's Golden Age. In Schjeldahl's estimation, a *fin-de-siècle* artist like Klimt ultimately failed to attain the "grandeur" of a painter like Picasso precisely because he remained tied to representations of the body and never fully explored alternative styles or cubism.

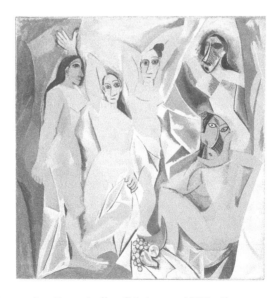

Figure I.2 Pablo Picasso, *Les Demoiselles d'Avignon*, 1907, oil on canvas. Acquired through the Lille P. Bliss Bequest, The Museum of Modern Art, New York.

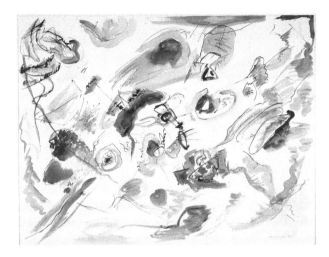

Figure I.3 Wassily Kandinsky, *Untitled*, 1910, watercolor and Indian ink and graphite on paper. Musée National d'Art Moderne, Centre Georges Pompidou, Paris.
Source: © 2016 Artists Rights Society (ARS), New York. Photo: © CNAC / MNAM / Dist. RMN-Grand Palais / Art Resource, NY.

Constructing the Viennese Modern Body: Art, Hysteria, and the Puppet offers an important corrective to this narrative of Austrian modernism. First and foremost, this book examines how representations of the human body remained a relevant and vigorously avant-garde trope in modern Viennese visual culture. In establishing this claim, the book reveals that the new style of figuration in *fin-de-siècle* Vienna was just as revolutionary as the fractured, fragmented, and de-compartmentalized body depicted in cubism or other competing forms of European modernism. As an artistic motif, the Viennese modern body could therefore be seen throughout the city's visual arts, theatrical and avant-garde cabaret performances, and even in medical documentation relating to corporeal pathology, particularly the hysterical body. Accordingly, the non-abstracted body became a focal point and a key exemplar of modernism in *fin-de-siècle* Vienna. The intriguing forms and expressive gestures of the Viennese modern body likewise attracted the attention of scholars and critics for over a century, and yet little consideration has been given to the manner in which expressionists were manipulating the pathological body as though it were a metaphorical puppet controlled by the hand of the modern artist. Just as hysteria laid claim to the theatricality of the pathological body, the puppet body served as a symbol of the expressionists' desire to communicate a theatrically rich gestural language to their viewers through the bodies of their sitters. A conundrum of the modern body was thus born in Vienna.

The Viennese Modern Body

What is the Viennese modern body? How was this modernized body visualized in *fin-de-siècle* Vienna, or elsewhere in Europe during the turn of the century? And why did it play such a significant role in the visual culture of the Wiener Moderne period (as it was called at the time)? In the realms of medicine and theater, it will be shown that the modern body tended to appear uniformly as a pathological or hysterical figure. The modern body that appeared in the visual arts did not, however, emerge through a common iconography, or within a unified artistic style. Instead, multiple permutations materialize in works by Oskar Kokoschka, Egon Schiele, Koloman Moser and their contemporaries. These expressionist artists were not the first, however, to utilize expressive gesture in a painting: one thinks immediately of the role that gesture played in works by the Italian baroque artist Caravaggio, or the French neo-classical painter Jacques-Louis David. The continued interest in corporeal gestures thus placed these young expressionists in a long artistic tradition focused on communicating meaning to the viewer through the body language of their sitters or subjects.

Within the current literature on Austrian modernism, the artistic body in Vienna has principally been subjugated to a Freudian psychoanalytic understanding of narcissism, sexual eroticism, depravity, and death. This is somewhat surprising given that *fin-de-siècle* Viennese artists did not openly acknowledge Sigmund Freud's theories as an inspiration for their images of "pathological" figures. Despite this conundrum, works by Kokoschka, Schiele, and Moser are often subjected to a psychoanalytic reading of their purported inner content.[2] Expressionist works have similarly failed to escape an art historical discourse centered on European abstract painting, a narrative that, as previously discussed, has tended to be dominated by figures like Picasso and Kandinsky. Rather than seeking to perpetuate a dichotomy that further pits Vienna against Paris, or Munich against Vienna, the present book instead illuminates how the modern body developed historically as a common theme in the visual culture of these European (art) cities, culminating in Vienna at the turn of the twentieth century.

In their book *The Making of the Modern Body: Sexuality and Society in the Nineteenth Century*, Catherine Gallagher and Thomas Laqueur convincingly analyze the manner in which the Industrial Revolution, colonialism, Victorian conservatism, and gender politics invariably shaped the human body in the 1800s. In the opening pages of their study, they state that:

> The human body itself has a history. Not only has it been perceived, interpreted, and represented differently in different epochs, but it has also been lived differently, brought into being within widely dissimilar material cultures, subjected to various technologies and means of control, and incorporated into different rhythms of production and consumption, pleasure and pain.[3]

Since any history of the modern body is contingent on the time, location, and individuals that bring it into being, a single conception of the Viennese modern body is invariably contestable. The pages that follow thus reveal how the modern body in *fin-de-siècle* Vienna was one that directly confronted and incorporated what I believe can be called "hystero-theatrical gestures" as a means of bringing material form to a body fashioned through the inner and outer vision of the artist, playwright, or physician. These hystero-theatrical gestures, or manifestations of theatrical movements inspired by clinically hysterical taxonomies, were of particular interest to symbolists, Secessionists, and expressionists who hoped to visually codify a body that represented their modern epoch. In speaking of the modern body in works by Schiele, the Viennese artist and writer Albert Paris von Gütersloh tellingly characterized it, in 1911, as "the morbidity, depravity, and obscenity of a figure."[4] As a challenge to cultural norms and academic conventions, the Viennese modern body was thus shaped by radical advances in modern psycho- and physiopathology, by experimentations in avant-garde theater, and by breaking with the healthy and naturalistic body exemplified by late nineteenth-century history painters, in particular Hans Makart. In other words, artists envisioning the modern body in Vienna were creating images that articulated non-academic figures that bordered on the pathological, the grotesque, and the puppet-like.

Constructing the Viennese Modern Body

In Kokoschka's *Hans Tietze und Erica Tietze-Conrat* (*Hans Tietze and Erica Tietze-Conrat*, 1909, Plate 1), the artist offers viewers a double portrait of two sitters: a married couple who were both prominent art historians in turn-of-the-century Vienna. Although neither of the Tietzes appears to exhibit any conspicuous type of pathology, the viewer is nonetheless aware that this articulation of the Viennese modern body is decidedly anti-classical and anti-academic. Both individuals, for instance, stare off into a void, as if lost in a trancelike state. Their respective stares suggest that they are perhaps incapable of seeing one another, or the viewer, with their physical eyes. Kokoschka's painting further depicts Erica Tietze-Conrat's right arm as being shorter, or ill proportioned, in relation to her left arm.

The use of foreshortening is one viable explanation for her asymmetrical, seemingly incongruent arms, and yet the flattened space of Kokoschka's canvas complicates this reading, suggesting that the background, middle ground and foreground of the painting have collectively dissipated into a single compacted space that repudiates or defies the traditional rules of symmetry and perspective. Without the semblance of depth or three-dimensional space, this two-dimensional painting presents the viewer with bodies that appear to be transfixed to, rather than emerging from, an abstracted color pattern. Hans Tietze's right shoulder literally dissolves into the surrounding space, calling further attention to the notion that these bodies do not reside in a naturalistically rendered, perspectival space, but instead occupy an artistic space that rejects the tenets of traditional, academic art.

The principle focus of the painting is instead the subjects' hands. Erica's flesh-toned hands initially appear to be anatomically correct, until the viewer notices that the artist has rendered the fingers of her left hand in such a way that they appear boneless and pliable. The tips of her fingers are frozen in a gesture that suggests they have either just touched (and then parted from) her husband's left hand, or are about to touch his fingertips. The language of their hands thus recalls the gesture of post-creation envisioned by Michelangelo centuries earlier in the *Creation of Adam* (c. 1511–12) on the ceiling of the Sistine Chapel. Even though the rendering of Adam's left hand in Michelangelo's fresco and Hans' left hand in Kokoschka's canvas are largely dissimilar, this comparison serves as a reminder that countless works in the history of European art have used corporeal gestures to communicate a particular narrative or meaning to the viewer.

In any case, Hans' left hand is disarming. Due to its central position on the canvas, one also notices that Hans' right hand appears to be pliable, as though his arm has been replaced with a prosthetic—a wired, wax appendage easily manipulated and stretched by the painter. With an action that also involves human fingers, and which specifically involves the body of the modern artist, Kokoschka scratched areas of the painted canvas with his fingernails, leaving noticeable disruptions and striations on the work's visual surface. Overall, this inspection of corporeal form in Kokoschka's painting reveals that the bodies of Hans and Erica Tietze are characteristic of the concept of the unnatural modern body frequently expressed in *fin-de-siècle* Vienna.

Egon Schiele's artistic interpretations of the modern body explored such oddities in their extreme, rendering his own physique or those of young women as emaciated living corpses—or lifeless dolls or puppets—that convey an iconography of the anti-classical human body.[5] In Schiele's canonical *Aktselbstbildnis* (*Nude Self-Portrait*, 1910, Plate 2) the body of the artist fills the picture plane, overwhelming the viewer with a body ridden with the semblance of decay. Schiele's mottled skin clings to his ribs and skeletal frame. The artist's grimace communicates his discomfort (or disgust) with his awkward body, while the emptiness of the eye sockets asks the viewer to question whether he or she is observing a living being, a resuscitated cadaver, or an inanimate marionette with elongated limbs. Schiele's hands become a central focus in *Nude Self-Portrait*, given that the artist's extremities are large and ill proportioned in relation to the rest of his body. Moreover, when one considers the darkness of the fingers on his right hand, his skin appears to be afflicted by disease, perhaps gangrene. If we read these blackened fingers as signs of a physiological skin disorder, then perhaps the dark augmentations to his thighs are further evidence of necrotic wounds corrupting his flesh.

As with Kokoschka's *Hans Tietze and Erica Tietze-Conrat*, the arms in Schiele's *Nude Self-Portrait* are out of proportion with the rest of the body, an artistic choice that gives the impression that they are not entirely human, but rather, puppet-like limbs. As read through Schiele's image, the Viennese modern body is corrupt, either because it reflects the sitter's internal turmoil, or highlights his physiological pathology. Regardless of the artist's motivations for depicting his body in this manner, the end result is a representation of the body that is in opposition to those in academic paintings of the same period. Instead, his body more closely resembles the gaunt figures in Klimt's *Faculty Paintings*—particularly the first two, *Philosophy* and *Medicine* (1900–07, Figures I.4 and I.5)—which, a decade earlier, had been notoriously condemned by academicians at the University of Vienna as works that illicitly flaunted grotesque, ugly, disease-ridden and pornographic bodies.[6]

Koloman Moser, a painter, illustrator and craftsman affiliated with the Vienna Secession and the Wiener Werkstätte (Viennese Workshops), was another expressionist who explored the Viennese modern body in painted form. Created in 1915, his near life-sized canvas entitled *Der Liebestrank–Tristan und Isolde* (*The Love Potion–Tristan and Isolde*, Plate 3) presents the viewer with a theatrical presentation of the tragic protagonists in Richard Wagner's opera *Tristan und Isolde* (1859). Iconographically similar to paintings by the Swiss symbolist artist Ferdinand Hodler, *The Love Potion* is just one example of Moser's continued interest in symbolist themes of star-crossed lovers, or of tragic heroes and heroines, all of which share an equally long history in the performing arts. Moser's Isolde, dressed in a peplos-like garment reminiscent of a medical patient's gown, offers a bowl of love potion to Tristan, who, according to the original medieval legend and the nineteenth-century opera, believes it to be poison. With her arms outstretched in front of her torso, eyes closed, and chin tilted slightly, Isolde is transformed into a somnambulist: the modern sleepwalker. Tristan's hand gestures, in turn, seem almost comical in relation to Isolde's gesture of self-guidance. He appears frozen in place, only turning his wrists outward in an expression of surprise or helplessness, perhaps explained by the fact that his sword has fallen to his feet. What ultimately makes Moser's bodies particularly

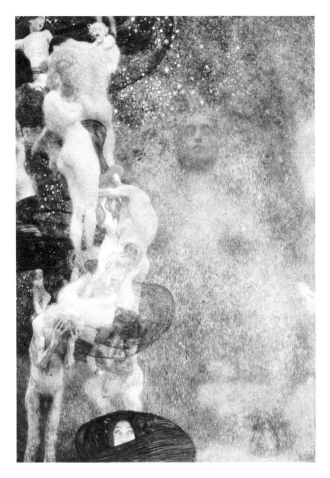

Figure I.4 Gustav Klimt, *Philosophy*, 1900–07, oil on canvas. Destroyed by fire in 1945 at Schloss Immendorf.
Source: Photo: Austrian Archives / SCALA / Art Resource, NY.

modern, however, is that his visual language appears to have been deliberately intended to reference clinical pathology by way of the female somnambulist.

Moser's painting, moreover, depicts subjects dressed in clothes that combine classical garments and modern attire, with Isolde wearing a curious peplos/medical gown and Tristan a tunic-like shirt and contemporary shorts. By contrast, the subjects in Kokoschka's double portrait of the Tietzes appear in contemporary clothing, and Schiele's self-portrait is nude. The blue highlights on Tristan's and Isolde's bodies—a color that complements the yellowish-orange tone of their skin—also signals to the viewer that these bodies, however more naturalistically rendered than the figures in Kokoschka's or Schiele's paintings, are not wholly academic. Rather than depicting them as conspicuously pathological bodies (though I argue later that Isolde's somnambulist gestures suggest just this), Moser's painting initially presents the viewer with a theatrical scene in which the protagonists express a narrative through painted gestures, just as actors utilize corporeal movements to convey meaning in an opera,

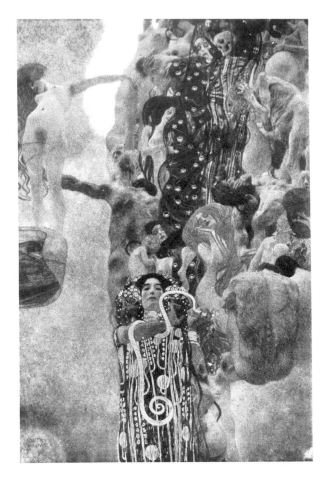

Figure I.5 Gustav Klimt, *Medicine*, 1900–07, oil on canvas. Destroyed by fire in 1945 at
        Schloss Immendorf.
Source: Photo: Foto Marburg / Art Resource, NY.

theatrical drama, or cabaret performance. As such, one clue to decoding the Viennese
modern body might be found in the understanding that expressionist artists were
collectively constructing these forms through references to theater and medical pathology, or, perhaps, a combination of both.

The Current Literature

In his seminal book, *Fin-de-Siècle Vienna: Politics and Culture* (1980), Carl E.
Schorske adopts a socio-historical methodology to analyze the crisis of liberalism
that he believed had struck the bourgeoisie, forever changing the nature of politics,
urban architecture, and artistic practice in the Austrian capital.[7] In the years following
Schorske's book, however, a number of scholars have expanded upon and challenged
this thesis. One of the first studies to adopt a revisionist approach to the field was
Steven Beller's *Rethinking Vienna 1900* (2001), in which he and other cultural historians provided groundbreaking insights and alternative narratives on the development of

modernism in *fin-de-siècle* Vienna, including examinations into the changing Viennese art market, the city's conceptualization of cosmopolitanism, the role of women, anti-Semitism, and Freudian psychology.[8] In a similar fashion, art historians like Alessandra Comini, Claude Cernuschi, Jane Kallir, Klaus Albrecht Schröder, Reinhard Steiner, and Patrick Werkner, to name only a few, have rightly explored psychological themes in Viennese expressionism, specifically the presumed inwardness, narcissism, and sexual preoccupations of painters like Kokoschka and Schiele. Building on *fin-de-siècle* reviews of their "grotesque" paintings,[9] Comini, in her pivotal book *Egon Schiele's Portraits* (1974), proposes that contemporary critics were, in fact, reinforcing the idea that young expressionist artists were exploring the modern body through "'pathological' portraits" as their contribution to European modernism.[10] Building on this assertion, Werkner later suggested that it was the discourse surrounding the hysterical body that may have served as "an important source of Viennese Expressionism."[11]

In their book *Madness and Modernity: Mental Illness and the Visual Arts in Vienna 1900* (2009), Gemma Blackshaw and Leslie Topp likewise examine the contorted body in Viennese expressionism, proposing that medical photographs of corporeal pathologies, rather than Freud's essays on various psychoses, directly impacted the iconographies of male bodies explored by Wiener Moderne artists.[12] Blackshaw's and Topp's research does much to underline the notion that scholarship on Viennese modernism has consistently suffered from relying on psychoanalytic arguments. They posit that such narratives grant too much authority to Freud's writings, and as a result, offer a superficial discussion of the manner in which expressionists may or may not have approached contemporary medical discourses in their respective works. The fact that Freud and the expressionists were working in the same (albeit small) city during a similar historical period does not clearly reveal that these two spheres were in direct dialogue with one another. In the final analysis, one is left with one of two possible conclusions: either that Freudian psychoanalysis offers the most culturally and historically relevant method of conceptualizing the content of pathological subjects in both painting and theater due to mere proximity; or that Freud's theories had little or nothing to do with the materialization of the modern body in the visual and performing arts in *fin-de-siècle* Vienna.

Klaus Albrecht Schröder, Reinhard Steiner, and Patrick Werkner each respectively observed that photographs of patients afflicted with nervous disorders in the Parisian psychiatrist Jean-Martin Charcot's *Iconographie photographique de la Salpêtrière*, or *IPS* (*Photographic Iconography of the Salpêtrière*, 1876–80) may have provided visual referents for expressionist portraits (particularly those by Schiele). In their research, Blackshaw and Topp contrastingly move the focus away from *IPS*, and instead examine Charcot's later journal, *Nouvelle Iconographie de la Salpêtrière: Clinique des Maladies du Système Nerveux*, or *NIS* (*New Iconography of the Salpêtrière: Clinic of the Diseases of the Nervous System*, 1888–1918), which concentrated on images of both male and female patients, rather than focusing exclusively on the female pathological body, which filled the pages of *IPS* (see, for example, Figure I.6).[13] In her earlier study, "The Pathological Body: Modernist Strategising in Egon Schiele's Self-Portraiture," Blackshaw similarly argued that the young expressionist was capable of fulfilling an avant-gardist maneuver involving the aesthetics of pathological bodies that Klimt painted into *Philosophy* and *Medicine* (Figures I.4 and I.5). Because Blackshaw was here invested in examining the practice of self-portraiture among Viennese male artists, it is understandable that her analysis is more concerned with photographic precedents that illustrate male patients with neurasthenia (or similar nervous disorders), rather than female subjects diagnosed with hysteria.[14]

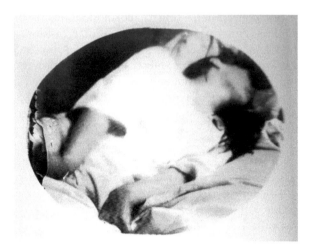

Figure I.6 Paul Régnard, *Tétanisme*, image of Augustine, hysterical patient of Jean-Martin Charcot, published in *Iconographie photographique de la Salpêtrière*, vol. II, c. 1878, photograph.
Source: Photo: © PVDE/Bridgeman Images.

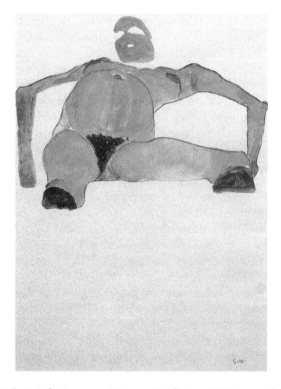

Figure I.7 Egon Schiele, *Nude Pregnant Woman Reclining*, 1910, gouache and black chalk on paper. Leopold Museum, Private Collection, Vienna.
Source: Photo: akg-images.

To illustrate that Schiele had access to photographs of pathological bodies in *NIS*, Blackshaw turns to a well-known anecdote in the scholarship on Schiele, which recalls that the artist was permitted, in 1910, to produce sketches from actual patients at the University of Vienna's Frauenklinik (Clinic for Women), which was then under the direction of his friend, Dr. Erwin von Graff (see Figure I.7). Prior to gaining his appointment in gynecology at the Frauenklinik, Graff had studied pathological anatomy.[15] Blackshaw thus argues, "this activity provides us with crucial evidence that Schiele was working in a clinic within a university which championed the pathological anatomy approach to psychiatry, and which held the complete run of the *NIS* journal."[16] Blackshaw's research has further shown that Schiele attended lectures on pathological expression conducted by a Dr. Kronfeld, who Schiele and his friend Erwin Osen, a fellow artist and mime, assisted by producing drawings that represented various types of expression witnessed on the faces or bodies of patients at the Steinhof Psychiatric Hospital, just outside Vienna.[17] Blackshaw consequently argues that certain images in *NIS* acted as descriptive archetypes for artists interested in the pathological body; and while her research does not prove definitively that Schiele actually worked from photographs in *NIS*, her analyses are compelling and subsequently lay the groundwork for research on the Viennese modern body.

In many ways, *Constructing the Viennese Modern Body* is a continuation of the existing literature, as well as expansion of the scholarship that has examined the emergence of the pathological body in *fin-de-siècle* Vienna. One of the most important contributions that the current book makes is that of moving this discussion into the realm of theater: be that the theater of pathological medicine, the theater of actors and actresses enacting hysterical gesticulations on dramatic stages, or the theater of the metaphorical marionette and pathological puppet. Within the pages of this book, I consider how—and for what reason—Viennese artists, actors, playwrights, directors, and writers experimented with the contorted, unnatural, and theatrical staging of corporeal form, and how this was an important articulation of modernism. My study examines the meaning that was given to expressive gestures in the visual and performing arts, as well as in psychological discourses examining the non-academic or pathological body. The research demonstrates that there was a clear vogue for hystero-theatrical gestures among both physicians and playwrights in *fin-de-siècle* Central Europe, the latter of whom adapted these clinical movements to the theatrical stage.

Even though modern psychological medicine had classified these movements as signs of clinical hysteria, examples of such artistic corporeal forms can be identified in concurrent French symbolist paintings, and in Austrian and German modernist theatrical and operatic performances. Such hystero-theatrical gestures were also the source of the symbolic body language adopted by Viennese modern painters, including Kokoschka, Schiele and Moser. The dramatic language of the painted modern body was further imbricated by another form of body language, namely that of inanimate puppets used in avant-garde marionette theater. The semiology of these *Puppen* (puppets, dolls, or marionettes in German) was thus commonly understood as a metaphor for the manipulated human body, for the corrupted nature of modernity itself, and for a body controlled by external forces.

In contrast to Schorske's *Fin-de-Siècle Vienna*, which treats psychoanalysis as a methodology with which to analyze the visual and performing arts in Vienna circa 1900, the present book treats psychoanalysis as a temporally restricted, cultural construct that developed in tandem with European modern art and theater, rather than a methodology to explain these areas of creativity. I thus argue that the historical development of Freudian psychoanalysis is more critical to our understanding of how the modern body was constructed throughout the modern period than the specific theories and techniques that it adopted. Key to my revisionist approach to Viennese expressionism is my interest in the changing nature of vision in modern Austrian society—a discourse that crucially implicates optical vision and inner/psychological visions in an artistic dichotomy that helped to develop the notion of the modern body in medical arenas, on theatrical stages, and on artistic canvases.

Eric R. Kandel's book *The Age of Insight: The Quest to Understand the Unconscious in Art, Mind, and Brain, From Vienna 1900 to the Present* (2012) is an example of recent, interdisciplinary studies that seek to bring together art, psychoanalysis, and neuroscience in order to discuss biological insights into the visual arts and artistic observations of the human brain.[18] Although Kandel's book and my own both reach beyond the field of art history in order to develop a richer understanding of expressionist paintings, my book is unique in that it avoids a discourse centered on neurobiology in favor of one focused on theater, and accordingly investigates the critical confluence of hystero-theatrical gestures in the visual and performing arts alongside (but without being subsumed by) the discipline of psychopathology that was emerging in Vienna between the 1890s and 1920s. By providing a discursive explanation of the appearance of these gestures in the dramatic and critical literature, in photographs of the theatrical "madwoman," and in turn-of-the-century theater journals, I show that these gestures became symbols of an entirely contrived (that is, *theatrical*) notion of hysteria.

My book also demonstrates how the work of Viennese playwrights like Arthur Schnitzler and Hugo von Hofmannsthal, and of visual artists like Kokoschka and Schiele, depicted pathological gestures as an effective means of communicating a language of the modern body, but one that was wholly artificial. In short, the trickeries of the artistic body thus served as effective manifestations of a corporeal pathology that could be brought to life on the theatrical stage and the artistic canvas. This book not only provides a new approach to the role of corporeal gesture in Austrian modern paintings, but it is also concerned with the manner in which Central European audiences responded to the appearance of these bodies and their movements in visual culture. As such, this study additionally demonstrates that the Viennese modern body was constructed through processes and discourses that could be observed not only in the Austrian capital, but throughout the German-speaking world at the turn of the century.

A Brief Synopsis

In this book, I explore the manifestation of expressive gestures of the Viennese modern body in figural paintings, modern dramatic performances, puppet theater, and through their theoretical explication in emerging medical research on hysteria. Chapter 1 provides an in-depth discussion of the historical context in which the modern body emerged at the turn of the century, with a particular focus on how the changing role of vision impacted how artists and their critics conceived and perceived these bodies. For example, in 1911, Archduke Franz Ferdinand condemned bodies in paintings by Kokoschka as pathological, diseased and ugly. For the young expressionist artist, however, the belief that the human body still held the power to excite contemporary viewers was the justification for a particularly avant-garde endeavor. In order to provide the theoretical framework for my discussion of modern vision and the body in Vienna, I begin Chapter 1 with an examination of Kokoschka's seminal essay "On the Nature of Visions" (1912). Through an examination of his thesis and subsequent notion of "the semblance of things," I investigate the tension between inner and optical vision within the wider context of visuality in Viennese modern art.

Historically, expressionism has been understood as a disparate, modern European style interested in the inner vision (*innere Sehen*) or visions (*Gesichte*) of the artist's imagination, as well as his personal musings and emotions. This conceptualization is largely owed to analyses of expressionism conducted by turn-of-the-century figureheads like Kandinsky, Hermann Bahr, and Wilhelm Worringer. Each of these individuals argued for the importance of breaking with a reliance on outer vision (*äußere Sehen*), favoring instead a deeper and more personal understanding of artistic form. As a result, critics and historians today tend to promote abstraction over figuration in the visual arts, particularly because Kandinsky and Worringer advocated abstraction as a modernist language at the turn of the century. In contrast to this formulation, Kokoschka's theory suggests that both inner and outer visions are key to understanding Viennese expressionism. His notion of "the semblance of things" articulates the interplay within this vision dialectic by highlighting the continual importance of daily visual stimuli—including corporeal gestures—to artists living and working in post-Secession-era Vienna. When read alongside other prevailing theories of expressionistic sight, it is clear that Kokoschka's dialectic contrasts sharply with conceptualizations of modern vision offered by Bahr, Kandinsky, and Worringer, as well as with those of Paul Fechter, Gustav Klimt, and Egon Schiele.

Chapters 2, 3 and 4 discuss the relevant inter-disciplinary and cross-national dialogues that were taking place between medical science, theater, and paintings of the modern body in Western and Central Europe at the *fin de siècle*. In contrast to theories popularized by more contemporary scholars, the second chapter argues that it was not Freud, nor his theories of hysteria or of the uncanny, that directly inspired depictions of the modern body in Viennese visual culture. Instead, I argue that it was the theater that initially responded to medical "performances" popularized by Charcot on the expressive potential of the pathological body. Chapter 2 consequently charts the emergence of the Parisian hysterical body in Charcot's medical theories and its transferal to the theatrical stage in Vienna.

Previous studies have suggested that Charcot's photographs of hysterical female patients (1877–80) may have provided visual referents, if not actual prototypes, for the contorted, unnatural, and diseased bodies in expressionist works. This literature is particularly significant for its analysis of hysteria as a constructed psychological disorder. In addition, the contemporary literature on Charcot's findings, as well as on Freud and Josef Breuer's *Studies on Hysteria* (1893–95), suggests that hysteria was a gendered disorder, insofar as this corporeal disease was believed to afflict the female rather than male body. I discuss how hysteria thus became the "fashionable disease," or *Modekrankheit*, of the *fin-de-siècle* woman, and how its hold on the female body allowed psychoanalysis to provide a medical justification for the trope of the femme fatale eternally present in literature, theater, and art.

Building upon this turn-of-the-century vogue for hysteria, Chapter 3 explores the concurrent interest in hystero-theatrical gestures in both the performing and visual arts of Central Europe. I chart the movement of these gestures from the Parisian clinic and cabaret to theatrical performances staged in Berlin, Munich, and Vienna. I argue that hystero-theatrical gestures, whether in the field of psychology or modern theater, were conceived as visible and dramatic manifestations of different classes of pathology. The potential for these gestures to communicate a language of the modern body was similarly explored by Austro-German directors and playwrights like Max Reinhardt and Hofmannsthal, and by performers like Gertrud Eysoldt, Tilla Durieux, and Anna Bahr-Mildenburg, who each participated in dramatizing the trope of the theatrically hysterical madwoman in German-speaking theater. I focus in particular on the critical reception of modern plays, especially the reaction to the premiere performances of Frank Wedekind's *Erdgeist*, Oscar Wilde's *Salomé*, and Hofmannsthal's *Elektra*. Each of these theater pieces featured actors deploying the gestures of the hysterical madwoman, as revealed in the language employed by critics on the three works. Because experimental or expressionist theater was often censored or restricted in *fin-de-siècle* Vienna, an examination of modern dramatic performances staged elsewhere helps to substantiate why visual art depicting the pathological body in the Austrian capital was regarded as avant-garde and shocking.

Chapter 4 turns from a broad focus on avant-garde drama in Central Europe to a more specific exploration of hystero-theatrical gesture in Viennese theater and its relationship to modernist painting. Although a strong distinction exists between "high" theater and "low" cabaret, where musical theater replaced classical drama, hystero-theatrical gestures appear to have been treated similarly in both arenas. That is to say, audiences were able to observe expressive "madwomen" (including Elektra, Isolde, and Salome) in both elitist and popular performances throughout the period. The visual and performing arts of *fin-de-siècle* Vienna often overlapped, since a number of modernist painters were also active in the city's Cabaret Fledermaus. Examining the appearance of "mad" movements on the dramatic stage, within scientific treatises, and in modernist canvases, thus provides a fuller and more accurate picture of the cross-disciplinary interest in hystero-theatrical gestures in *fin-de-siècle* Vienna. Kokoschka again serves as a key figure in this chapter, since his particular artistic ventures deliberately blurred the boundary between painting and theater.

Chapter 5 summarizes and synthesizes themes explored in the previous chapters through an investigation of the body in Viennese literature, centered on modern puppets and marionette theater. More specifically, the chapter explores the crisis of semantic language that pervades this literature, and suggests that corporeal gestures in paintings became effective and alternative modes of communication for Austrian artists and writers. Contemporary critics and writers were quick to discuss the importance of an expressive language of signs and gestures in their review of various artworks, in poetry, and in their theoretical analyses of the metaphorical puppet body. In turn, they were additionally swift to examine the emergence of the grotesque and uncanny aspects of the *Puppe* as an inhuman doppelgänger. I therefore argue that the language of the uncanny puppet served as a metaphor for the human body in Schiele's various self-portraits, in Kokoschka's paintings of his "sex doll," and in literary works by Hofmannsthal, Gütersloh, Heinrich von Kleist, and Rainer Maria Rilke.

Finally, Chapter 6 examines the modern, pathological body alongside the bodies of puppets, marionettes, and dolls intended as doppelgängers for their human counterparts. The chapter presents a number of visual analyses of modern bodies in Viennese expressionist paintings and their relationship to the inanimate (though equally expressive) gestures and movements of a *Puppe*. I initially examine the conceptual link between three seemingly disparate aspects of the pathos of modernity: the expressionist body, psycho-physiologic pathology, and the theatrical marionette as a corporeal metaphor. Accordingly, I investigate the choreography of the Viennese marionette theater alongside the contorted gestures painted concurrently by Viennese expressionists. I argue that such hystero-theatrical bodies were critically recognized as representing the hysteric, enacting through their movements a psychopathology that could be mapped onto the modern body. Case studies included in this chapter tease out various *fin-de-siècle* connotations of the *Puppe*, including those found in "puppet" plays penned by Kokoschka and Arthur Schnitzler, and in paintings by Kokoschka and Schiele, which collectively highlight the artistic interest in the marionette as a metaphorical foil for human corporeality and the modern condition.

This book ultimately considers the manner in which artists, actors, playwrights, and psychiatrists collectively experimented with the theatrical staging of the modern body in Viennese visual culture. By envisioning modern painting as a fusion of figuration and gestures, Viennese artists abstracted the body from its traditional academic form by adopting a new visual vocabulary centered on theatricality and pathology. Just as young female hysterics became puppets to their medical physicians, *fin-de-siècle* Viennese artists positioned their subjects as manipulated marionettes. In other words, as the contemporary discourse on hysteria was being formulated as a gendered disorder, theatrical and painted bodies were being codified within the taxonomies of the "fashionable disease" of the early twentieth century. Through optical vision and observation, and not simply through inner vision and emotions, these artists forever changed the nature of visual culture in Vienna, bringing the new, modern body to the attention of its public.

Notes

1 Peter Schjeldahl, "Golden Girl: The Neue Galerie's new Klimt," *The New Yorker*, July 24, 2006, n.p.
2 One example of this literature is Rosa J. H. Berland, "The Exploration of Dreams: Kokoschka's Die Träumenden Knaben and Freud," *Source: Notes in the History of Art* 27, no. 2/3, Special Issue on Art and Psychoanalysis (Winter/Spring 2008): 25–31.
3 Catherine Gallagher and Thomas Walter Laqueur, eds, *The Making of the Modern Body: Sexuality and Society in the Nineteenth Century* (Berkeley: University of California Press, 1987), vii.
4 For Gütersloh's quote, see Albert Paris von Gütersloh, *Egon Schiele* (Vienna: Brüder Rosenbaum, 1911), 4.
5 Gemma Blackshaw has similarly suggested that Schiele's self-portraits provide images of the pathological body. See Gemma Blackshaw, "The Pathological Body: Modernist Strategising in Egon Schiele's Self-Portraiture," *Oxford Art Journal* 30, no. 3 (2007): 377–401.
6 Hermann Bahr, the well-known *fin-de-siècle* Viennese critic, theater director and writer, documented the various attacks and public criticisms directed at Klimt's infamous *Faculty Paintings*. See Hermann Bahr, ed., *Gegen Klimt: Historisches, Philosophie, Medizin, Goldfische, Fries* (Vienna: Eisenstein & Co., 1903).
7 Carl E. Schorske, *Fin-de-Siècle Vienna: Politics and Culture* (New York: Knopf, 1980).
8 Steven Beller, ed., *Rethinking Vienna 1900*, vol. 3, *Austrian and Habsburg Studies* (New York: Berghahn Books, 2001).
9 See sources listed in Chapter 1, notes 1 and 5–8.
10 Alessandra Comini, *Egon Schiele's Portraits* (Berkeley: University of California Press, 1974), 44.

11 Patrick Werkner, "The Child-Woman and Hysteria," in *Egon Schiele: Art, Sexuality, and Viennese Modernism*, ed. Patrick Werkner (Palo Alto: The Society for the Promotion of Science and Scholarship, 1994), 69.

12 Gemma Blackshaw and Leslie Topp, eds, *Madness and Modernity: Mental Illness and the Visual Arts in Vienna 1900* (Farnham: Lund Humphries, 2009).

13 Blackshaw, "The Pathological Body," 383–84. See also references in Chapter Two, note 7.

14 Blackshaw, "The Pathological Body," 382–88.

15 This anecdote is repeated throughout the scholarship on Schiele, and first appears in Fritz Karpfen, ed., *Das Egon Schiele Buch* (Vienna: Verlag der Wiener Graphischen Werkstätte, 1921), 22.

16 Blackshaw, "The Pathological Body," 392. Blackshaw also addresses Kokoschka's purported interest in pathological corporeality, as witnessed in his 1908 drawing *The Lunatic Girl*, and his 1909–10 paintings of Adolf Loos' mistress, the English dancer Bessie Bruce, who was being treated for tuberculosis at a Swiss sanitarium near Montreux, which Kokoschka visited at Loos' expense. In addition to Blackshaw, Claude Cernuschi also discusses Schiele's visits to the Frauenklinik, as well as the iconography of Kokoschka's *The Lunatic Girl* alongside the taxonomy of "insane patients," in Claude Cernuschi, *Re/casting Kokoschka: Ethics and Aesthetics, Epistemology and Politics in Fin-de-Siècle Vienna* (Madison: Fairleigh Dickinson University, 2002), 44.

17 Blackshaw, "The Pathological Body," 392.

18 Eric R. Kandel, *The Age of Insight: The Quest to Understand the Unconscious in Art, Mind, and Brain, From Vienna 1900 to the Present* (New York: Random House, 2012).

1 "The Semblance of Things"
Re-Visioning Viennese Expressionism

Someone should break every bone in that man's body![1]
——Archduke Franz Ferdinand, referring to Oskar Kokoschka, 1911

This astonishingly severe declaration, uttered by the heir to the Austro-Hungarian Empire, was perhaps the most politically charged of all the adverse critiques directed toward modern artistic representations of the body in *fin-de-siècle* Vienna. According to anecdotal evidence, Ferdinand, who was known for his moral earnestness, expressed this damning sentiment at a private viewing of the February 1911 Hagenbund exhibition held in the Austrian capital.[2] The reason for his hostility was the inclusion in the exhibition of more than twenty paintings by the young Viennese expressionist artist and playwright Oskar Kokoschka. While obviously extreme in his desire to maim (if only metaphorically) the artist, the archduke was not alone in his contempt for Kokoschka's images. Indeed, individuals throughout the Viennese art world were both repulsed and intrigued by the contorted, strange, and "pathological" bodies in his paintings.[3]

One such image was Kokoschka's *Portrait of Lotte Franzos* (1909, Plate 4), which was included in the Hagenbund exhibition. In the painting, a young woman with a wavy, bobbed haircut is pictured in three-quarter pose, wearing a pale dress. She appears demure, or lost in thought, as her eyes are cast downward and away from the viewer. Unconventionally, the woman is surrounded by thick, blurred outlines painted in blues, purples, and yellows, giving the illusion that these colorful auras were radiating directly from her body. Her face, neck, and hands are mottled and distorted, giving the impression that her skin has been afflicted by an extreme form of eczema or lined with deep wrinkles. The fingers of her left hand, in particular, are bent into unnatural angles, suggesting that the woman may also suffer from broken appendages, arthritis, or other disfigurements.

Franzos, a friend of Kokoschka's and herself an artist and art historian, as well as the wife of a prominent Viennese lawyer, was reportedly far from pleased when she saw the finished portrait, a reaction shared by local critics who viewed the canvas two years later at the Hagenbund.[4] The prominent Austrian art historian Josef Strzygowski was one such detractor who vehemently denounced Kokoschka's paintings and artistic vision. In an article published in the Viennese newspaper *Die Zeit* (*The Times*) on 9 February 1911, Strzygowski declared:

Here is Oskar Kokoschka. [...] With Koko-rays from his psyche he X-rays those persons who have the misfortune of coming under his paintbrush. What a putrid smell emanates from the picture of Frau Dr. L. Fr.! [... Here one] envisions off-putting pictures of syphilis and paralysis.[5]

Although Franzos was not openly named in Strzygowski's review, the inclusion of her initials makes clear that the critic was referring to her portrait. Writing as though Kokoschka's mind were capable of physically penetrating the bodies of his subjects, Strzygowski argued that the artist's subjects (including Franzos) were contaminated by his inner vision, the results of which might be confused for the telltale signs of venereal disease or some other illness. By suggesting that Franzos' portrait might actually smell bad, Strzygowski was claiming that Kokoschka's paintings were not only damaging to the bodies of his sitters, but were also a danger to their viewers, who were at risk of smelling rotten flesh, or figuratively contracting the diseases emanating from his artistic subjects.

Another Viennese critic, Karl Schreder, expressed similar disdain toward Kokoschka's paintings at the Hagenbund. In his review for Vienna's *Deutsches Volksblatt* (*German People's Paper*), also published on February 9, Schreder wrote that Kokoschka:

> paints "portraits," including well-known local figures. These gruesome pictures, whose faces seem to bear the disfigurement of a corrupting disease or the rotting process of decay, appear as if they have risen from a foul-smelling crypt or madhouse.[6]

Schreder further argued that some of Kokoschka's sitters appeared to have "crippled hands," or to have been afflicted by leprosy—no doubt a reference to the "corrupting disease" that Schreder believed was the cause of their visual disfiguration.[7] The critic Franz Grüner, writing for Karl Kraus' polemic newspaper *Die Fackel* (*The Torch*), likewise argued that individuals depicted in Kokoschka's Hagenbund portraits seemed as though they suffered from "severe disease and, having known years of imprisonment, were afflicted with repulsive physical and psychological ailments."[8] Grüner's critique was published more than two weeks after Strzygowski's and Schreder's reviews, so it is possible that his contempt for Kokoschka's canvases was merely an echo of the damning sentiments already offered by his colleagues. Regardless of the origins of Grüner's opinions, his article essentially summed up prevailing public opinions of Kokoschka, namely that the artist painted grotesque bodies rife with disease and decay.

Bearing in mind the negative criticism leveled against Kokoschka's paintings in the Hagenbund exhibition, there is an undeniable irony in Ferdinand's aggressive proclamation, given that the archduke proposed to leave Kokoschka's body in the same state that he and the critics found so repulsive in the artist's representations of "crippled hands" and disfigured bodies. It would be inaccurate, however, to presume that Ferdinand's sentiments were in any way insincere, despite there being no actual threat to Kokoschka's wellbeing. To be sure, Ferdinand only figuratively proposed a breaking of bones, and yet—in a very real sense—Kokoschka's images signaled a definitive break with art history, as well as a rupture with contemporary conceptualizations of artistic vision. It is clear that the artist's decision to distance his aesthetics from depictions of the academic body in favor of images of the newly emerging modern body—a body that appeared as though it were riddled with disease—was undoubtedly jarring to the archduke's sight and traditional sensibilities. Without a doubt, Kokoschka's art had disturbed the vision of *fin-de-siècle* Vienna, for his was a revelation of the pathological body.

As stated in the introduction to this book, the literature on Viennese expressionism has tended to analyze the movement alongside a Europe-wide interest in more dominant, non-figurative styles, or by adopting a psychoanalytic methodology. Moreover, the current scholarship on the Wiener Moderne has promulgated the notion that artists associated with this particular style were wholly concerned with expressing inner emotions and feelings. In contrast to the existing literature, this volume examines how artists affiliated with expressionism did not in fact abandon the aesthetics of the outer body for the inner mind. The current chapter consequently examines the radical nature of Kokoschka's theory of vision (which embraced both optical and inner vision) and how this model of expressionistic sight (which continually favored figuration over pure abstraction) helped to construct artistic representations of the Viennese modern body in the early twentieth century (see, for example, Plates 1–4). Importantly, this chapter explores how Kokoschka's novel conceptualization of artistic vision diverged or converged with contemporaneous theories of expressionistic sight offered by his interlocutors in the German-speaking art world, namely Hermann Bahr, Paul Fechter, Wassily Kandinsky, Egon Schiele, and Wilhelm Worringer.

On the Nature of Visions

Oskar Kokoschka visually and theoretically explored the changing role of vision in *fin-de-siècle* Vienna more than any other Austrian artist or playwright of his period. Kokoschka's personal conceptualization of artistic vision is not only evident in a number of his paintings, including those displayed at the 1911 Hagenbund exhibition, but also in his seminal essay "Von der Natur der Gesichte" ("On the Nature of Visions"), which he first delivered as a public lecture in 1912 at Vienna's Akademischen Verband für Literatur und Musik (Academic Association for Literature and Music). In this quasi-manifesto on visual culture and modern aesthetics, Kokoschka theorized the dialectical nature of expressionistic vision, one informed by inner visions, as well as their binary opposite: optical sight. In conceiving of this dialectic of vision, Kokoschka declared:

> Without intent I draw from the outside world the semblance of things; but in this way I myself become part of the world's imaginings. Thus in everything imagination is simply that which is natural. It is nature, vision, life.[9]

Kokoschka, who was twenty-six years old at the time, spoke with the authority of an artist who had long recognized the stakes involved in defining one's art (and one's self) as avant-garde within the cultural milieu of *fin-de-siècle* Vienna. As a burgeoning painter-playwright, he equally understood the importance of establishing a unique, theoretical basis in which to root the iconography of his developing style. Kokoschka's essay therefore persists as a foundational text in the conceptualization of the relationship between inner emotions and optical vision in Viennese expressionism. At the close of his treatise, Kokoschka acknowledged that the catalyst for his work, the inspiration for the visions of his inner imagination, was drawn from the "semblance of things" that he observed and collected from the daily, optical stimuli of his immediate surroundings. More precisely, Kokoschka argued that the awareness of these inner visions, or *Gesichte*, did not materialize through a state of mere remembrance on the part of the viewer, but operated on "a level of consciousness" that allowed the viewer to experience visions within his or her own self.[10]

Kokoschka further posited that this awareness on the part of the viewer was part and parcel to the act of living, or of collecting images optically from the material world:

> The effect is such that the visions seem actually to modify one's consciousness, at least in respect of everything that their own form proposes as their pattern and significance. This change in oneself, which follows on the vision's penetration of one's very soul, produces the state of awareness, of expectancy. At the same time there is an outpouring of feeling into the image, which becomes, as it were, the soul's plastic embodiment [...] The life of the consciousness is boundless. It interpenetrates the world and is woven through all its imagery.[11]

This passage is significant not only for its contextualization of emotive feeling in the image-forming process, but also of the supposed psychological effect that visions have on the mind of the agent. Kokoschka, however, suggests that this effect transpires not through involuntary psychic activity, but through the active awareness (or consciousness) of the viewer in whom the vision arises. But here Kokoschka also indirectly proposes two different ways of thinking about consciousness. On the one hand, he posits that consciousness is one's awareness of the external world and its visual stimuli. On the other, he quite specifically defines consciousness as "the source of all things and of all conceptions. It is a sea ringed about with visions."[12] In this sense, consciousness is not merely an awareness on the part of the agent, but rather, it is something akin to his or her "inner core," or fundamental understanding of all things external and internal.[13]

One might infer that the simple act of remembering a material image is an essentially thoughtless act, given that, according to Kokoschka, this process occurs beyond the consciousness (or "awareness") of the agent who creates, experiences, and draws inspiration from the vision in question. What is more, if the agent lacks consciousness on both levels, then the vision will fail to materialize, insofar as Kokoschka implies that an unconscious vision is indistinguishable from a mere memory of the outside world. Should the viewer fail to acknowledge the presence of the vision, the self will be denied this particular image of the soul. The suggestion that consciousness sets meaning into a vision is therefore seemingly contradictory, insofar as visions are typically understood to be psychic phenomena; and yet the conscious awareness of *Gesichte* is patently fundamental to Kokoschka's conceptualization of the semblance of things. Rather than arguing that Kokoschka's theory is inconsistent—given that his formulation of artistic vision argues for the centrality of both inner and outer processes in the development of this sensorial construct—the present chapter proposes that this rather radical handling of the role of opticality in the development of expressionism implicitly explains expressionistic sight as a process formed through the dialectical tension that arises from these two prevalent, though oppositional views of artistic vision. This multivalent understanding of vision and its relationship to the historiography of expressionism has, until now, eluded scholarship on this particular movement.

Binaries of Vision I: Kokoschka, Worringer, and Fechter

To appreciate the uniqueness of Kokoschka's position in the debate over the role of physical sight in Viennese expressionism, it is important (and necessary) to recognize how his paradigm of vision differed from more dominant theories put forward in the German-speaking art world (namely Austria and Germany) at the beginning of the twentieth century. From a historical perspective, inner vision overwhelmingly dominated this discourse, thereby positioning physical vision as a contestable and peripheral construct. Charles Townsend Harrison has rightly suggested that this historical bias toward inner, expressive vision highlights the attitudes held by many expressionist artists, critics, historians, and theoreticians of the period, who "assumed that the demand for fidelity to appearances was in conflict with the demand for fidelity to feeling."[14] Harrison's analysis neatly summarizes turn-of-the-century notions of vision (again, both inner and optical) and their function in a work of art. More significantly, however, it underscores the manner in which scholars have tended to approach expressionism as a style that was entirely devoted to revealing the artist's inner emotions so as to completely, or at least openly, reject any allegiance to purely optical processes.[15]

The supremacy of inner vision was subsequently endorsed and propagated in the vast majority of turn-of-the-century writings on German expressionism, including the immensely influential book *Abstraktion und Einfühlung* (*Abstraction and Empathy*, 1908), written by the Munich-based art historian Wilhelm Worringer. In the book's opening pages, Worringer—in contrast to Kokoschka's later writings—readily admonishes "the visible surface of things" in the external world when compared to iconographies employed in abstract and "primitive" painting.[16] Worringer further argues that an autonomous work of art should be devoid of any connection to this visible surface (which he called "nature") so as to denounce the historical importance placed on natural beauty in determining the aesthetic value of a work of art. For Worringer, the aesthetics of natural beauty and the laws or dogma of art were autonomous principles. Rather than perpetuating the idea that realism or naturalism is the highest attainable goal in the domain of the plastic arts, his theory instead posits that the movement toward abstraction, and away from realism, was an evolution that continued throughout the history of artistic production. Thus, on the matter of the psychological inner vision of the artist, Worringer writes:

> Now what are the psychic presuppositions for the urge to abstraction? We must seek them in these peoples' feeling about the world, in their psychic attitude toward the cosmos. Whereas the precondition for the urge to empathy is a happy pantheistic relationship of confidence between man and the phenomena of the external world, the urge to abstraction is the outcome of a greater inner unrest inspired in man by the phenomena of the outside world; in a religious respect it corresponds to a strongly transcendental tinge to all notions.[17]

As with Kokoschka's theorization of the semblance of things in the outside world and their relationship to the inner visions of the artist, Worringer here argues that the external phenomena of the world play a role in formulating the "inner unrest" of the modern artist. In this respect, Kokoschka's theory might be seen as being aligned with Worringer's principles of abstraction, suggesting that the latter was not fundamentally attacking the "visible surface" of external phenomena in his treatise. As underscored by Harrison's earlier assessment, however, this impression is deceptive, as Worringer's theory ultimately favors the "inner unrest" of modern painting, arguing that the feelings, psychic attitudes, and inner emotional responses of the corresponding agent unequivocally take precedence over the "happy" (in other words the "superficial" and "non-transcendental") visual stimuli of the external world. Although the principal aim of Worringer's book was to question the hegemonic classifications that surrounded abstraction and realism (or what he calls "empathetic art"), he essentially articulated and helped to establish as doctrine a number of the foundational principles of German expressionist painting, including the supremacy of inner vision over the mere opticality that surrounded the critical rhetoric of this style in the early twentieth century. Worringer's denunciation of the visible surface of things also allowed him to develop a theory of (German) expressionism that opposed (French) impressionism and the latter's reliance on optical vision and natural beauty. For Worringer, this visible surface, or *sichtbare Oberfläch*—which could equally refer to the superficiality of corporeal sight—had to be destroyed, abandoned, transcended, or at the very least challenged, in order to move beyond realism's non-instinctive approach to painting. By contrast, the importance given to psychological images in Kokoschka's (Austrian) model did not seek to overshadow the significance placed on the semblance of things in depicting visions from the outside world.

Similar attitudes to Worringer's thoughts concerning the hegemony of inner vision in the construction of the tenets of expressionistic sight can be found in a slightly later book entitled *Der Expressionismus* (*Expressionism*, 1914), written by the Berlin art and theater critic Paul Fechter. Although not as well known today as *Abstraction and Empathy*, Fechter's *Expressionism* was perhaps the earliest work to uniformly discuss modern artists like Kokoschka and Kandinsky in terms of a collective "German" expressionist style. Fechter, like Worringer, was quick to admonish impressionism in favor of expressionism's anti-decorative approach to art production, and adopted—in an avant-gardist manner typical of the period—the belief that the latter style had the ability to convey "emotional sensations" and spiritual truths to Germanic peoples.[18] He did not, however, fill his book with a lengthy debate on the advantages of inner vision over physical optics, though he did offer the following observation: "The depiction of the outside world will be left to photography and cinema; in its place enters the emotion-filled vision of the artist."[19] What is most interesting about this passage is Fechter's belief that impressions of the outside world should be left to mechanical forms of optical reproduction, such as the camera, whereas a work of art, in drawing upon the emotions and inner vision of the artist, must derive from the artist's soul or imagination. Even though Fechter never specifically mentions the "visible surface of things," he nevertheless makes clear that descriptions of the outside world amount to mere mimesis when compared to the emotional catalysts of expressionist painting.

The rather negative connotation attached to the "visible surface" in German expressionism, as initially proposed by Worringer and later adopted by Fechter, thus stands in stark contrast to Kokoschka's later theory of the semblance of things within Viennese expressionism. According to Kokoschka, these appearances, which subsist as recollections of the outside world gathered through physical sight, are the origins of inner, expressionistic visions. One can confidently deduce that, according to Kokoschka's notion of the semblance of things, optical vision cannot be abandoned in favor of inner vision, since the latter invariably relies on the former and would not be possible without it. With this equation in mind, it appears that Kokoschka quite deliberately uses the unusual German word *Gesichte* to refer to "visions" in order to suggest that such phenomena are linked to both inner and optical processes. A more common choice might have been to use the word *Visionen* or *Traumbilder* ("dream pictures"), or even to add the modifier *innere* to *Gesichte* to denote images that originate in the mind's eye and therefore exist in distinction from an optical visualization of the outside world. Instead, Kokoschka's use of *Gesichte*, which is more or less a German equivalent of the English "faces," creates a rather deliberate double entendre with the word *Gesicht*, which, in its formal but uncommon meaning, refers to physical vision or optical sight, and in its more common usage refers to an individual's face or visage.[20] Thus the very semantics employed by Kokoschka to connote the dualism of *Gesicht(e)* or vision(s) reflects the same dialectic set out in his prescriptive essay on modern painting.

The subtleties and nuances between these different Austro-German ideas on vision, sight, and visions are important, as they highlight the dialectical nature of the semblance of things, and reinforce the contention that the interplay between inner and outer vision was a key component of Kokoschka's understanding of expressionistic sight. In his manifesto on vision, this tension is made clear when he contends that inner visions (*innere Gesichte*; *Visionen*; *Traum*) are plastic embodiments of the soul and the self, and are otherwise unattainable without the aid of optical sight (*Sehen*; *Gesicht*). However, since *Gesicht* is typically used to denote an individual's face, it is equally apparent that the substance and content of *innere Gesichte* are largely dependent on the *Gesicht* and the human eye, which capture their underlying images. Given the role of opticality in the construction of visions, Kokoschka does not negate the importance of outer over inner vision, but instead suggests that these two modes of seeing exist in a symbiotic, and thus inextricable, relationship. It is through this relationship, then, that the semblance (or inner vision) of a thing (observed through outer vision) is able to inform the content of an expressionist painting by providing a plastic embodiment of the artist's soul. Moreover, this re-evaluation of artistic vision negates the hegemony of inner vision and emotive feeling in determining expressionist iconographies. Significantly, this power struggle between outer vision (emphasized in impressionism) and inner vision (so central to symbolism and expressionism) was due largely to the impact of other influential early twentieth-century texts on art, such as Worringer's *Abstraction and Empathy*. Kokoschka's essay, on the other hand, quite remarkably stands apart for its support of the part played by physical opticality in the creation of the iconography and semiology of expressionism, particularly when viewed alongside Worringer's and Fechter's respective denigration of optical vision's role in this developing style.

Binaries of Vision II: Kokoschka, Bahr, and Kandinsky

Kokoschka's theory of artistic vision was not only unique in relation to German historiographies of expressionism, but also stood apart from theories developing in his native country in the early twentieth century and from the French models of the mid-nineteenth century. In 1914, two years after Kokoschka delivered his lecture *On the Nature of Visions* at the Akademischen Verband, the prominent Viennese theater director, art critic, and playwright Hermann Bahr completed the manuscript of his widely read book *Expressionismus* (*Expressionism*, first published in 1916). Regarding the nature of visions, Bahr unassumingly states that, "every history of painting is invariably the history of vision."[21] This dogmatic statement, from a section of the book entitled "Sehen" ("Vision"), is succeeded by the following thoughts on the dialectical nature of expressionistic vision:

> And if the beholder vehemently retorts that the painter should express nothing but what he sees, the expressionist assures him: We too only paint what we see!

But on this point they cannot agree, as they cannot agree on the meaning of vision. When they speak of vision, each of them means something different. What is vision? Every history of painting is invariably the history of vision. Technique changes when vision changes; and technique changes because vision [or the mode of seeing] has changed. It changes in order to oblige the changes of vision. But vision changes according to man's relationship to the world, since man views the world according to his position towards it.[22]

Although it is unclear whether Bahr was responding to Kokoschka's ideas on the awareness of visions, given that Kokoschka also stated that their "history can never be delimited," Bahr's assessment of the changing modes of vision in the early twentieth century does appear to have something in common with Kokoschka's understanding of inner and outer vision, as well as with the ideas of the Swiss-German art historian Heinrich Wölfflin, who, like Bahr, was interested in the role that the history of vision had played in the history of art.[23] Bahr's use of the word *Sehen* undeniably implies the use of one's physical eyes to observe natural forms, though Kokoschka's dialectic should not be forgotten here. For Bahr, vision above all implies the inner imagination of the expressionist artist and the belief that art could perform a spiritual function for the creator, as well as the receptive viewer, of a particular work. Contrary to Bahr's seeming interest in optical *Sehen* in the preceding passage, his theories in *Expressionism* ultimately suggest that a total reliance on physical vision will lead the modern artist dangerously back to the *passé* art of the impressionists.[24] In Bahr's formulation of expressionism, this new style openly confronts and challenges its opposite, impressionism, which Bahr tellingly considers "the final word in classical art."[25] Like Worringer, Bahr implies that this inversion of the physical eye was accomplished through the expressionists' favoring of the mind's eye, so that their style could distance itself from the opticality of impressionism. Moreover, Bahr's analysis of expressionism reinforces the hegemony of inner vision as a natural byproduct of symbolism, while simultaneously highlighting the avant-garde nature of an artistic movement free from any strict adherence to the pitfalls of classical models of optical sight, such as mimesis, proportion, perspective, and the effects of light.[26]

One can further surmise, as in Worringer's earlier history of expressionism, that Bahr believed that impressionism was inextricably, and thus regrettably, tied to optics, whereas Austrian modern art necessarily rejected French physical vision in favor of a deeper and more personal approach to creating art.[27] Bahr's diatribe against impressionism was not, however, a prevalent attitude among artists affiliated with the Vienna Secession, such as Gustav Klimt, who continued to favor, to varying degrees, the opticality employed by impressionists and the brushwork of the post-impressionists. Instead, Bahr's notion shares a greater affinity with Worringer's denunciation of impressionism, given that the contemporary critical literature surrounding German (more than Austrian) modernism more vehemently rejected the French tradition of impressionism in favor of "Germanic" expressionism.[28] Robert Jensen, whose research has investigated the art market in *fin-de-siècle* Vienna and subsequent promotional strategies employed by Kokoschka and Egon Schiele, has even suggested that this break was instituted as a marketing ploy to distance Viennese expressionism from the "'major' artistic language of Parisian modernism."[29] Regardless, however, of the motivation for expressionism's opposition to impressionism, the end result was that a strong dichotomy was created between these two distinct styles. And rightly so, given that Kokoschka's dialectical model makes clear that impressionism's solitary understanding of vision (that is, as optical) was in conflict with expressionism's interest in the duality of artistic vision, at least in Vienna circa 1900.

Kokoschka's personal musings on the interplay of physical sight, mental images and the spiritual nature of vision(s) also highlights the commonalities and disconnects that exist between Kokoschka's theory and the ideas espoused by other expressionists, particularly the Munich-based Der Blaue Reiter (The Blue Rider) group, which Kandinsky founded with Franz Marc in 1911. As previously mentioned, Kandinsky's thoughts on the spiritual foundation of expressionism, as articulated in writings like *Über das Geistige in der Kunst* (*Concerning the Spiritual in Art*, 1911) and *Über die Formfrage* (*On the Question of Form*, 1912), share certain affinities with Kokoschka's model of expressionistic sight, though Kandinsky's texts, like Worringer's *Abstraction and Empathy*, tend to elevate inner vision in relation to the spirit, while relegating optical vision to a lesser role. This belief likewise resonates throughout Bahr's concurrent analysis of expressionism, which maintains that impressionism separates man from his spirit, and in so doing stops the impressionist from truly expressing himself.[30] Building on Johann Wolfgang von Goethe's earlier observations on the relationship between vision and romantic painting, Bahr concluded:

> The eye of the impressionist only beholds, it does not speak; it hears the question, but does not answer. Instead of eyes, impressionists have another set of ears, but no mouth [...] But the expressionist tears open the mouth of humanity; the time of its silence, the time of its listening is over—once more it seeks to give voice to the spirit's reply.[31]

Kandinsky's and Bahr's respective analyses of the inner spirit both suggest that the expressionist (whether German or Austrian) is privileged with the responsibility of creating works of art through the use of emotions, as opposed to visual observation, and can either abuse this advantage through vanity and greed, or exalt it through the plastic embodiment of the spirit's inner meaning. In this regard, Kandinsky's interest in the primacy of inner meaning can be related to Kokoschka's rhetoric on visions, in that both men believed that an outpouring of feeling originating in the soul of the artist could reciprocally produce images of these inner meanings.[32] When speaking of the obstacles that hinder artists from moving toward this goal and the spiritual life of art, Kandinsky reminds his readers that the secret "power of 'vision'" will undoubtedly rescue the artist from such fetters.[33] By contrast, Kokoschka argues that the full potential of a vision, and that which leads to the physical embodiment of the soul's yearning, must be recognized on a purely conscious level. Carl Schorske tellingly referred to this process as Kokoschka's "vision-consciousness."[34] As such, Kokoschka's understanding of vision essentially maintains that the search for the material form of inner content is attainable only through the synthesis of optical and inner vision, rather than the hegemonic displacement of the one by the other. The result was a vision dialectic that was specific to expressionistic sight, as well as images from the artist's imagination that were linked to the Viennese modern body.

This discussion of the artist's body and its relation to the mind is subsequently found in Kokoschka's ideas concerning the role of the spirit, the soul, and the body in the image-forming process. Concerning the spiritual in a work of art, Kokoschka writes:

> The enquiring spirit rises from stage to stage, until in encompasses the whole of Nature. All laws are left behind. One's soul is a reverberation of the universe. Then too, as I believe, one's perception reaches out toward the Word, towards awareness of the vision.[35]

In this quote, the artist's reference to "the Word" is an allusion to an earlier section of the essay in which he quotes directly from the New Testament: "'The Word became flesh and dwelt among us.'"[36] When read together, these two passages suggest that one's conscious perception of a vision is made complete when the Word (or the spirit) inhabits the body (or flesh) of the artist. The body is thus a container or vessel for the soul, which, in turn, nourishes itself from the spirit that allows the mind to become aware of, and then interpret, the nature of the vision. Just as the substance and content of *innere Gesichte* are dependent upon the *Gesicht* and its physical eyes to acquire the images on which they are founded, so the mind relies on the body to provide it with a "plastic embodiment" of the soul. The "problem," then, with Kokoschka's articulation of expressionism, as argued by detractors like Franz Ferdinand, was that the bodies in his paintings were "ugly" and "grotesque," and thus visible markers of the corrupted nature of the artist's own soul, as well as of the potentially pathological state of his sitters' inner nature. One need only recall Lotte Franzos' own disapproval of Kokoschka's portrayal of her body (see Plate 4), a condemnation that tellingly suggests that viewers might have mistaken her soul as being equally diseased.

Binaries of Vision III: Kokoschka and Klimt

Although the well-known Austrian Secession and symbolist artist Gustav Klimt was not an expressionist, his infamous *Fakultätsbilder* (*Faculty Paintings*, 1900–07) were nevertheless caught in the Viennese discourse on modern vision and the body. When anachronistically filtered through Kokoschka's dialectical theory, the figures that materialize in the *Faculty Paintings*, and particularly those seen in the first two canvases, *Philosophy* and *Medicine* (Figures I.4 and I.5), presented *fin-de-siècle* viewers with glimpses of Klimt's vision of modern bodies. Klimt scholars have consistently noted that the artist's 1894 government commission to paint three large-scale canvases for the ceiling of the grand hall in the new University of Vienna building (1877–84) marked a decisive juncture in the artist's career. Commissioned by the Austrian Minister of Education, Johannes Wilhelm Rittér von Hartel, the paintings were intended to represent the academic faculties of philosophy, medicine, and law, but sparked immediate controversy in the Viennese art world when conservative critics and faculty members lambasted the paintings for being too "ugly," "heinous" and overly "risqué" for their sacred temple of knowledge.[37] Following a lengthy and heated anti-Klimt campaign, which began in the local press in spring 1900, and culminated in spring 1905, Klimt withdrew from the project altogether.[38]

In one particularly damning review of the *Faculty Paintings* published on 29 March 1901, the critic Karl Schreder, who, as we have already read, also disparaged Kokoschka's portraits at the 1911 Hagenbund exhibition, wrote:

> [The modern artist] throws sand in the eyes of a gullible public. Unfortunately, many allow themselves to be blinded without seeing through the humbug that is being carried out in the sacred name of "art." Klimt did not satisfactorily fulfill his duties to visually illustrate "philosophy" and "medicine." Rather, as a "new artist," he abandoned the conventional route of allegory, taking instead the path of incomprehensibility. Nothing is worse for a work of art than when it is not understood by the general public.[39]

Although Schreder's words were meant to undercut the agenda and artistic prowess that Klimt displayed in the *Faculty Paintings*, the critic's sentiments also reveal the sense of a disruption to receptive vision caused by works that some believed displayed controversial images. Schreder chastises both Klimt, for failing in his task to produce intelligible art, as well as the public, for being so easily duped by the aesthetics of the "new artist." Schreder's belief that "nothing is worse for a work of art" than to be incomprehensible to the masses, is not only a deeply anti-avant-garde notion, but also highlights the degree to which optical vision still enjoyed supremacy over inner artistic vision in the conservative critical press.

Given that Klimt ultimately abandoned the government commission, is it therefore fair to assert that he simply failed to act as a modernist capable of defending—or worse, was guilty of abandoning—his vision of the modern body?[40] This seems unlikely, as this new body was firstly present and critically recognized in Klimt's *Faculty Paintings*, and only later in expressionist canvases. In truth, the public interest over the controversy in the local press serves to reiterate the relevance of a discourse centered on the dialectics of vision in *fin-de-siècle* Vienna. The centrality of artistic vision, as discussed by Austrian artists and their critics, thus reveals a wide spectrum of opinions on what constituted vision in the Austrian capital, which included (but were not necessarily limited to): optical or physical modes of seeing; artistic or inner vision; psychological or pathological vision; theatrical or dramatic vision; and finally, receptive vision, as offered by critics and the public alike. The very real consequences of the disruption to receptive vision are all the more visible in Klimt's confrontation with the short-sighted consideration afforded to his *Faculty Paintings* in Vienna circa 1900.

The polemic against Klimt's paintings notwithstanding, critics like Peter Altenberg—a well-known poet and writer associated with the Jung Wien (Young Vienna) literary group, of which Bahr was also a member—wrote favorably about the artist's modernist vision. Altenberg tellingly declared:

> Gustav Klimt, as a visual painter, you are simultaneously a modern philosopher, a wholly modern poet! As you paint, you suddenly transform yourself, almost fairytale-like, into the most modern man, which perhaps you are not in the actual days and hours of life.[41]

Here, Altenberg specifically uses the phrase *"erschauender Maler"* to describe Klimt as a "perceptive" or "visual" painter who utilized his physical sight to create modern works of art, given that *erschauender* literally denotes an "onlooking" painter, rather than a "visionary" artist. Yet the idea that Klimt is also a "forward-looking" painter is also evident in the passage, particularly when Altenberg insists that Klimt was at once a visual artist, poet, and philosopher when he painted. What is more, the concept of the "onlooking" artist consequently reinforces the idea that Klimt, who was at the forefront of Viennese modernity, was incorporating expressive bodies into his canvases as a means of creating visual poetry; in other words, creating paintings that focused on both inner and outer modes of vision. Klimt's interest in the representation of the non-academic body, as witnessed in the dialogue surrounding the *Faculty Paintings*, thus perfectly represents the dual tension that was felt between optically "seeing" and comprehending a work of art, and the more forward-minded desire to conflate physical sight into artistic vision at the *fin de siècle*.

Following the height of the controversy surrounding the *Faculty Paintings*, Klimt, along with other founding members of the Vienna Secession, including Josef Hoffmann and Koloman Moser, left the Secession in 1905 to form the Klimtgruppe (Klimt Group). In order to broadcast their arrival on the Viennese art scene, and also to highlight the fact that their vision for Viennese modern art had shifted from that of the Secession, members of the Klimt Group famously organized two major exhibitions: the Kunstschauen (art shows) of 1908 and 1909. It is interesting that the pavilion for the 1908 Kunstschau showcased an entire room devoted to the artwork of children, just as the Secession had done in 1902 with an exhibition titled *Das Kind als Künstler* (*The Child as Artist*).[42] The inclusion of the "children's" gallery at the Kunstschau suggests that the Klimt Group was as overtly devoted to the notion of youthfulness as its predecessor (the Secession) had been, though Klimt and younger artists like Kokoschka and Schiele nevertheless had converging ideas on how youthfulness should be expressed in art. Examining this idea alongside Altenberg's conceptualization of Klimt's "perceptive vision" (again, a vision that is both "of the body," as well as emotively perceptive), one might analyze whether or not Klimt himself can be said to embody the trope of the creative man-child, which was so prevalent in the writings of Jung Wien members and in the younger expressionists' fixation on self-portraiture.

Klimt, of course, was a prominent modernist painter in Vienna, but unlike the subsequent generation of expressionists, he was not transfixed by images of the self, nor was he particularly interested in depicting the man-child in his paintings. Instead, women—both real and allegorical—were, and remained, the focus of Klimt's oeuvre. This is evident in the canvases he exhibited at the first Kunstschau, and in his well-known *Judith II (Salome)* (1909, Figure 1.1), which Klimt exhibited one year later at the second Kunstschau.[43] During his opening remarks at the 1908 exhibition, Klimt reinforced the notion that he was still deeply committed to carrying out his artistic vision, declaring: "It is in vain that our opponents attempt to combat the modern movement in art, to declare it dead. For theirs is a struggle against growth, against becoming—against life itself."[44] In hindsight, it is interesting that Klimt chose to relate modern art to the dichotomy of life and death, as though he were acutely aware of the fact that his avant-garde bodies were being codified as manifestations of disease and death. This notwithstanding, his statement makes clear that he perceived himself not as neglecting his larger agenda but as a visionary devoted to Viennese modernism.

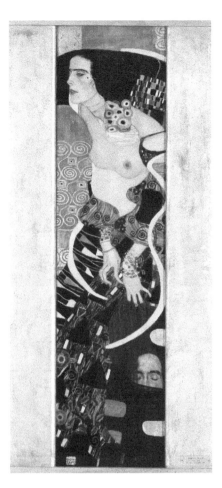

Figure 1.1 Gustav Klimt, *Judith II (Salome)*, 1909, oil on canvas. Galleria d'Arte Moderna di
　　　Ca'Pesaro, Venice.
Source: Photo: Cameraphoto Arte, Venice / Art Resource, NY.

The 1908 Kunstschau was moreover the first professional platform for many of the
young artists who later became associated with Viennese expressionism. Kokoschka's
breakthrough piece for the show—*Die Träumenden Knaben* (*The Dreaming Youths*,
1907–08), which he dedicated to Klimt—was appropriately deemed to be an expressive fairytale for adults, combining literary prose with color lithographs of androgynous
bodies in fantastical landscapes. Filled with the angst of adolescence, these images, particularly one lithograph entitled *Die Erwachenden* (*The Awakening*, Figure 1.2), signaled
that Kokoschka was attempting to push the discourse surrounding youthfulness from
childlike "primitivism" to the realm of pubescent sexuality. Kokoschka's early modernist
vision was thus focused on depictions of the adolescent teenage body, both male and
female. The bodies that populate *The Awakening* visually and symbolically embrace androgyny and, in turn, communicate a language of the (de)sexualized puppet body. For
this reason, *The Awakening* is discussed at greater length in Chapter 6, a chapter that is
specifically focused on the metaphorical marionette alongside the Viennese modern body.

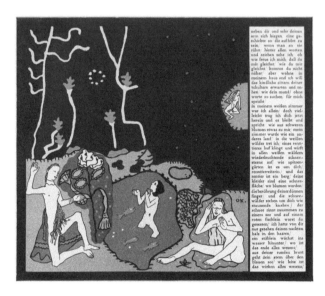

Figure 1.2 Oskar Kokoschka, *The Awakening*, from *The Dreaming Youths*, 1907, printed 1908, color lithograph. Wien Museum Karlsplatz, Vienna, Austria.

Source: © 2016 Fondation Oskar Kokoschka / Artists Rights Society (ARS), New York / ProLitteris, Zürich. Photo: Erich Lessing.

By 1909 Kokoschka had nevertheless begun to take issue with Klimt's symbolist style, as well as with Austrian art nouveau/Viennese Jugendstil, arguing that these styles only emphasized the decorative surface of a work of art. Jugendstil had, in fact, borrowed heavily from the aesthetics of foreign schools, namely French art nouveau, impressionism and symbolism, Belgian naturalism, the English Pre-Raphaelite movement, and German Jugendstil.[45] These non-native styles therefore remained at the periphery of the more avant-garde iconographies of expressionism, and as such, the dichotomies between inner and outer vision, between expressionism and impressionism, further suggest that these binaries relied upon one another in order for their meanings to be understood in *fin-de-siècle* Vienna. It would be incorrect then, to conceive of Viennese Jugendstil as a "new style" of art, which the French term art nouveau implies, or as a style "of the youth," as literally translated in the German. Instead, the Secession's embrace of Jugendstil as an alternative to Viennese historicism and the Vienna Academy's classical-realism legitimized the movement's claims to modernity through the belief that it had tapped into the eternal wellspring of youthful creativity, and by extension, youthful genius. It is all the more clear that youthful vision—as a key component of Viennese modernism—remained the one constant in the fluid transition from Secessionism to expressionism. In other words, the players changed, but the game remained the same. Expressionism thus developed out of Austrian art nouveau and symbolism as an emancipated movement, given that many of the Secessionists who had initially embraced Jugendstil as Vienna's contribution to modernism later became expressionist painters, playwrights, and poets.

As previously analyzed by Claude Cernuschi, the expressionist distrust of the ornamental surface of things aligned Kokoschka with the prominent Viennese architect and polemicist Adolf Loos, whose essay "Ornament und Verbrechen" ("Ornament and Crime," 1908) argued for a style of art and architecture centered on austerity and practicality, rather than excessive decoration.[46] Cernuschi suggests that Loos' artistic patronage of Kokoschka, who the architect saw as an ally who propagated his theories, was built on a system of reciprocity, given that the younger artist was simultaneously seeking to replace his previous artistic "father" (Klimt) with a new, more radical one (Loos). To support this claim, Cernuschi has examined how Kokoschka's style began to change in 1909 when the artist, now a member of Loos' intellectual circle, rejected the "decorative patterning, and flattened surface" of the Secession style, in favor of "an art of physical immediacy, [and] visual distortion."[47] Cernuschi's assertion brings to the fore the notion that Kokoschka's vision dialectic might additionally parallel the relationship between physicality and psychology—or between the body (optics) and embodiedness (inner visions)—by suggesting that these two phenomena work in harmony to bring material form to the inner content of a vision. It is important to remember, however, that the aesthetics of the Klimt Group had initially fostered Kokoschka's early articulations of modernism. As such, his interest in the semblance—or visible surface—of things reinforces the notion that his development as an expressionist was formed around the dialectical tension that existed between Klimt's "older" style and Loos' "newer" aesthetic. In replacing Klimt's style with his own, Kokoschka thus asserted that Klimt's Secessionist/symbolist vision, although certainly perceived as "modern" right at the turn of the century, had become *passé* by 1909.

Schiele's Expressionistic Vision

Kokoschka was not the only young artist in Vienna to grapple with the changing nature of vision in the emerging expressionist style. Schiele, Kokoschka's contemporary and artistic rival, was likewise drawn to the tension that existed between inner and optical sight and the expressive possibilities that such a binary could provide for his avant-garde renderings of the human body. As with Kokoschka's *The Dreaming Youths*, which showcased adolescent figures shaped by the artist's desire to portray inner (psychological) and outer (biological) bodily changes (see Figure 1.2), Schiele's oeuvre was similarly focused on different ways of viewing the subject in modern art. In her seminal book *Egon Schiele's Portraits* (1974), Alessandra Comini asserts that "the elusive element which this Expressionist artist sought in his portraiture accurately mirrors the collective cultural quest of his time: the inner self-psychological man."[48] Comini reminds her readers that the human figure was "the most persistent motif in the art of Egon Schiele," and in choosing the body as his muse, Schiele, according to Comini, sought to uncover "a lie—that is what the façade had become. Truth lay underneath and could only be exposed by probing, or even attacking, the psyche."[49] In this regard, Comini's sentiments fall in line with Harrison's earlier remarks concerning the manner in which the extant literature on the development of expressionism, and not on Schiele's images alone, has favored the primacy of inner visions of the psyche over the outer, superficial façade. The question that remains is whether or not Schiele's writings on vision reinforce the hegemony of inner vision over optical sight, or, conversely, reflect a belief similar to Kokoschka's dialectical model, in which both inner and outer vision were harnessed by the expressionist artist to construct the Viennese modern body.

Before delving into the specifics of this matter, it is first important to grasp the differences in the ways in which Kokoschka and Schiele presented their respective writings on modern vision to the art world at large. Having gained admission to the Akademie der bildenden Künste Wien (Vienna Academy of Fine Arts) in 1906, Schiele was quickly recognized by his peers as an exceptional talent. This point is historically significant because unlike Kokoschka, who at the time was enrolled at the Wiener Kunstgewerbeschule (Vienna School of Arts and Crafts, now the Universität für angewandte Kunst Wien, or the University of Applied Arts Vienna), Schiele gained his initial reputation at Vienna's more "prestigious" art school. Schiele nevertheless became dissatisfied with his training at the Academy, due to its focus on traditional methods, and consequently sought out Klimt in 1907 as a surrogate master instructor. Klimt subsequently introduced Schiele to the Wiener Werkstätte, where the young artist worked alongside fellow students like Kokoschka, as well as with more established artists like Koloman Moser and Klimt himself. In 1908 Schiele participated in his first exhibition in Klosterneuburg, a suburb of Vienna. After completing his third year at the Academy in 1909, he left the institution to form the short-lived Neukunstgruppe (New Art Group), which he organized with other young Viennese artists, poets and composers; Kokoschka joined the group in 1911.[50] Under Schiele's leadership, the group publicly referred to themselves as *Neukünstler*, or "New Artists," and asserted their avant-gardist stance in a collective exhibition organized at the Kunstsalon Pisko in 1909.[51] Like the Secession and Klimt Group before them, the New Artists did not share a single artistic style but instead were unified through their common disdain for the Academy and its outmoded practices. Kimberly Smith has recently noted that Schiele's decision to form the "anarchist" group and cut ties with the Academy before establishing himself as a well-known artist risked jeopardizing his ability to secure wealthy patrons affiliated with the prestigious institution; additionally, it endangered his future potential as a skilled artist in the Austrian capital.[52] Schiele's decision was nevertheless successful, since his radical stance gained him notoriety in the city, attracting the attention of Vienna's scandal-seeking journalists, who gleefully attended the Pisko show in order to denounce his "ugly" and "morbid" art.[53] Following their January 1912 exhibition, the New Art Group quietly disbanded, and Schiele, as well as Kokoschka, emerged as independent members of the modern art scene in Vienna.

As discussed earlier, Kokoschka revealed his modernist ideas in his 1912 public lecture "On the Nature of Visions," which, along with the later publication of the transcript, served as a formal, quasi-manifesto designed to explain the distinctiveness of his post-Klimt, expressionist period. Schiele, by contrast, routinely expressed his ideas on art, vision, and the modern body in less formal poems and aphorisms composed between 1909 and 1910, and in personal letters penned between 1910 and 1918. A number of his poems were later published, between 1914 and 1916, in the leftist Berlin magazine *Die Aktion: Wochenschrift für Politik, Literatur, Kunst* (*The Action: Weekly Journal for Politics, Literature, Art*), which also reproduced his drawings throughout the period.[54] While a number of these poems refer to a dualism of vision like that discussed in Kokoschka's lecture, it is important to note that Schiele never developed a comprehensive theory of modern vision, as Kokoschka had. It is true that Schiele had previously written the manifesto for the New Art Group, but Kokoschka was unique in contributing to the contemporary debate on the role of vision in Viennese expressionism with anything approaching a manifesto on expressionistic sight. Schiele was instead content to reflect upon this question in non-dogmatic, poetic contemplations.

Schiele's friend and promoter, the Viennese writer and art critic Arthur Roessler, published a number of Schiele's writings, including previously unpublished letters and poems, following the artist's death in 1918.[55] One letter, sent to Roessler in January 1911 when Schiele was twenty years old, reveals some of the artist's thoughts on artistic vision. Schiele writes:

> I, eternal child, I sacrificed myself for others, those who I pitied, those who were far away, or who looked at me but did not see. I brought gifts, sent glances and flickering, quaking air currents toward them; I scattered opportunities before them and did not speak. Before long a few recognized the facial expressions of inner vision and then they asked no more.[56]

In referring to himself as an "eternal child," Schiele chose terms that recall the language of the Secession, Jugendstil, Jung Wien, and the "child" pavilion at the 1908 Kunstschau. His words reinforce the idea that his personal vision was guided by youthful curiosity, by pubescent angst, by childlike innocence, or even adolescent voyeurism. Equally, Schiele positions himself as a martyr, as an individual who must sacrifice himself to those who look, but do not see. His prose conveys the idea that he, the avant-garde artist, is compelled to aid his viewers by helping them to see the "real" Egon Schiele. If this is the case, then Schiele could be said to privilege inner vision over corporeal sight, as he seems to suggest that one's optical vision is only able to discern façades, whereas one's inner vision is capable of penetrating the psyche. Were this the end of his thoughts on the act of seeing, one might be tempted to conclude that Schiele, like Worringer, Bahr, or others, was consistently interested in the supremacy of inner visions over optical sight. However, in the following sentence Schiele states that a wordless language of meanings had been conveyed to a few of Schiele's onlookers when they "recognized the facial expressions [*die Mimik*] of inner vision [*des Hineinsehens*]." When one translates the unusual German word *Hineinsehen*, we see that the term literally implies a vision that is capable of "looking into something," though I would argue that Schiele's compound noun equally implies "inner vision," and is thus similar to Kokoschka's use of the uncommon word *Gesichte* to connote "visions." But as in Kokoschka's dialectical model of expressionistic sight, Schiele's musings seem to place equal weight on *die Mimik*, or facial expressions, as a means to communicate meaning to his viewers. That is to say, were his viewers incapable of using their physical eyes to view his physiognomy, then they would fail to register the glimpses of his inner psyche.

In a poem from 1909–10 entitled "Visionen" ("Visions"), which was later published in *Die Aktion* in 1914, Schiele wrote rather existentially on the role of visions, while simultaneously demonstrating a poetic fondness for the language of synesthesia:

> Everything was dear to me; I wanted to look lovingly at the angry people, to challenge their eyes to remain so, and to the envious I wanted to give them gifts and tell them that I am worthless. [...] The white pale girls showed me their black feet and red garters and spoke with their black fingers. But I thought about vast worlds, about finger flowers and wet mornings. If I myself was there, I was hardly aware. I saw the park: yellow-green, blue-green, red-green, quaking-green, sunny-green,

violet-green, and listened to the blossoming orange flowers. [...] I thought about my colorful portrait visions and it seemed to me as if I had once spoken only to them.[57]

In the poem, Schiele uses certain words to describe both inner and outer modes of vision. He "looks lovingly" in the hope that others will return his affectionate gaze, yet there is also an implied desire to control the eyes of the "angry people." When speaking of the pale girls in the park, the description of their white skin and black fingers and feet evokes a striking visual contrast that can only be gleaned through optical sight, and Schiele states that the girls communicate to him, and each other, through a sign language of gestures. Next, the artist describes the park, and the impression left on the reader is that Schiele is overwhelmed by the colors he sees there, by the sunshine on the grass, and by the wind as it rustles through the grass and the nearby trees. The final effect is a synesthetic experience that permits the artist to "hear" the flowers blossom on a nearby orange tree. But then Schiele turns from the sphere of optical sight and physical sensations to an inner world where he converses with subjects in his expressive "portrait visions," or *Porträtvisionen*, as if they were themselves capable of speaking. The broader implication is that Schiele's artistic imagination has brought material form to figures that had long occupied his mind's eye, that are not necessarily portraits of known or actual persons, but perhaps bodies that only exist in the artist's inner psyche.

Schiele returns to the image of the pallid girl (in "Visions") in a subsequent poem entitled "Das Porträt des Stillbleichen Mädchens" ("Portrait of a Silent Pale Girl") written sometime between 1909 and 1910.

A pollution of my love, yes. I loved everything. The girl came, I found her face, her consciousness, her worker's hands; I loved everything about her. I had to portray her, because of how she looked and how close she was to me. — Now she is gone. Now I encounter her body.[58]

In the text, Schiele again implies that the avant-garde artist must harness both outer and inner vision in order to create a modern portrait. He writes that he found the girl's face with his physical eyes, and also her consciousness, perhaps within the depths of his own psyche. His motivation for portraying her as a subject in his art is undeniably her physical appearance ("because of how she looked") yet, remarkably, it is only after she has departed ("now she is gone") that Schiele is able to truly "see" her body, to encounter it with new eyes. The crux of the poem therefore seems to reside in the idea that Schiele's outer vision, which was captivated by the young girl, was a prerequisite to the creation of the image, but it was his inner vision that allowed him to fully grasp the expressive, eternal qualities of the girl's body, either as a subject in his artwork or as an apparition in his mind. In this regard, the silent pale girl may not have been a "real" girl at all, but only one of Schiele's *Porträtvisionen*.

I think it is incorrect to assume that Schiele wrote or conceived of his poems as literal descriptions of his artwork, and yet it is nevertheless fruitful to ponder whether or not an image like *Sitzender Frauenakt mit geneigtem Kopf und erhobenen Armen* (*Seated Female Nude with Tilted Head and Raised Arms*, 1910, Plate 5) was created as a "portrait vision" of one of the pale girls in Schiele's "Visions," or the quiet girl in "Portrait of a Silent Pale Girl." The subject in Schiele's watercolor drawing is depicted with ruddy-pale skin, and her arms, hands and fingers conspicuously communicate an esoteric sign language to the viewer, just as the fingers of the girls in "Visions" spoke to one another and to Schiele. What is more, the girl's body in *Seated Female Nude with Tilted Head and Raised Arms* is the only thing that the viewer encounters, given that the sitter, as with most of Schiele's portraits, is the sole component of the composition. As I discuss in later chapters of this book, the awkward geometry of the female body, which recalls the language of androgynous figures in Kokoschka's *The Dreaming Youths*, with their over-sized, outstretched limbs, uncannily embodies the semiotics of a puppet or mario-nette's body. In Schiele's drawing, the female nude visually and metaphorically becomes a "living" doll or puppet manipulated by the artist's optical sight (his fondness for her bodily form) and inner visions (his ability to encounter her body even when she is physi-cally absent). The girl is thus a portrait of a human figure, yet simultaneously an artistic vision of a human body controlled by the artist-as-puppet-master: that is, as ultimate creator of a figure that has its referent in the material world (a human body), as well as the world of the artist's imagination (an idea of a body).

Like Kokoschka, Schiele eventually became disillusioned with Klimt's style, even though Klimt had served as one of his unofficial teachers during his pre- and post-training at the Academy, and at the 1908 and 1909 Kunstschau exhibitions. In a letter written around 1910, Schiele summarized his thoughts on his former mentor: "I went by way of Klimt until March. Today I believe I am someone entirely different."[59] In the extant scholarship on Schiele, this statement has often been regarded as the moment that Schiele rejected Klimt, just as Kokoschka had done when joining the circle of Adolf Loos in 1909.[60] I want to propose, by contrast, that rather than be-ing an outright dismissal of Klimt's style, Schiele's statement was instead a comment on how his changing artistic vision had transformed him into an independent artist whose success was no longer contingent on Klimt's guidance or more considerable reputation. Schiele's newer, "younger" vision had thus led him down a different path from Klimt, who had nevertheless profoundly inspired his compositions prior to 1910.

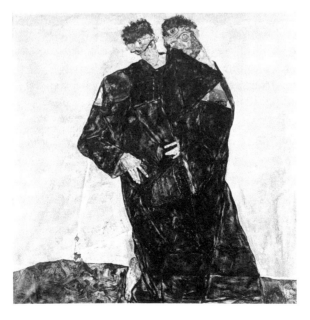

Figure 1.3 Egon Schiele, *The Hermits*, 1912, oil on canvas. Leopold Museum, Vienna.
Source: Photo: Erich Lessing / Art Resource, NY.

For a view of this complex relationship in painted form, it is useful to turn to Schiele's *Die Eremiten* (*The Hermits*, 1912, Figure 1.3), which was created two years after the young artist's purported "break" from Klimt. The image is a double portrait of Schiele and Klimt, their bodies joined together and cloaked in black monks' cowls or, more probably (due to the decorative patches on the shoulders), the long, stylized smocks that Klimt wore while painting. If the garments were intended to be cowls, then Schiele may be suggesting that the two artists had become isolated from society or the Viennese art world, as the title certainly implies. Alternatively, if Schiele chose to cover their bodies in two of Klimt's painting smocks, then the symbolism of their robes may be a hint that Schiele, in 1912, still felt a strong affinity toward Klimt, something which the closeness of their forms appears to substantiate. Regardless, the iconography of the painting undeniably depicts Schiele as the leader, given his position as the foregrounded figure. This artistic decision symbolically forces Klimt to cling to Schiele's body for support and, in a somewhat ironic fashion, the visual arrangement seems to suggest that Klimt must now look to Schiele for guidance.

Perhaps the most striking element of *The Hermits* is the fact that Schiele's eyes are open, while Klimt's are closed. Schiele, with his head cocked downward, pierces the viewer with his stare, while Klimt, with his head on Schiele's shoulder, appears to be sleeping or lost in reverie. Given the dichotomy between their closed and open eyes, I suggest that the visual language of *The Hermits* highlights the dialectics of vision that constructed artistic bodies in Viennese expressionism. More specifically, Klimt's eyes indicate that his vision of modern art—of Secessionstil, Jugendstil, or symbolism—has metaphorically fallen asleep, or may even be dead. By contrast, Schiele's penetrating stare shows that he is wide awake and ready to open Vienna's eyes to the vision of expressionist bodies. In speaking about the painting, Schiele referred to the image as a "vision," rather than a mere portrait.[61] Thus, when he wrote in "Visions" that he "wanted to look lovingly at the angry people, to make their eyes do the same," it is interesting to wonder if he was anticipating the condemnation of the new expressionist style (like that offered by Franz Ferdinand) in order to help viewers truly "see" a modern work of art. For Schiele, "seeing" is therefore not merely an appreciation of the visible surface of the canvas, but the ability to be able to look into the soul, psyche, and imagination of the young artist.

A personal letter from Schiele to Dr. Oskar Reichel dated June 1911 seemingly reinforces this reading. In it, the artist states:

> Painting is a skill. [...] I became aware and I quickly counted, observed every cipher and tried to see. The painter can also look. But seeing [or vision] is something more.[62]

Given that Schiele repeatedly asserted his ability to "see" the truth of modern art and the ciphers of the world, it is not surprising that unreceptive critics who did not understand—or wish to understand—Schiele's vision argued that he was an artist who squinted, rather than an individual who saw the world in full.[63] This critical denunciation of his optical sight was unquestioningly intended as a disparaging pun on Schiele's name, since *schielen* in German literally means "to squint," yet the artist himself drew upon this clever double entendre during his lifetime in at least one poem, entitled "Empfindung" ("Sensation," c. 1915). In the text, Schiele writes: "High, great winds made my spine cold / and I squinted there. On top of a scratchy wall I saw / the whole world."[64] It is clear that to "squint" and to "see" are here synonymous with the artist's unique vision (and perception) of the semblance of things that inhabit his world. Squinting or not, Schiele thus makes evident that he, like Kokoschka, was cognizant of the fact that the dialectics of expressionistic vision were paramount to their developing style(s).

Conclusion

Diverging notions of artistic vision in the early twentieth century helped to create the dichotomy that undeniably exists between Kokoschka's understanding of the formative tenets of expressionistic sight and the other prevailing theories of artistic vision offered by Bahr, Fechter, Kandinsky, and Worringer, who respectively reinforced the dominance of inner vision over optical sight. Whereas Kandinsky continued to argue that the inner spirit exists as the driving force for the creative energy leading to avant-garde work, Kokoschka instead maneuvered away from a discussion of the supremacy of spiritualism—or the mystical/psychic processes—in order to give equal weight to both psychological and physiological functions. In Kandinsky's theory this privileging of inner feeling is reinforced and made apparent, in contrast to Kokoschka's attempt to balance the two divergent concepts. This is possibly due to the fact that Kokoschka presupposed that the outer and inner conditions of the human spirit do not materialize as a dialectic of opposition, as in Kandinsky's handling of vision, but as a necessary dualism. Schiele's writings, though certainly not as theoretical as Kokoschka's treatise, similarly adopted the standpoint that modes of seeing in Viennese expressionism were contingent upon the manifestation of both psychic and optical sight. The inner and outer condition, as well as consciousness and unconsciousness, were therefore all needed in order to successfully arrive at form. In the case of Viennese expressionism, this subject matter took the shape of modern bodies.

To be sure, Kokoschka's notion of vision (singular) was a physiological operation, while visions (plural) were primarily of the mind. It can be observed, then, that the allegiance to optical sight and the reciprocal criticism of it were closely allied ideas within the developing history of expressionism in both Germany and Austria. While certainly not the only difference between the two Germanic schools of expressionism, this formulation of artistic vision ostensibly persists as the greatest disparity between Kokoschka's theory of expressionistic sight and the theories offered by his contemporaries in the *fin-de-siècle* German-speaking art world. More important still, Kokoschka's dialectic of vision provides an alternative theory of art focused on the Viennese modern body, even as other modes of artistic creation were turning toward abstraction and non-representational forms, particularly French cubism or Kandinsky's style of German expressionism.

In discussing the iconography of the Viennese modern body in the introduction to this book, I made use of three important case studies: Kokoschka's *Hans Tietze and Erica Tietze-Conrat* (1909, Plate 1), Schiele's *Nude Self-Portrait* (1910, Plate 2), and Koloman Moser's *The Love Potion—Tristan and Isolde* (1915, Plate 3). In returning to these images, it is important to note that each of the paintings involves a disturbance of vision on the part of the figure(s) being depicted. In Kokoschka's *Hans Tietze and Erica Tietze-Conrat*, it is apparent that neither of the sitters is optically connected to one another or to the viewer. Instead, their vacant stares and puppet-like hand gestures suggest that they look, but do not see. Schiele's *Nude Self-Portrait*, by contrast, robs the artist's body of its eyes entirely, leaving only vacant space or empty sockets where his visual organs ought to reside. Such a maneuver seems to suggest that the modern body, at least in Schiele's *oeuvre*, must convey a sense of bodily disfigurement—in this case blindness—while simultaneously implying that the modern artist can still "see" (or "squint") even without his optical sight. Finally, in Moser's *The Love Potion*, the female protagonist is rendered incapable of utilizing her eyes to guide her body toward her would-be lover, and instead must rely on her haptic sense to get her bearings and find her way to Tristan. As such, it is clear that these works collectively call attention to the relationship between optical sight and inner vision that became a unifying element in an art movement that embraced such a wide array of styles. The desire in all of these images to depict disrupted vision is therefore not coincidental. Rather, the shared interest in the changing nature of artistic vision signals that each of these Viennese artists was caught up in a discourse centered on dualisms, particularly on the tension between abstraction and figuration, and on outer and inner ways to see art.

Given the overwhelming focus on the abnormal, diseased, or pathological body in *fin-de-siècle* Viennese art, it is not surprising that much of the current literature on expressionist bodies has likewise been preoccupied by psychoanalytic interpretations of developing sexuality or of angst-ridden figures, due largely to Freud's concurrent extrapolations on childhood, adolescence, and puberty in his much-discussed *Drei Abhandlungen zur Sexualtheorie* (*Three Essays on the Theory of Sexuality*, 1905).[65] The male body—and particularly the body of the young male artist—found fruition with the expressionists, and it is equally evident that their focus on the expressive female body was indebted to Secessionstil and to Klimt's post-1905 canvases. The next chapter of this book turns to the discourse surrounding turn-of-the-century notions of hysteria and psychosexual trauma as concepts that visually altered modernism in Vienna. Just as the man-child was equated with artistic vision, male genius, and the modern painter in both symbolism and expressionism, the woman-child—drawn from the depictions of psycho-pathological bodies offered by Viennese expressionist artists—became synonymous with two other *fin-de-siècle* artistic fixations: the femme fatale and the hysterical patient. It was, after all, turn-of-the-century critics like Grüner, Strzygowski, and Schreder who suggested, as early as 1911, that the subjects of Kokoschka's paintings were better suited to the madhouse, clinic, or ward for the criminally "insane." The following chapter thus makes clear that while Freud's writings may not actually have provided direct inspiration for the psychological portraits created by Kokoschka and his compatriots, the larger European discourse on the psychosexual, hysterical body—be that male or female—ultimately found fruition in the re-visioning of the modern body carried out by Viennese expressionism at the beginning of the twentieth century.

Notes

1 Franz Ferdinand, quoted in Edith Hoffmann, *Kokoschka: Life and Work* (London: Faber and Faber, 1947), 86. Hoffmann writes that Ferdinand declared: "Dem Kerl sollte man die Knochen im Leibe zerbrechen." Peter Altenberg also discusses this anecdote in Peter Altenberg, "Authentisch," *Simplicissimus* 16, no. 36 (1911): 621. See also Werner J. Schweiger, *Der Junge Kokoschka: Leben und Werk 1904–1914* (Vienna: Brandstätter, 1983), 195.

2 Regarding Franz Ferdinand's reaction, see the sources in note 1. For a contemporary account of his staunch morality, see Leo Valiani, *The End of Austria-Hungary* (New York: Alfred A. Knopf, 1973), 9.

3 Peter Selz has noted that Kokoschka's early works were "shocking" to contemporary audiences. See Peter Selz, *German Expressionist Painting* (Berkeley: University of California Press, 1957), 161. These shocking paintings, and others, were more recently the focus of a contemporary exhibition at Frankfurt's Schirn Kunsthalle. See Tobias G. Natter and Max Hollein, eds. *The Naked Truth: Klimt, Schiele, Kokoschka and Other Scandals*, trans. Elizabeth Clegg (Munich: Prestel, 2005).

4 Gemma Blackshaw mentions Franzos' "dismay" at seeing her portrait, in Gemma Blackshaw, *Facing the Modern: The Portrait in Vienna 1900* (London: National Gallery Company and Yale University Press, 2013), 30.

5 Josef Strzygowski, "Junge Künstler im Hagenbund," *Die Zeit* 10, no. 3010 (February 9, 1911): 1. The original German reads: "Da ist dieser Oskar Kokoschka. [...] Mit diesen Koko-Strahlen seiner Psyche durchleuchtet er auch die Personen, die das Unglück haben, unter seinen Pinsel zu geraten. Welcher faule Geruch geht von dem Bilde der Frau Dr. L. Fr. aus! [...] Man lasse ihn gewisse Orte mit abschreckenden Bildern von Syphilis und Paralyse ausmalen."

6 Karl Schreder, "Kunstuntergang im 'Hagenbund'," *Deutsches Volksblatt* 23, no. 7941 (February 9, 1911): 1. The original German reads: "Er malt 'Porträts,' darunter solche stadtbekannter Persönlichkeiten. Wie aus Tollhäusern oder aus mephitischen Grüften emporgestiegen, erscheinen diese grauenvollen Bildnisse, deren Antlitze entweder die Entstellungen zerstörender Krankheiten oder eines zersetzenden Verwesungsprozesses zu tragen scheinen."

7 Schreder, "Kunstuntergang im 'Hagenbund'," 1. The original German reads: "Und wie grausig sind nur die durchwegs verkrüppelten Hände, teils angeschwollen, teils halb verfault, als hätte die Lepra ihre entsetzlichen Verwüstungen begonnen."

8 Franz Grüner, "Oskar Kokoschka," *Die Fackel* 12, no. 317/318 (February 28, 1911): 18. The original German reads: "Kein Betrachter tritt vor seine Bilder, der nicht sofort anmerken würde, daß die Dargestellten aussehen wie nach schwerer Krankheit, nach mehrjähriger Kerkerhaft, mit abstoßenden physischen und, versteht sich, psychischen Gebrechen behaftet und dergleichen mehr."

9 Oskar Kokoschka, "On the Nature of Visions," in Hoffmann, *Kokoschka: Life and Work*, 287. The English translation of Kokoschka's text, arranged by Hedi Medlinger and John Thwaites in 1947, was the earliest published version of the artist's essay, which was later transcribed into German by Kokoschka himself in 1956. In the later version, the German text reads: "ich ziehe aus der Welt absichtslos etwas als Dinge empor. Dann aber werde ich nichts mehr sein, als eine, Ihre Einbildung." See Oskar Kokoschka, "Von der Natur der Gesichte," in *Oskar Kokoschka: Schriften 1907–1955*, ed. Hans Maria Wingler (Munich: Langen Müller, 1956), 341. Although the content remains unaltered in the later version, its more awkward construction inclines me to use the earlier (English) version of Kokoschka's lecture. What is more, this version was definitively approved by Kokoschka, who had already been living in England for nine years and was fluent in English when he collaborated with Hoffmann on her book.

10 Kokoschka, "On the Nature of Visions," 285.

11 Kokoschka, "On the Nature of Visions," 285.

12 Kokoschka, "On the Nature of Visions," 287.

13 Kokoschka, "On the Nature of Visions," 286.

14 Charles Harrison, "Abstraction," in *Primitivism, Cubism, Abstraction: The Early Twentieth Century*, eds. Francis Frascina, Charles Harrison, and Gill Perry (New Haven: Yale University Press, 1993), 208. In many ways, Harrison's examination of expressionism builds on Peter Selz's scholarship in this area, as Selz was arguably the first late twentieth-century art historian to provide an overview of the historical, critical discourse surrounding the role of vision in German expressionism. See Peter Selz, *German Expressionist Painting* (Berkeley: University of California Press, 1957), 3–11.

15 In addition to Harrison's analysis, Robert Jensen has equally argued that a review of the primary, critical literature and secondary, biographical scholarship collectively shows that, "expressionist rhetoric sacrifices the artist's conscious agency to compulsive psychological forces." See Robert Jensen, "A Matter of Professionalism: Marketing Identity in *Fin-de-Siècle* Vienna," in *Rethinking Vienna 1900*, ed. Steven Beller (Oxford: Berghahn Books, 2001), 199.

16 Wilhelm Worringer, *Abstraktion und Einfühlung: Ein Beitrag zur Stilpsychologie,* Third edn (1908; Munich: R. Piper & Co., 1911), 1. The original German reads: "die sichtbare Oberfläche der Dinge."

17 Worringer, *Abstraktion und Einfühlung,* 16–17. The original German reads: "Welches sind nun die psychischen Voraussetzungen des Abstraktionsdranges? Wir haven sie im Weltgefühl jener Völker, in ihrem psychischen Verhalten dem Kosmos gegenüber zu suchen. Während der Einfühlungsdrang ein glückliches pantheistisches Vertraulichkeitsverhältnis zwischen dem Menschen und den Aussenwelterscheinungen zur Bedingung hat, ist der Abstraktionsdrang die Folge einer grossen inneren Beunruhigung des Menschen durch die Erscheinungen der Aussenwelt und korrespondiert in religiöser Beziehung mit einer stark transzendentalen Färbung aller Vorstellungen."

18 Paul Fechter, *Der Expressionismus* (Munich: R. Piper & Co., 1914), 28. Fechter employs the phrase: "Seelisch-Sensuellen in ein allgemein geistiges Weltgefühl."

19 Fechter, *Der Expressionismus,* 27. The original German reads: "Die Darstellung der Außenwelt wird der Photographie und dem Kino überlassen; an ihre Stelle tritt die gefühlerfüllte Vorstellung des Künstlers." Fechter uses the German words *Vorstellung des Künstlers* to connote artistic vision, though this phrase could equally be translated as the "imagination of the artist."

20 Carl Schorske has briefly commented on the semantics of the word *Gesicht*, noting that "the German word *Gesicht* denotes both 'vision' or 'image' and 'visage' or 'face,' thus embracing both the subjective and the objective side of visual perception. The double meaning is integral to Kokoschka's conception of the artist's consciousness, but compels us in English to stress now one side, now the other, of the complex." See Carl E. Schorske, *Fin-de-Siècle Vienna: Politics and Culture* (New York: Vintage Books, 1981), 340n.

21 Hermann Bahr, *Expressionismus* (1916; Munich: Delphin-Verlag, 1919), 51. The original German reads: "Alle Geschichte der Malerei ist immer Geschichte des Sehens." R. T. Gribble alternatively translates this passage as: "The history of painting is nothing but the history of vision—of seeing," in Hermann Bahr, "Expressionism," in *Art in Theory, 1900–1990: An Anthology of Changing Ideas*, eds. Charles Harrison and Paul Wood (Oxford: Blackwell Publishers, 1992), 117.

22 Bahr, *Expressionismus,* 50–51. The original German reads: "Die Technik verändert sich erst, wenn sich das Sehen verändert hat. Sie verändert sich nur, weil sich das Sehen verändert hat. Sie verändert sich, um den Veränderungen des Sehens nachzukommen. Das Sehen aber verändert sich mit der Beziehung des Menschen zur Welt. Wie der Mensch zur Welt steht, so sieht er sie."

23 Kokoschka, "On the Nature of Visions," 286. Bahr's theorization is curiously similar to Heinrich Wölfflin's understanding of vision's history in his work *Kunstgeschichtliche Grundbegriffe* (*Principles of Art History*, 1915), in which he states: "Vision itself has its history, and the revelation of these visual strata must be regarded as the primary task of art history." See Heinrich Wölfflin, *Principles of Art History: The Problem of the Development of Style in Later Art*, trans. M. D. Hottinger (New York: Dover Publications, 1950), 11.

24 Bahr, *Expressionismus,* 92.

25 Bahr, *Expressionismus,* 92. The original German reads: "Der Impressionismus ist ja nur das letzte Wort der klassischen Kunst."

26 Even though "classical" here can be read as the academic treatment of optical models developed during the Renaissance, Bahr's use of the word "classical" primarily connotes the flawed tenets of impressionism and its failure to break with the notion of optical truth.

27 Building upon the contemporary literature on Viennese expressionism (including Bahr's work), Carl Schorske reasserts that this style was primarily concerned with exploring the inner feelings and psychological forces of Viennese artists, writers, and intellectuals. See Schorske, *Fin-de-Siècle Vienna.*

28 For a discussion of German expressionism's strong opposition to French modern art, including impressionism, developed in the first decade of the twentieth century, see Geoffrey Perkins, *Contemporary Theory of Expressionism* (Bern: Peter Lang, 1974); and Jensen, "A Matter of Professionalism," 203.

29 Jensen, "A Matter of Professionalism," 20–23.

30 Bahr, *Expressionismus,* 112–13.

31 Bahr, *Expressionismus*, 113. The original German reads: "Das Auge des Impressionisten vernimmt bloß, es spricht nicht, es nimmt nur die Fragen auf, antwortet aber nicht. Impressionisten haben statt der Augen noch ein paar Ohren, aber keinen Mund ... Aber der Expressionist reißt den Mund der Menschheit wieder auf, sie hat lange genug nur immer gehorcht und dazu geschwiegen, jetzt will sie wieder des Geistes Antwort sagen."

32 Concerning Kokoschka's relationship to Kandinsky and the latter's subsequent (and more popular) texts on expressionism, it is known that both men were good friends and collaborated on a number of Blaue Reiter projects in 1912, the same year in which the two writers both published their respective essays. For Kandinsky's theories concerning the spiritual in art, see Wassily Kandinsky, *Über das Geistige in der Kunst: Insbesondere in der Malerei* (Munich: R. Piper & Co., 1912). With regard to Kokoschka's and Kandinsky's joint involvement in Der Blaue Reiter, see Klaus Lankheit, "A History of the Almanac," in *The Blaue Reiter Almanac*, ed. Klaus Lankheit (New York: Da Capo Press, 1974), 32, 34.

33 Kandinsky, *Über das Geistige in der Kunst*, 9. The original German reads: "Kraft des 'Sehens.'"

34 Schorske, *Fin-de-Siècle Vienna*, 342.

35 Kokoschka, "On the Nature of Visions," 286.

36 Kokoschka, "On the Nature of Visions," 286.

37 Hermann Bahr documented the various contemporary attacks and public criticisms directed at Klimt and the *Faculty Paintings*. For these negative reviews, see Hermann Bahr, ed., *Gegen Klimt: Historisches, Philosophie, Medizin, Goldfische, Fries* (Vienna: Eisenstein & Co., 1903), 13–59. See also Schorske, *Fin-de-Siècle Vienna*, 226–67; and Peter Vergo, "Gustav Klimts 'Philosophie' und das Programm der Universitätsgemälde," *Mitteilungen der Österreichischen Galerie* 22/23, no. 66/67, Klimt-Studien (1978/79), 69–100.

38 For details surrounding the commission, see Bahr, *Gegen Klimt*. Klimt's friend and patron Berta Zuckerkandl, who was also an art critic for the local press, interviewed the artist on April 12, 1905 following his withdrawal from the Ministry commission. Klimt's words, as paraphrased by Zuckerkandl, are reproduced and translated in Berta Zuckerkandl, "The Klimt Affair," in *Gustav Klimt: The Ronald S. Lauder and Serge Sabarsky Collections*, ed. Renée Price (Munich: Prestel, 2007), 459–61.

39 Karl Schreder, quoted in Bahr, *Gegen Klimt*, 57. The original German reads: "...streut einer leichtgläubigen Welt Sand in die Augen. Leider lassen sich viele dadurch blenden, ohne den Humbug zu durchschauen, der mit dem geheiligten Namen 'Kunst' getrieben wird. Klimt hat seine Aufgaben, die 'Philosophie' und die 'Medizin' bildlich darzustellen, nicht befriedigend gelöst. Indem er als 'Neuer' die hergebrachten Wege der Allegorie verließ, begab er sich auf die Pfade der Unverständlichkeit. Nichts aber ist schlechter für ein Kunstwerk, als wenn es von der Allgemeinheit nicht verstanden wird."

40 This understanding of Klimt's *Faculty Paintings* is offered in Gemma Blackshaw, "The Pathological Body: Modernist Strategising in Egon Schiele's Self-Portraiture," *Oxford Art Journal* 30, no. 3 (2007): 399.

41 Peter Altenberg, in "Ansprache," quoted in Johannes Dobai and Fritz Novotny, *Gustav Klimt*, ed. Friedrich Welz (Salzburg: Galerie Welz, 1967), 70. The original German reads: "Gustav Klimt, als erschauender Maler bist Du zugleich ein moderner Philosoph, ein ganz moderner Dichter! Indem Du malst, verwandelst Du Dich urplötzlich, ja fast märchenhaft, in den, modernsten Menschen, der Du vielleicht im realen Dasein des Tages und der Stunde gar nicht bist!"

42 Peter Vergo, *Art in Vienna, 1898–1918: Klimt, Kokoschka, Schiele and their Contemporaries* (London: Phaidon, 1993), 180. Schorske also discusses the "Art of the Child" exhibition, which occupied the first room of the Kunstschau pavilion, in Schorske, *Fin-de-Siècle Vienna*, 327. For a discussion of the 1902 Secession exhibition, see Ludwig Hevesi, "Das Kind als Künstler," in *Altkunst-Neukunst: Wien 1894–1908*, ed. Otto Breicha (1909; Klagenfurt: Ritter Verlag, 1984), 449–54.

43 Jane Kallir, *Egon Schiele: Life and Work* (New York: Harry N. Abrams, 1996), 56.

44 Gustav Klimt, quoted in *Katalog der Kunstschau Wien 1908* (Vienna: Holzhausen, 1908). For an English translation, see Vergo, *Art in Vienna*, 179–80.

45 See, for example, Schorske, *Fin-de-Siècle Vienna*, 214.

46 Claude Cernuschi, *Re/casting Kokoschka: Ethics and Aesthetics, Epistemology and Politics in Fin-de-Siècle Vienna* (Cranbury: Associated University Presses, 2002).

47 Cernuschi, *Re/casting Kokoschka*, 25.

48 Alessandra Comini, *Egon Schiele's Portraits* (Berkeley: University of California Press, 1974), 1.

49 Comini, *Egon Schiele's Portraits*, 1, 6.

50 Comini, *Egon Schiele's Portraits*, 30.

51 For a contemporary review of the exhibition, see Arthur Roessler, "Neukunstgruppe. Ausstellung im Kunstsalon Pisko," *Arbeiter Zeitung* no. 336 (December 7, 1909): 21.

52 Kimberly A. Smith, *Between Ruin and Renewal: Egon Schiele's Landscapes* (New Haven: Yale University Press, 2004), 21.

53 Comini, *Egon Schiele's Portraits*, 48.

54 Egon Schiele, "Skizzen," *Die Aktion* 4, no. 9 (February 1914): 234; Egon Schiele, "Gedichte," *Die Aktion* 4, no. 15 (April 1914): 323; Egon Schiele, "Die Kunst der Neukünstler," *Die Aktion* 4, no. 20 (May 1914): 428; Egon Schiele, "Zwei Gedichte," *Die Aktion* 5, no. 3/4 (January 1915): 37–38; Egon Schiele, "Ährenfeld," *Die Aktion* 5, no. 31/32 (August 1915): 398; Egon Schiele, "Abendland," *Die Aktion* 6, no. 35/36 (September 1916): 493.

55 Schiele's letters, poems and aphorisms were published posthumously in Arthur Roessler, ed., *Briefe und Prosa von Egon Schiele* (Vienna: Buchhandlung Richard Lányi, 1921).

56 Roessler, *Briefe und Prosa von Egon Schiele*, 48. The original German reads: "Ich ewiges Kind,—ich brachte Opfer anderen, denen, die mich erbarmten, denen, die weitweg waren oder mich Sehenden nicht sahen. Ich brachte Gaben, schickte Augen und flimmernde Zitterluft ihnen entgegen, ich streute ihnen überwindbare Wege vor und—redete nicht.— Alsbald erkannten einige die Mimik des Hineinsehens und sie fragten dann nicht mehr."

57 Roessler, *Briefe und Prosa von Egon Schiele*, 22–23. The original German reads: "Alles war mir lieb; ich wollte die zornigen Menschen lieb ansehn, damit ihre Augen gegentun müssen, und die Neidigen wollt' ich beschenken und ihnen sagen, daß ich wertlos bin. [...] Die weißen bleichen Mädchen zeigten mir ihren schwarzen Fuß und das rote Strumpfband und sprachen mit den schwarzen Fingern.—Ich aber dachte an die weiten Welten, an Fingerblumen und nasse Morgen. Ob ich selbst da bin, hatt' ich kaum gewußt.—Ich sah den Park gelbgrün, blaugrün, rotgrün, zittergrün, sonniggrün, violettgrün, und horchte der blühenden Orangeblumen. [...] Ich dachte an meine farbigen Porträtvisionen und es kam mir vor, als ob ich einmal nur mit jenen allen gesprochen hätte."

58 Roessler, *Briefe und Prosa von Egon Schiele*, 21–22. The original German reads: "Eine Pollution meiner Liebe,—ja. Alles liebte ich. Das Mädchen kam, ich fand ihr Gesicht, ihr Unbewußtes, ihre Arbeiterhände; alles liebte ich an ihr. Ich mußte sie darstellen, weil sie so schaut und mir so nahe war.—Jetzt ist sie fort. Jetzt begegne ich ihrem Körper."

59 A facsimile of the letter can be found in Elisabeth Leopold et al., *Egon Schiele: Letters and Poems 1910–1912 from the Leopold Collection* (Munich: Prestel, 2008), 57. The original German reads: "Ich bin durch Klimt gegangen bis März. Heute, glaub ich, bin ich der ganz andere."

60 See, for example, Reinhard Steiner, *Egon Schiele, 1890–1918: The Midnight Soul of the Artist* (Cologne: Taschen, 2000), 21–30.

61 Christian M. Nebehay, *Egon Schiele, 1890–1918: Leben, Briefe, Gedichte* (Salzburg: Residenz Verlag, 1979), 320.

62 Roessler, *Briefe und Prosa von Egon Schiele*, 144. The original German reads: "Malen ist ein Können. [...] Ich bin wissend geworden und habe schnell gezählt, habe jede Ziffer beobachtet und zu ersehen versucht. Schauen kann auch der Maler. Sehen is aber doch mehr."

63 Alessandra Comini and Kimberly Smith have both examined the literature on Schiele's "squinting." See Comini, *Egon Schiele's Portraits*, 41; and Smith, *Between Ruin and Renewal*, 187.

64 "Empfindung" was one of two poems published in Schiele, "Zwei Gedichte," 37–38. The original German reads: "Hohe Großwinde machten kalt mein Rückgrat / und da schielte ich. Auf einer krätzigen Mauer sah ich / die ganze Welt."

65 Sigmund Freud, *Three Essays on the Theory of Sexuality*, ed. James Strachey, trans. James Strachey, Revised ed. (1905; New York: Basic Books, 2000).

2 "The Woman Emerges"
Medical Vision and the Spectacle of Hysteria

The longer we have been occupied with these phenomena the more we have become convinced that the splitting of consciousness is present to a rudimentary degree in every hysteria.[1]

—Josef Breuer and Sigmund Freud, 1893

In a whole series of cases the hysterical neurosis is nothing but an excessive overaccentuation of the typical wave of repression through which the masculine type of sexuality is removed and the woman emerges.[2]

—Sigmund Freud, 1909

The theoretical constructs that helped to define notions of vision and consciousness in *fin-de-siècle* German and Austrian literature and visual culture were of paramount importance to artistic opticality and the development of Oskar Kokoschka's conceptualization of "the semblance of things." The dialectic that developed between inner and outer vision, and the tension that existed between vision and consciousness were not, however, confined to the realm of the fine arts, as is clear from the overwhelming interest paid to these topics in medical treatises and avant-garde theater performances produced in Vienna at the turn of the century. Although vision and consciousness were handled by the visual and performing arts and psychiatric medicine as separate theorizations of a similar quandary—that is, the need to understand inner stimuli and their effect on corporeal form—artistic and psychological vision were generally recognized as allies in Viennese literature on the modern, pathological body. Hysteria, or "hysterical phenomena," as Sigmund Freud and Josef Breuer referred to this presumed neurological disorder, accordingly became the common denominator in the physiological manifestation of pathological female bodies in medical and artistic discourses. After becoming the *Modekrankheit*, or "fashionable disease," at the turn of the century, hysteria and its hold on the female body allowed psychological medicine to "scientifically" reinforce the age-old trope of the femme fatale then in vogue throughout modern European literature, painting, and the performing arts.[3] However, it was the aesthetics—rather than the psychic trauma—of these medical phenomena that made the pathological or hysterical female into the principal muse of Viennese theater of the period. The pathological body was in turn embraced by a number of Austrian symbolist and expressionist artists, including Kokoschka, Gustav Klimt, and Egon Schiele. This motif was clear for all to see in Klimt's *Philosophy* and *Medicine* (1900–07, Figures I.4 and I.5) and *Judith II (Salome)* (1909, Figure 1.1), in Kokoschka's *Portrait of Lotte Franzos* (1909, Plate 4), and in Schiele's *Seated Female Nude with Tilted Head and Raised Arms* (1910, Plate 5), to name only a few of the many works centered on representations of the pathological body produced in *fin-de-siècle* Vienna.

In view of the above, this chapter investigates psychological theories concerning vision and consciousness in order to examine the earliest visual manifestation of pathological bodies (those appearing in late nineteenth-century medical photographic journals) and the manner in which the aesthetics of the hysterical female body became fertile ground for visual artists, playwrights, and actors associated with the Jung Wien Group, the Vienna Secession, the Klimt Group, and the expressionist movement. Although this examination does not rely on psychoanalysis for its methodological basis, a clear understanding of the history of the discipline is critical, revealing that Parisian, rather than Viennese, notions of hysteria provided the basis for the earliest articulations of hystero-theatrical gestures and dramatic movements inspired by the disorder. At the forefront of this discourse was the French neuropathologist Jean-Martin Charcot, whose studies on the expressive choreography of hysterical attacks were conspicuously transferred to the stage in Paris by actresses and cabaret dancers. It is equally clear that when these hystero-theatrical gestures later appeared in avant-garde theater in Vienna, playwrights were forging (perhaps unknowingly) a conceptual link to Charcot's diagnosis of hysteria as a disorder *of the body*, rather than to Freud's later conceptualization of hysteria as a psychological disturbance *of the mind*.

One question that deserves some attention from the outset is why a lengthy review of psychological discourses surrounding turn-of-the-century notions of hysteria is relevant to an examination of Viennese visual culture, particularly when numerous scholars have already viewed expressionist iconographies through the blurry lens of Charcotian or Freudian psychology.[4] It is certainly true that if visual artists were aware of the advances being made in the field of neuropathology, then they were likely looking to findings associated with the Vienna General Hospital, since this was the medical center affiliated with the University of Vienna, and the site of Freud's medical experimentations in the early twentieth century. Historians of Viennese culture, most notably Carl Schorske, have also reinforced the supposed interconnections between Freud's theories and symbolist and expressionistic paintings by Klimt, Kokoschka and Schiele, while maintaining the importance of political and social arenas in constructing images of the pathological body.[5] The literature on Schiele, in particular, almost uniformly argues that there was an immediate connection between the sexually taboo bodies in his artwork and those that "emerge" in Freud's respective ideas on human sexuality, sexual development, and psychosexual trauma. Because a number of scholars, mainly historians of expressionist art, have regarded psychoanalytic theory as the catalyst for artistic production in *fin-de-siècle* Vienna, alternative avenues of dialogue have been slow to explain the presence of the modern body in the city's visual and material culture.

As stated in the introduction, Gemma Blackshaw and Leslie Topp have offered one such corrective, arguing that Freud's understanding of psychoanalysis had little connection to images of the mentally ill in *fin-de-siècle* Viennese visual culture. In fact, they suggest that Freud's "anti-utopian" approach to corporeal form was not of interest to visual artists until the 1920s, since his theories rejected all analyses of the visible/external body as an effective form of treatment.[6] Blackshaw's and Topp's assertion is supported by scholarship that specifically charts the appearance of pathological bodies at the *fin de siècle*, given that numerous art historians have suggested that the visual referents, if not actual prototypes, for the contorted, unnatural, and diseased bodies in expressionist paintings may have been provided by Charcot's photographs of hysterical patients.[7] Also significant is Georges Didi-Huberman's book *Invention of Hysteria: Charcot and the Photographic Iconography of the Salpêtrière* (2003), which provides an analysis of female hysteria as a constructed, rather than preexisting, psycho-physiological disorder.[8]

Building on the existing scholarship that examines the aesthetics and theatricality of medical hysteria, this chapter also demonstrates that hysteria—in both Parisian and Viennese conceptualizations of the disorder—was principally a gendered "disease," given that it was historically believed to be visible on (or apparent in) the female, rather than the male, body. Turn-of-the-century notions of hysteria were, in essence, responding to earlier corporeal conceptions of hysterical attacks, which suggested that these putative bouts were caused by a detached or floating uterus. This hypothesis was challenged by Charcot in the 1870s and 1880s, as well as by Freud in the 1890s, although the latter continued to prescribe "uterine massages" to some of his hysterical female patients as a supplemental treatment to psychoanalysis. This notwithstanding, some men in *fin-de-siècle* Europe were also diagnosed with hysteria, and it is clear that in Viennese expressionism, male artists were capable of symbolically transplanting the theatricality of this predominantly female disorder onto the male body, and often their own bodies.[9] In terms of iconography, this maneuver is perhaps most explicit in Schiele's *Nude Self-Portrait* (1910, Plate 2), in which the theatrics of hysteria have been conspicuously mapped onto a body that appears emaciated, elongated, and diseased.

It is one thing to acknowledge that visual artists, like Schiele, were incorporating the iconography of pathological bodies borrowed from the realm of medicine. But it is quite another to analyze why artists, actors, and playwrights felt that modern medicine was of interest to the realm of theatrical simulacra, inner imagination, and artistic creativity. Klimt, for instance, had friends who were medical doctors, and he likewise studied clinical patients in order to gain a greater understanding of anatomy, as did countless artists who trained in European art academies from the fifteenth to early twentieth centuries. Are we then to presume that a formal study of anatomy at the academy was supplanted by a study of pathological bodies in the clinic, and thus surmise that the clinic became the new, more modern art academy? I do not deny that visual artists were incorporating these iconographies in order to be seen as avant-garde, but I believe that what is more important in this narrative is the idea that their artistic activities were designed to showcase a uniquely Viennese, non-academic body to their viewers. In this regard, and in line with Alastair Wright's recent extrapolations on the role of pathology in Henri Matisse's early French canvases, the vanguard in Vienna was driven by the desire to show contemporary society the "new" body, as filtered through a modern sensibility.[10] The result was a body deemed malformed, grotesque, and even ugly by some critics, but one that nonetheless definitively and stylistically signaled a break with the older traditions associated with academic painting and Austrian historicism. Furthermore, artistic representations of this new body suggested that modern medicine could provide a language of inner expression that the artist could visually transplant onto the bodies of their subjects, either their own or those of others.

The discussion that follows in this chapter is thus a critical re-evaluation and extension of the extant literature, and pays particular attention to the overarching role that hysteria—more than any other neuro-physiological disorder of the turn of the century—played in depictions of the modern body in Viennese visual culture, and not simply the visual arts. I forego an argument based purely on the search for iconographic origins or prototypes in favor of an investigation that focuses instead on the socio-historical meanings afforded to pathological gestures (*Gesten* or *Gebärden* in German), specifically those associated with the cult of hysteria, and how these medical movements were discussed in the critical literature, be that medical, theatrical, or poetic. What these bodies and gestures meant to their historical audiences is, in my opinion, the more critical question at hand. As such, Charcot's photographs form only one very exclusive and specific facet of the materialization of expressive, corporeal gestures in post-Secession Vienna. By investigating the parameters of medical observations of hysterical women, I set the stage for a more culturally based understanding of the iconography of pathology, or hystero-theatrical gestures, in Vienna. This analysis does not, therefore, focus exclusively on the historical reception of *fin-de-siècle* paintings but seeks to understand the specifics of scientific discourses on hysteria, as well as the role that gestures played in the avant-garde drama that developed before, alongside, and in relation to, the visual arts. By examining Charcot's notions on the aesthetics of hysteria, rather than just Freud's Viennese formulation of the disorder, I lay the groundwork for an explanation of the way in which modern medicine's attempt to scientifically classify (and thus typify) the hysterical woman became particularly appealing to the semiotics of theater because she, like the artifice of a dramatic character, was nothing more than a caricature, a prop, and a staging of what hysteria had to look like at the turn of the century. To begin, let us first consider the discourse surrounding the "scientific" formulation of hysteria, its etiology, and its importance to Viennese consciousness and vision circa 1900.

Studies on Hysteria

In their introductory essay to *Studien über Hysterie* (*Studies on Hysteria*, 1893–95), Josef Breuer and Sigmund Freud suggested that the most fundamental element of the disorder known as hysteria was the presence of abnormal states of consciousness.[11] This position was also expressed in a subsequent study, *Zur Ätiologie der Hysterie* (*The Etiology of Hysteria*), which Freud wrote without Breuer's help in 1896.[12] Accessed through hypnotic suggestion, these abnormal states were understood as the result of pathogenic thoughts caused by psychic trauma to the patient and her consciousness. The manner and method in which physicians were capable of gaining access to the origins of this mental trauma, as formulated in Freud's and Breuer's analysis, ultimately persisted as the foremost distinction between their theory and those proposed by French psychologists like Charcot, Hippolyte Bernheim, and Pierre Janet. For Freud and Breuer, the normality of consciousness became disturbed and thus rendered abnormal through the presence of hysteric hallucinations.[13] One of the major side effects, or "physical mechanisms," of hysterical attacks was therefore the disturbance of vision. This was apparent on an optical, physiological, and mental level as hysteria, which blurred and distorted vision, disturbed the patient's consciousness with recurrent hallucinations and ultimately revealed itself in the body of the hysteric through epileptic fits.

These findings were largely based on Breuer's case history of a patient named Bertha Pappenheim (known by the pseudonym "Anna O.") and Freud's analysis of Fanny Moser ("Emmy von N."), which together form the bulk of the findings in *Studies on Hysteria*. According to Breuer's and Freud's research, hysteria was not simply a threat to corporeal vision, but, as is revealed by Breuer's notes regarding Anna O., was just as much a disruption of the unconscious, or *Unbewusste*, and its mental faculties. The fact that Breuer and Freud believed that hysteria literally split consciousness into two states further supported their conclusion that the unconscious was linked with these attacks. More precisely, this division of consciousness meant that the patient could experience normal psychic (or conscious) activities in a primary state, while simultaneously being inflicted by hallucinations, memory loss, and a "lack of inhibition and control" in a secondary, abnormal state.[14] At present, I want to focus on the first two afflictions: hallucinations and memory loss, while the third, the loss of inhibition and control, will be crucial to the second section of this chapter and my analysis of the characterization, construction, and reinforcement of hystero-theatrical gestures and the trope of the femme fatale, as they applied to the hysterical woman both in psychological discourses and theatrical productions.

Breuer's and Freud's understanding of this secondary, abnormal state of consciousness was fundamentally derived from an earlier study on hysterical attacks presented by Charcot in 1887.[15] As analyzed by Breuer and Freud, Charcot's formulation of hysteria suggested that the onset of all major attacks could be distinguished in four phases of manifestation classified as the epileptoid phase, the phase of large movements, the hallucinatory phase, and the phase of terminal delirium.[16] The Viennese formulation of hysteria suggested moreover that the splitting of consciousness was grounded in the third phase—which Charcot had earlier described as the one in which *attitudes passionelles* (suggestive body postures and gestures) presented themselves—since it was through hallucinations that the disruption to physical *and* psychic vision occurred.[17] It is telling that Breuer and Freud embraced Charcot's third principle—which dealt exclusively with mental faculties—while dismissing the first two stages based purely on physical symptoms. In so doing, the Viennese psychologists were able to offer their own theory of hysteria as a psychic disorder fundamentally rooted in mental trauma, and simultaneously distinguish and distance themselves from the French hypothesis that psychic trauma could physically manifest itself in the body of the pathological patient. Even though Freud's and Breuer's findings were certainly understood as novel concepts for their time, one cannot deny that their analysis of consciousness and its role in hysteria was still largely indebted to Charcot's prior understanding of the disorder. In response to his treatment of the hysterical patient "Madame D." Charcot wrote:

> This woman, whom we have been able to hypnotize, rediscovers in her hypnotic sleep the memory of all the facts that have transpired until the present, and all these memories thus unconsciously recorded are revived in hypnosis, associated, uninterrupted, so as to form a continuous course and a second self, but a latent, unconscious self, which strangely contrasts with the official self.[18]

By positing that a second self was revealed through hypnosis, Charcot essentially offered Freud and Breuer a pre-established model for their formulation of split consciousness. In Charcot's study, the self, rather than consciousness, undergoes the split, the result of which is not only the emergence of a primary and secondary self, but also of a conscious and unconscious self. Freud and Breuer, by contrast, argued that this division occurs within consciousness alone, since the emphasis on unconscious processes and their role in psychoanalysis had not yet been developed in *Studies on Hysteria*. This difference notwithstanding, the task facing Charcot, as well as Freud and Breuer, was to reunite these halves into, for Charcot, the "singular self" or, for Freud and Breuer, the patient's "consciousness."

To a certain extent, and for the purpose of the present study, the distinction between the "singular self" and "consciousness" is somewhat immaterial, given that the studies conducted by Charcot, Freud, and Breuer collectively reiterate the importance of consciousness and hypnotism in *fin-de-siècle* psychopathology. Having been legitimized by Charcot as a valid scientific process in 1882, hypnotism (or mesmerism) was thus rescued from its previous position in the realm of pseudo-science and charlatanism and granted the highest level of medical competency by becoming the treatment commonly used to treat a series of turn-of-the-century afflictions.[19] Charcot and Freud both adopted the belief that hypnotism could induce an "artificial hysteria," though their disparate views on hypnotic vision subsequently caused another major split between the Parisian and Viennese theories of this disorder.[20] Charcot believed that hypnotic vision could be used as a cathartic tool to help patients forget traumatic events that damaged the nervous system, and could in turn diminish (or even eradicate) their hysterical attacks.[21] He consequently felt that the cure for hysteria lay in the simple act of forgetting the memory or trauma that caused the hysterical episode to present itself in the first place.

This form of treatment remains in direct opposition to modern psychology's understanding of how best to treat reactions arising from a traumatic life event. Importantly, the anti-Charcotian process of "non-forgetting" was originally proposed by Freud in his formulation of psychoanalysis and its emphasis on recollection and association. While certainly dissimilar from the current approaches of cognitive behavioral therapies, Freud's later psychological research on hysteria, as published in his 1900 case study of the hysteric patient "Dora," is nevertheless more in line with present-day therapies than Charcot's or Janet's "school of forgetting."[22] In this regard, we can say that Freud's understanding of hypnotic vision focused exclusively on identifying and healing mental traumas in the psychological life of a patient, while Charcot was more interested in forgetting mental trauma in order to improve the physical mechanics of hysterical attacks.

Although this emphasis on mental trauma persisted as the driving force behind most of Freud's psychoanalytic theories, the difference of opinion regarding the origins of hysteria appears to be the result of conflicts that developed between the Viennese and Parisian doctors, rather than being based purely on contrasting scientific research on corporeality, consciousness, and hypnotic vision. Having traveled to Paris in 1885 to study neuropathology with Charcot, Freud quickly become discouraged by his derisive manner and began to work independently on case studies of female patients and their hysterical gestures at the Salpêtrière mental hospital (for semblances of these gestures, see Figures I.6, 2.1–2.3).[23] Having undoubtedly hoped to pioneer new theories of psycho-physiological therapy alongside Charcot, or at least to be regarded as his equal, Freud instead concluded that "Charcot, who is one of the greatest of physicians and a man whose common sense borders on genius, is simply wrecking all my aims and opinions."[24] One of these opinions—a belief that, as previously discussed, marked the major difference between the Viennese and Parisian theories of hysterical attacks—was that hysteria was a psychological disorder caused by mental trauma rather than an illness caused by lesions of the nervous system that were visible through the contortions of the suffering body. Unsatisfied with the research he had conducted at the Salpêtrière, Freud left Paris in 1886 and, according to his personal letters, returned to Vienna depressed and disheartened.[25] Yet despite his negative experiences with Charcot, Freud nonetheless completed the first German translations of Charcot's writings on hypnosis, hysteria, and the nervous system, which effectively introduced these French texts to the Viennese medical community.[26] Since he included his own notes on the original findings alongside the translations, Freud was thus able to criticize Charcot's research by highlighting the uniqueness of his own theories of hypnotism and hysteria in his native city.

Among the works that Freud brought back from Paris were the three volumes of *Iconographie photographique de la Salpêtrière*, or *IPS* (*Photographic Iconography of the Salpêtrière*) published by Charcot and his team between 1876 and 1880.[27] As the title suggests, the work was an attempt to catalog the iconography of hysterical attacks at the Salpêtrière in order to preserve the physical behaviors associated with this gendered affliction for scientific posterity. With the assistance of D. M. Bourneville and photographer Paul Régnard, Charcot offered Paris the first published "scientific" photographs of female hysteria, but not the first images of mental disorder ever recorded via the medium of photography. In fact, as early as 1851, the British physician Hugh W. Diamond had photographed "mad" women at the Surrey County Asylum in Springfield, England, with the intention of reproducing these images in the *Photographic Journal* (the journal of the Photographic Society of Great Britain), for which he was a contributing writer.[28] Similarly, by 1873 clinicians at the San Clemente Hospital in Venice, Italy were cataloguing their patients via photographs.[29] Local doctors then used this archival registry as a tool to record and study the appearance of every female patient treated in the hospital.[30] Unlike Diamond or Charcot though, the physicians at San Clemente did not publish their photographs in medical journals or take steps to visually document the onset of pathologies on the bodies of their wards. The photographs taken at the Surrey County Asylum and San Clemente Hospital do, however, demonstrate the burgeoning interest in psychopathological disorders that existed by the second half of the nineteenth century, yet Charcot's images were undeniably the most extensive and widely disseminated images of clinically interned women produced during this period, and the first to be made available to medical and lay audiences alike.

Even more crucial is the realization that *IPS* narrowed the rather broad and generic definition of "lunacy" to a more defined examination of hysteria—a disorder, according to nineteenth-century physicians, that presented itself in specific symptoms. Charcot reiterated that these symptoms were visible in four presenting phases of the disorder, while Breuer and Freud maintained that the physical mechanisms of hysteria were merely aspects of a larger psychological (rather than corporeal) pathology. To clarify, it is not that Charcot did not believe that hysteria affected the mental faculties of his patients. Rather, he argued that this disorder *first* affected the patient's nervous system, with memory being affected only in the aftermath of a shock or trauma to the body.[31] Freud, by contrast, suggested that the physical followed the mental, though it was clearly through the physical ailments of hysteria and not necessarily the manifestation of mental trauma that he and Breuer were first introduced to the nature of hysterical attacks; ironically, then, it was through Charcot's photographs that the Viennese physicians concluded that the Parisian had misdiagnosed the disorder. As such, the importance of the photographs in Charcot's *IPS* to the ideas subsequently outlined by Freud and Breuer in *Studies on Hysteria*, which did not reproduce images of hysterical symptoms, is undeniable. In his defense of Freud's formulation of psychoanalysis and early theories on hysteria, Harold Blum reminds us that prior to the physician's attempts to provide a treatment, hysterical patients were relegated to the margins of Austrian society.[32] Blum calls further attention to the fact that before Freud these patients went untreated since psychopathology (including hysteria) was not a public health concern. In this regard, Freud's work on hysteria, *sans* photographs, brought the hysterical woman to the foreground of Viennese modern culture and allowed the hysterical body to be recognized and positioned, both corporeally and metaphorically, as the new and modern body.

In *The History of Sexuality* (1978), Michel Foucault offers few ideas on the history of hysteria, and yet it is through his limited conceptualization of the disorder that the strongest parallel can be drawn to the pathological bodies in Viennese expressionism.[33] Undoubtedly working from scientific texts on hysteria, though never specifically citing Freud's or Charcot's understanding of this psychopathology, Foucault bases his formulation on hysteria's biological, physical, and thus gendered implications. That is to say, rather than focusing on hysteria as a disease caused by mental trauma, or by a shock to the nervous system, Foucault suggests that hysteria was historically understood as, and thus seen to embody, the "movement of sex."[34] In drawing this conclusion, Foucault makes a number of things clear. First, he calls attention to the idea that the discourse surrounding hysteria is not simply a discussion of modern pathological science or gender-based symptoms, but is in fact a discourse centered on sexual identity and the most "incurable" of the causes of hysteria: a woman's biological sex. Secondly, Foucault's focus on the movement of sex is surprisingly more indebted to ancient theories of hysteria as a physiological disorder, in which the uterus (or *hystera* in Greek) was believed to be an irrational animal that roamed the female body at will, causing disease and hysterical fits as a result of its corporeal journey.[35] As early as 1618 the French physician Charles Le Pois had suggested that hysteria was perhaps a disease of the brain, rather than uterine animism, though theories of the wandering uterus were still being discussed well into the early twentieth century.[36] This spurious and laughable account of hysterical symptomology is alarmingly also recognizable in Freud's notes on the treatment of Fanny Moser ("Emmy von N."), who was temporarily cured of "mild hysterical states" when a gynecologist "put her uterus right by massage."[37] As such, and contrary to his assertions that the cure for hysteria lay in psychiatric therapy, it appears that even Freud continued to believe, at least to a small degree, that physical treatments were necessary to cure hysteria's gender-based attack of this female sex organ.

Interestingly enough, when the first theories of hysteria as a non-uterine disorder were developed in the seventeenth century, they simultaneously lost all connection to sexual desire, which had previously been present in most of the ancient formulations of the affliction, as well as in Freud's post-1896 theories.[38] This de-sexualized formulation was by all accounts the stance adopted by Charcot when he began his experiments on hysteric patients at the Salpêtrière; and even though it was largely Freud who re-introduced the role of sex in hysteria's symptomology, we cannot fail to recognize that Charcot's experiments and photographs were themselves constructed around the sex of hysteria. Mark Micale has recently suggested that the symptoms of hysteria offered physicians, writers, and dramatists a metaphorical language for the "detached and mobile womb, sexual and maternal deprivation, demonic possession, pathological femininity, defective heredity, clinical exhibitionism, [and] a dysfunctional doctor-patient relationship."[39] Micale's assertions not only highlight the widespread aesthetic appeal of *fin-de-siècle* psychopathological medicine in the fields of science, literature, and drama, but also implicate the modern physician in the construction of the sexualized hysteric and her pathological femininity. More than simply being female, the hysterical woman was believed to be biologically predisposed to become the madwoman, *la bête noire*, *la femme fatale*, whose spastic epileptic movements (often codified as erotic gesticulations) mutually repulsed and excited the male viewer.[40] This sexual tension is perhaps best visualized in the two most famous formulations of medical hysteria to have been documented at the turn of the century: Charcot's "Augustine," and Freud's "Dora."

Embodying Hysteria: Augustine and Dora

When Charcot dedicated himself to the monumental task of documenting the symptomology of hysterical attacks in *IPS*, the result was a collection of photographs that offered his viewers a modern depiction of hysteria while satisfying his desire to combine experimental procedures with the creation of an archive for educational purposes.[41] That is to say, he employed the fairly new technology of photography in order to catalog physical taxonomies and present a greater understanding of hysteria to other physicians and future students. Like the scientific investigations of today, Charcot's process was aimed at documenting hysteria as he conducted controlled experiments, and at charting the progress of the malady over a period of time. Or this, at least, was his intention, since he first needed a patient who could exhibit the specific symptoms of hysterical attacks while simultaneously serving as the ideal aesthetic muse. The obvious problem was finding a willing subject who could demonstrate these symptoms "at will" and for the length of time required to capture an image in the artificial environment of the photographer's studio. The answer to Charcot's great dilemma came in the form of a fifteen-year-old patient given the pseudonym "Augustine," who quite literally came to embody female hysteria in *fin-de-siècle* Paris.

As previously analyzed by Georges Didi-Huberman, the photographs of Augustine in *IPS* can be read as a catalog of artifice, as well as documents that reveal the intricate and complicated interplay between male doctors, male photographers, and female patients at the Salpêtrière.[42] This institution was not only the foremost hospice for madwomen, or *bêtes noires*, as they were commonly referred to throughout this period, but by the end of the nineteenth century was also the largest mental ward of its kind in all of France.[43] Didi-Huberman further claims that the Salpêtrière of Charcot's time was more than a mere asylum or mental clinic; it was, in end effect, a formidable city of incurable women.[44] This, by all accounts, was the world Charcot governed: a microcosm of incorrigible women with the incurability of a pathological disorder that was based, as it were, on their biological gender. In 1872 Charcot was named Professor of Pathological Anatomy at the Salpêtrière and, in 1881, just one year after the publication of the third volume of *IPS*, he became the director of the Clinical Chair of Diseases of the Nervous System, a post, according to journalist and playwright Léon Daudet, that reinforced Charcot's position as "the Caesar" of the medical profession.[45] It was in this environment that Charcot unlocked the secrets of the mind, and more importantly, the aesthetic significance of Augustine's pathological hysteria.

When Augustine was first admitted to the Salpêtrière sometime between 1876 and 1878, Charcot wrote:

> She is a coquette. [...She] is tall, well-developed (neck a bit thick, ample breasts, underarms and pubis covered with hair), with a determined tone and bearing, temperamental, noisy. No longer behaving in the least like a child, she looks almost like a full-grown woman, and yet she has never menstruated.[46]

In this conflation of scientific reporting with an almost lascivious description of Augustine's countenance and physical appearance, Charcot describes a patient who was both specimen and woman—a beholder of maladies, as well as a woman to behold. She was also the coquette: a woman who targets men with flirtations that, while insincere, are nevertheless enticing. She was a woman, and yet not a woman; she was sexual, and yet de-sexualized. In a very real sense, Charcot suggests that he had not simply discovered the body or sex of hysteria, but had uncovered the ideal patient in Augustine, as she was also the aesthetic embodiment of the child-woman, a favorite and equally familiar end-of-the-century motif utilized by artists, playwrights, poets, and now physicians.[47]

According to V. Penelope Pelizzon, Augustine—whose identity is known to us only through her alias—also endures as the "photogenic starlet of the Salpêtrière," and the "pinup girl for epileptic hysteria," as envisioned by Charcot.[48] In line with this assertion, Didi-Huberman concludes that Charcot's interest in Augustine's presumed hysterical afflictions did not stem from a purely scientific—and thus objective—perspective, but also from the male desire to behold, gaze upon, and consume the spectacle of the hysterical woman in motion.[49] He argues that in constructing these images, Charcot merely reinforced the age-old belief that hysteria was caused by a shifting of the uterus to an improper position in the female body.[50] Rather than presenting the reality of hysteria, the photographs in *IPS* instead illustrate Foucault's assertion that the disorder was historically understood as the movement of sex, and more precisely, the movement of female sexuality. In this respect, the female body in motion could be construed as sexual, and by incorporating the movements of the disordered hysterical woman into the performing and visual arts (as Charcot did with documentary photography), artists and playwrights could simultaneously reveal sex in its modern iteration. The movements of the body therefore mirrored the wandering uterus itself, suggesting that the sexual woman moves because her reproductive organs move her. Charcot's construction of the hysterical woman, as embodied by Augustine, should therefore be recognized as the first medical articulation of the femme fatale, however artificial this construction may be. She could neither escape the guilt of her sex, nor her femininity.

It thus appears that this handling of femininity in relation to the hysterical body was largely a Parisian understanding of the psychopathological disorder, since Charcot was principally interested in disseminating images that revealed the physicality of hysteria manifest on the body of the female patient (Figures I.6, 2.1–2.2). Charcot's understanding of the pathology consequently enabled him to restate the hypothesis that hysterical symptoms were the physical markers of lesions to the

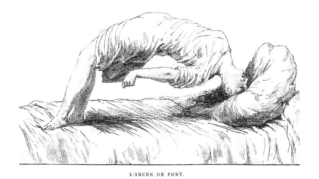

L'ARCHE DE PONT.
D'après l'Iconographie photographique de la Salpêtrière, par Bourneville et P. Regnard.

Figure 2.1 French School, *L'arche de pont*, in *Iconographie photographique de la Salpêtrière*, c. 1884, print. Bibliothèque de la Faculté de Médecine, Paris, France.
Source: Photo: Archives Charmet/Bridgeman Images.

nervous system, and in so doing, he reinforced the veracity of his photographs and clinical illustrations, since corporeal symptoms could be physically recorded. As noted earlier, Freud encountered these photographs and drawings in Paris and personally treated patients whose hysterical symptoms were recorded in *IPS*.[51] Although his correspondence does not specify whether he personally attended to Augustine, who was ostensibly Charcot's "exclusive" intellectual property during the period, Freud nevertheless frequented Charcot's well-attended Tuesday Lectures at the Salpêtrière. Choreographed to demonstrate how hysteria afflicted a woman's body, these educational lectures-cum-medical performances involved Charcot hypnotizing a patient and then having her reveal the physicality of hysterical attacks by acting out the various markers of her illness (see, for example, Figure 2.2).[52] Augustine's demonstrations at the Tuesday Lectures, which illustrated her uncanny ability to be afflicted "at will" by these symptoms, and provide Régnard's camera lens with the timeliest evidence of these attacks, were by all accounts rehearsed routines. If anything, they did more to reveal the artifice of hysteria than the scientific accuracy of the disorder. It is important to note that demonstrations of hypnotic hysteria had been conducted before Charcot's serious interest in hypnotism, which he did not publicize until 1882.[53] Prior to this date, any attempt to seek scientific recognition of the practice was a purely experimental and, within the larger field of neuroscience, hypothetical procedure. Indeed, if we recall that hypnotism was already regarded as a form of "artificial hysteria," then it is not so bold to surmise that nineteenth-century male attendants at the Tuesday Lectures were privy to the artificial nature of the demonstrations prior to attending. Viewers may therefore have been cognizant of the theatricality of the act, since hypnotism, as outlined by Charcot, was part and parcel of hysteria's incarnation as a performance or spectacle.

Having witnessed the exhibition of Augustine's contrived movements and gestures at the Salpêtrière, Freud returned to Vienna, where he struggled over his own conceptualization of hysteria for the following decade. In so doing, he moved away from

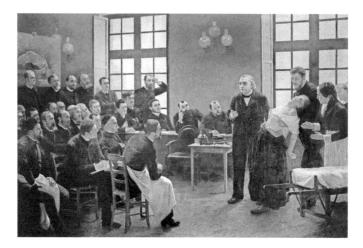

Figure 2.2 Pierre Aristide André Brouillet, *A Clinical Lesson at the Salpêtrière*, 1887, oil on canvas. Paris Descartes University, Paris.
Source: Photo: Erich Lessing / Awwrt Resource, NY.

analyzing hysteria as a disorder associated with the division of consciousness and hysteric hallucinations (as he had with Breuer in *Studies on Hysteria*), and came to understand it initially as a disorder brought about by past sexual abuse and resultant mental trauma, and finally as a disorder associated with the interaction between repression and infantile sexuality. Freud proposed the latter in his 1900 case study of the patient "Dora," though the notion that hysteria was principally driven by sexual motives persisted into his post-1900 studies, including *Drei Abhandlungen zur Sexualtheorie (Three Essays on the Theory of Sexuality*, 1905), "Hysterische Phantasien und ihre Beziehung zur Bisexualität" ("Hysterical Fantasies and Their Relation to Bisexuality," 1908), and "Allgemeines über den hysterischen Anfall" ("General Remarks on Hysterical Attacks," 1909). In many respects, Dora became Freud's Augustine—a woman who could illustrate his theories on hysteria, and thus one whose hysterical symptoms were conveniently explained by her doctor's formulation of her maladies.[54]

Born Ida Bauer, "Dora" was treated by Freud in Vienna in late 1900, even though the results of her treatment were withheld from the medical community until 1905, so as to maintain her anonymity.[55] Although Freud concealed her identity by referring to her as a young woman from a "remote provincial town" in Austria, Bauer was in reality the daughter of a wealthy Jewish textile manufacturer in Vienna.[56] The fact that both Bauer and Freud were prominent Viennese Jews has been the subject of considerable study on the role of Jewish culture and anti-Semitism in the Austrian capital. According to Harold Blum, had Bauer's actual identity been revealed, her situation would have been made worse, since her social position would have left her to be regarded as a mentally ill Jewess. "At that time and place," writes Blum, "being a woman and being Jewish were both psychosocially denigrated situations. This is relevant to the constant references to illness—to body illness and to being defective—which appear in the case."[57] Blum's assertion seems to suggest that *fin-de-siècle* attitudes toward Jews and women predisposed Bauer, at least in the eyes of her would-be detractors, toward mental and physical degeneracy, or that the inverse was true: that her degeneracy was caused by her cultural or familial heritage, as well as her gender. Because Augustine's cultural heritage was never revealed, the only "flaw" that could account for her presenting with hysteria was her sex, though one could argue that her role as a pseudo-actress was far more important to Charcot's studies (and the physicality of hysteria in *IPS*) than any legitimate diagnosis of hysterical symptoms.[58] The theatricality of Bauer's performance was never an issue, as the true drama was that which unfolded in the hallucinations and traumas that she relived privately on Freud's couch, rather than on the public stage of the Salpêtrière, or in front of Régnard's camera.

Two questions relevant to the discourse surrounding hysteria in *fin-de-siècle* Vienna emerge here: Did being hysterical unequivocally mean being female? And were these concepts always understood as synonymous, as they had been in Paris in the late nineteenth century? By all accounts, it appears they were. Yet despite this, Breuer's and Freud's initial prognosis of hysterical symptoms in *Studies on Hysteria* suggests otherwise, since both physicians treated cases of male hysteria.[59] In fact, even Charcot had diagnosed male hysterics, but not until 1881, when his hospital's outpatient clinic was first opened to male patients.[60] During his residence at the Salpêtrière, Freud had only witnessed hysterical symptoms on the bodies of female patients, just as the pages of *IPS* only represented female hysterics. It was not until 1888 that medical photographs documenting male hysterics first appeared in scientific publications, including the Salpêtrière's bi-monthly journal *Nouvelle Iconographie de la Salpêtrière: Clinique des Maladies du Système Nerveux*, or *NIS* (*New Iconography of the Salpêtrière: Clinic of Maladies of the Nervous System*), which Charcot's team produced between 1888 and 1918.[61] Unlike *IPS*, *NIS* was not specifically focused on hysteria, but instead concentrated on neuropathology and psycho-physiological diseases symptomatized on both male and female bodies. Similarly, in 1893, Freud and Breuer also posited that the splitting of consciousness—a process that was associated with both men and women and was therefore gender-neutral—was a cause of hysteria.

Freud's position on the etiology of hysteria did not, however, solidify into hard doctrine as Charcot's had. Rather, one can chart several dramatic changes in the Viennese physician's attitudes toward the nature of hysterical symptoms and their progenitors, particularly when we compare his 1895 findings in *Studies on Hysteria* with those described throughout, and following, his treatment of "Dora" Bauer.[62] In his 1909 essay "General Remarks on Hysterical Attacks," Freud is quite explicit that the cause of hysteria can no longer be rooted in processes of cognition, but should instead be understood in relation to the patient's repression of psychosexual fantasies. Not surprisingly, his (re)vision of hysterical symptoms was very much in line with his post-1900 theories of psychoanalysis, particularly those which concentrated on repression, association, and the interpretation of dreams.[63] To this end, he wrote:

> If it is true that the causes of hysterical disorders are to be found in the intimacies of the patients' psycho-sexual life, and that hysterical symptoms are the expression of their most secret and repressed wishes [and desires], then the complete exposition of a case of hysteria is bound to involve the revelation of those intimacies and the betrayal of those secrets.[64]

At the close of the essay, Freud concluded that "the hysterical neurosis is nothing but an excessive overaccentuation of … repression through which the masculine type of sexuality is removed and the woman emerges."[65] This understanding of hysteria as a purely female disorder essentially reinforced Freud's earlier essay on hysteria's relationship to bisexuality, in which the latter term was understood as a balance between male and female traits, or types, of sexuality present in all humans.[66] Hysteria was thus the direct result of every masculine trait being suppressed by a patient's femininity. If a man were to be diagnosed with hysteria during this period, one can infer that his female "type" of sexuality had repressed his masculine traits. Given that a man's biological sex cannot be suppressed (and nor can a woman's, for that matter), this gendered neurosis could not, according to Freud's later writings of 1908/09, fully afflict male patients. It is therefore easy to see how Freud's early twentieth-century understanding of hysteria, rather than his late nineteenth-century conceptualization of the disorder, supported the idea that the hysteric female could be regarded as a femme fatale. Medically speaking, her disorder unavoidably caused her over-accentuated femaleness to dominate her masculine type of sexuality, thus allowing the woman to emerge.[67]

What, then, had become of the duality of consciousness that was once present in every case of hysteria, as outlined by Freud and Breuer in *Studies on Hysteria*? This question is rooted in the understanding that Freud's later theory repositioned hysteria in the female mind, rather than in a universal or collective human mind, meaning that its symptoms could be transmitted only onto the female body. This is consistent with Freud's departure from hypnotism in the early twentieth century as an effective form of treatment and his move toward free association, where patients could talk through their problems, emotions, and, most importantly, their psychosexual dream scenarios. In his essay "Hysterical Fantasies and Their Relation to Bisexuality" (1908), Freud discusses the manner in which a patient's fantasies and daydreams are linked to the neurotic symptoms of hysteria, which, given their typically erotic nature, presented at the onset of adolescence and puberty.[68] In this construction of hysteria, Freud seems to reject all previous studies involving the visible body, or at least hysteria's ability to be mapped only onto the body of the female hysteric, and instead turns to an examination of the subject's neuro-erotogenic zones. Perhaps that is why Freud reinforced Charcot's self-attributed identity as a *visuel*, or one who learns through his eyes.[69] Monique David-Ménard has further pointed out that the psychic process developed by Freud might alternatively be conceived as the "history of the subject's symbolization of her own body."[70] Her analysis calls attention to the fact that while Freud's later formulation of hysteria may largely be anti-visual, it nonetheless has implications for the corporeal body of the female patient. Moreover, David-Ménard states that hysterical symptoms relied on expressive postures or gestures for meaning to be generated from the original traumatic event. Interestingly though, she concludes that "the hysteric has no body, owing to a lack, in her history, of symbolization of the body."[71] According to David-Ménard, when the hysteric repeated or continued her gestures or motions, her performance unequivocally corroborated Freud's post-1908 understanding of hysteria as a disorder caused by psychosexual trauma to her mind, rather than her corporeal form.[72]

In many respects, the drama of the hypnotized patient was replaced by the outpouring of emotions enacted during talk therapy sessions in Freud's office. Accordingly, and regardless of the distance he had taken from Charcot's ground-breaking theories on hysteria, Freud's dialectical understanding of hysteria in the first decade of the twentieth century suggests that this neurosis was a gender-based disorder, just as it had been in Paris two decades earlier when *IPS* was first published. From a cursory glance then, it appears that Freud's (re)visioning of the theory of hysteria undermines his earlier assertions that the unconscious processes at work in the mind of the hysteric were capable of revealing the patient's disorder. By later favoring a psychosexual, gender-based diagnosis, and thus distancing himself from a diagnosis based on the duality of consciousness, Freud argued that hypnotic visions were simply those performative acts of charlatanism that they had been prior to Charcot's legitimization of their medical efficacy. In this regard, Freud simply applied his earlier views on hypnotic vision to his later formulation of hysterical fantasies in a further attempt to root hysteria (and in this instance, bisexuality) in the mind of a patient who was not only female, but overtly sexual. The end result was that the clinical hysteric became the femme fatale, and the femme fatale became the modern madwoman.

A Third Option

Although investigations into the historical discourse surrounding hysteria in *fin-de-siècle* Vienna typically revolve around Charcotian neuropathology and Freudian psychoanalysis, a third option does exist. Among Freud's interlocutors working in the city around the turn of the century, the Austro-German psychiatrist Richard von Krafft-Ebing remains a relevant, if somewhat understudied, pioneer in the advancement of alternative theories on clinical hysteria. Leslie Topp's research into the development of *fin-de-siècle* Viennese architecture, including that of the modern sanatorium, has done much to elevate Krafft-Ebing's advances in understanding the etiology of hysteria and its consequent effect on the type of buildings that were being constructed in and around the Austrian capital throughout the period.[73] Although Topp's analyses provide an excellent review of the psychiatrist's theories, a brief examination of his work in this chapter is important to explaining his theory of hysteria, which was dissimilar from Charcot's or Freud's findings. Initially published in 1885, Krafft-Ebing's hugely successful book *Über gesunde und kranke Nerven* (*On Healthy and Diseased Nerves*) outlined, as the title implies, ideas concerning nervous disorders. In addition to identifying hysteria as a nervous condition, rather than a serious mental illness, Krafft-Ebing more importantly linked the mental health of his patients to their psyches and environments.[74] An interesting distinction is established here, given that Krafft-Ebing asserted that hysteria was an entirely corporeal disorder, rather than the neurophysiological pathology described by Charcot, or the psychosexual ailment proclaimed by Freud. Krafft-Ebing instead argued that hysteria, or the exhaustion of the body, occurred when one's nervous strength became overexerted or overstimulated by external factors.[75]

Environment was particularly important to Krafft-Ebing's research, as he believed that patients suffered primarily from physical, rather than mental, disorders, which could only be effectively treated by leaving modern civilization (read here as the modern, urban city) for the ideal environment of the sanatorium.[76] His notion that modernity was directly responsible for the increase in corporeal diseases at the turn of the century was not necessarily a novel concept, given that other *fin-de-siècle* neurologists (Topp cites the American physician George Beard) also advanced the idea that pathologies were stimulated by one's environment.[77] To combat the unhealthy effects of modern life in Vienna, Krafft-Ebing and his colleague Anton Löw consequently established the Purkersdorf Sanatorium, a rural health retreat for those affected by urbanism. Founded in 1890 as a sanatorium for nervous ailments and pathologies, including neurasthenia—or nervous exhaustion—Purkersdorf was appropriately situated in the surrounding Wienerwald (Viennese woods), which reportedly had an abundance of fresh, healthy air.[78] Krafft-Ebing's focus on the rural environment as a place of corporeal revitalization is yet another distinction between his thoughts on hysteria and those advocated by Charcot and Freud, who treated their patients exclusively within urban settings. Krafft-Ebing further surmised that it was not simply a lack of fresh air that made urban life in Vienna particularly unhealthy, but also that the miasma, or toxic "bad air" found in the city's theaters and concert halls, was particularly harmful to one's nervous system and overall health.[79] Medical doctors and scientists had largely dispelled the miasma theory by the late nineteenth century, yet Krafft-Ebing's prescription to leave Vienna nevertheless demonstrates how older, erroneous theories concerning the spread of disease in Europe were slow to dissipate. He likewise revealed his bias against the trappings of modern, bourgeois entertainment (such as theatrical and musical performances) for the benefits of the bucolic air that surrounded his sanatorium.

Like his contemporaries, Krafft-Ebing turned to hypnotic suggestion as a legitimate scientific treatment for hysteria within the controlled environment of the sanatorium. Published in 1893 under the title *Hypnotische Experimente* (*Hypnotic Experiments*), his treatise follows the models of Charcot's personal treatment of Augustine and Freud's private sessions with Dora, given that a single female patient, Fräulein Cl. Piegl, served as the basis for his studies on the healing potential of hypnosis.[80] Believing hypnotism to be "empirical psychological research," Krafft-Ebing subjected Piegl to a number of hypnotic experiments throughout the year of the book's publication. Given that *Hypnotic Experiments* argues for the legitimacy of this "scientific" treatment, Krafft-Ebing's treatise lacks much of the sensationalistic luster present in Charcot's or Freud's writings. Instead, the physician's book explains that Piegl presented with "marginal childhood illnesses and common cases of headaches," and most importantly, had parents who possessed healthy nerves.[81] One should not, however, assume that Krafft-Ebing's formulations of hypnotism and hysteria were completely devoid of gender bias, as his experiment with a female patient ultimately led to his conclusion that her hysteria may have been prompted by her sexual excitement, or by overstimulation of her nerves.[82] Unlike Freud, Krafft-Ebing never conceived of hysteria as a purely mental neurosis involving the patient's psychological processes. Rather, he believed that if the patient could be removed from her stimulating situation—be it one of sexual excitement, or the unhealthy air in a modern theater—she could be cured of her hysterical fits.

Conclusion

This discussion of psychological theory, the gender of hysteria, and the medical formulation of the femme fatale is particularly relevant to a further exploration of vision in *avant-garde* theater, in the iconography of the modern body, and in the appearance of hystero-theatrical gestures in Viennese modernism. First and foremost, Freud's re-evaluation of hypnotism as overly corporeal allowed this pseudo-medical practice to be easily adapted to the realm of theater; and where hypnotism went, hysteria followed. But this was already the case in Paris when Charcot was unlocking the secrets of psychopathology within the walls of the Salpêtrière. Given the historical circumstances that led hysterical madwomen to become particularly amenable to artists, actors, and dramatists working at the turn of the century, I next chart the visual movement of hystero-theatrical gestures through German and Austrian cabaret and theater culture to their somewhat concurrent, though often later arrival in Viennese expressionist art.

In this account, the term "hystero-theatrical gesture" is intended as a marriage of the concept of clinical hysteria to the notion of professional, artistically choreographed theatrical movements, though these gestures should not exclusively be understood as purely *of the theater*, as they also materialized in early medical depictions of hysterical afflictions. Let us return briefly to images from the medical world by looking at a photograph of Augustine from *IPS*, an illustration of a female patient exhibiting the "arche de pont" (or the arch of hysteria), André Brouillet's 1887 painting *Une leçon clinique à la Salpêtrière* (*A Clinical Lesson at the Salpêtrière*), and Jean-François Badoureau's sketch of a hystero-epileptic attack (also from *IPS*) (Figures I.6, 2.1–2.3). Each of these images reveals characteristics of hystero-theatrical gestures: spastic arms and limbs; tightly drawn fists, or strangely articulated finger gestures; the patient's head thrown back, rendering her unconscious or fixed with a demonic grimace; and the slightly erotic, voyeuristic quality of a naked or provocatively dressed female body. The aestheticized hysterical madwoman, now positioned as an artistic femme fatale exhibiting pathological gesticulations, subsequently provided playwrights, directors, and visual artists in Vienna with a rather unique language of the modern body.

In terms of Viennese visual art, Klimt's *Medicine* and *Judith II (Salome)* (Figures I.5 and 1.1), Schiele's *Nude Self-Portrait, Nude Pregnant Woman Reclining* and *The Hermits* (Plate 2, Figures I.7 and 1.3), and Kokoschka's *Portrait of Lotte Franzos* (Plate 4) all exhibit signs of the pathological body. In Klimt's *Medicine*, appropriately titled to represent the faculty of the school of medicine at the University of Vienna, the nude female figure in the upper-left portion of the canvas ostensibly "performs" a variation of the arc of hysteria or catalepsy (where the back is arched and the eyes closed), previously enacted by patients at the Salpêtrière (see Figures 2.1 and 2.2). Schiele's *Nude Pregnant Woman Reclining* might similarly be said to adopt such an arch, yet takes the semblance of pathology to the extreme: in this instance, the pregnant body reads more like a decapitated and dissected cadaver than a body brimming with life. Klimt's heroine in *Judith II (Salome)* also mirrors the finger gestures of a clinically hysterical woman, as do Schiele's fingers in *The Hermits*, especially as witnessed in Badoureau's drawing of a hystero-epileptic attack (Figure 2.3).

Schiele, whose *oeuvre* includes numerous self-portraits, was ostensibly interested in transplanting the "female" disorder of hysteria onto his own male body, a point made clear in *Nude Self-Portrait*, which, when compared to Badoureau's image, exhibits the facial grimace and ecstatic body gestures of a female hysteric. Finally, and as previously discussed in Chapter 1, Kokoschka's *Portrait of Lotte Franzos* had been identified by contemporary Viennese critics as showcasing a diseased figure, even suggesting that Franzos' flesh appeared as though it were peeling off of her body in smelly, putrid pieces. Writers like Karl Schreder and Franz Grüner had independently reinforced the idea that Kokoschka's paintings conveyed the sense that his sitters had either been entombed in crypts and madhouses, or afflicted by physical and psychological ailments. One might further note that the "broken" and unnaturally

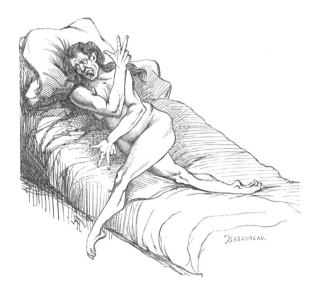

Figure 2.3 Jean-François Badoureau, *Hystero-epileptic attack: period of contortions*, in *Iconographie photographique de la Salpêtrière*, after a drawing by M. Richer, 1876, pen and ink on paper. Private Collection.
Source: Photo: Bridgeman Images.

positioned fingers of Franzos' hands are in dialogue with the finger gestures recorded in Badoureau's expressive illustration. When juxtaposed with this (French) drawing of a hysterical attack, Franzos' pathological appendages reinforce the belief already held at the *fin de siècle* that her portrait was riddled with sickness.

Having thus identified the appearance of a few hystero-theatrical gestures in Viennese modern artworks, the question remaining is how and when Austrian artists came to know, or directly study, the actual taxonomies of the pathological body. To illustrate how the adoption of hystero-theatrical gestures in Vienna's art world transpired, the next chapter contextualizes the appearance of the hysterically theatrical woman, a trope found in Charcot's medical publications, in French cabaret productions of the late nineteenth century, and in the Austro-German modern theater of the early twentieth century. These findings subsequently reinforce Blackshaw's and Topp's conclusion that Charcotian, rather than Freudian, notions of hysteria were more closely connected to the iconography of pathology in Viennese expressionism. A new observation made by the present study, however, is the understanding that Charcot's popularization of hysteria as a *Modekrankheit*, as well as his corresponding photographs of this particularly female disorder, seem to have primarily affected avant-garde theater, not modern painting, as witnessed in numerous performances by the popular French actress Sarah Bernhardt. Chapter 3 therefore examines why Parisian and not Viennese notions of hysteria were closer to the manifestation of expressive, corporeal gestures in modern theater. It will be shown that the aestheticization of the hysterical femme fatale on the theatrical stage became a means of transplanting the medically pathological female body to the realm of the arts. Rather than being strongly rooted in the medical specificity of Charcot's or

Freud's theories on hysteria, the hystero-theatrical gestures adapted by these dramatic performances, as originally borrowed from medical visions of the female hysteric, were, like the disorder itself, nothing more than a semblance of hysteria.[83]

Notes

1 Josef Breuer and Sigmund Freud, *Studies on Hysteria*, ed. and trans. James Strachey (1895; New York: Basic Books, 2000), 12.

2 Sigmund Freud, "General Remarks on Hysterical Attacks," in *Dora: An Analysis of a Case of Hysteria*, ed. Philip Rieff (1909; New York: Collier Books, 1963), 124.

3 The term *Modekrankheit* was first used in relation to hysteria by the theater critic Friedrich Brandes in his article "Dresdener Uraufführung der Salome von Wilde-Strauss," *Deutsche Tageszeitung*, December 11, 1905, n.p. The original German reads: "Hysterie ist jetzt die Modekrankheit." Because the *Deutsche Tageszeitung* was a conservative anti-Semitic newspaper, Brandes' review of Strauss' *Salome* is essentially damning, criticizing the opera's "Jewish" characters. Without analyzing the term *Modekrankheit*, Mark Micale similarly discusses the Parisian "culture of hysteria" that developed around this popular *fin-de-siècle* disorder. See Mark S. Micale, "Discourses of Hysteria in Fin-de-Siècle France," in *The Mind of Modernism: Medicine, Psychology, and the Cultural Arts in Europe and America, 1880–1940*, ed. Mark S. Micale (Stanford: Stanford University Press, 2004), 71–92, esp. 72. Brandes' comments are discussed in greater length in Chapters 3 and 4 of my book.

4 For literature examining the "link" between Freudian psychoanalysis and Viennese expressionism, see Richard H. Armstrong, "Oedipus as Evidence: The Theatrical Background to Freud's Oedipus Complex," *PsyArt: An Online Journal for the Psychological Study of the Arts* 2, no. 6a (January 1999): n.p.; Claude Cernuschi, *Re/casting Kokoschka: Ethics and Aesthetics, Epistemology and Politics in Fin-de-Siècle Vienna* (Madison: Fairleigh Dickinson University Press, 2002); Mario Erdheim, "Psychoanalyse Jenseits von Ornament und Askese: Zur Entdeckungsgeschichte des Unbewußten," in *Ornament und Askese: Im Zeitgeist des Wien der Jahrhundertwende*, ed. Alfred Pfabigan (Vienna: C. Brandstätter, 1985), 230–41; Wolfgang Georg Fischer, *Egon Schiele 1890–1918: Desire and Decay*, trans. Michael Hulse (Cologne: Taschen, 2004); Danielle Knafo, "Egon Schiele's Self-Portraits: A Psychoanalytic Study in the Creation of a Self," in *The Annual of Psychoanalysis*, ed. Chicago Institute for Psychoanalysis (Chicago: Chicago Institute for Psychoanalysis, 1991), 59–90; Carl E. Schorske, *Fin-de-Siècle Vienna: Politics and Culture* (New York: Knopf, 1980); Klaus Albrecht Schröder, *Egon Schiele: Eros and Passion*, trans. David Britt (Munich: Prestel, 1989); Reinhard Steiner, *Egon Schiele, 1890–1918*, trans. Michael Hulse (Cologne: Taschen Verlag, 2000); Patrick Werkner, ed., *Egon Schiele: Art, Sexuality, and Viennese Modernism* (Palo Alto: The Society for the Promotion of Science and Scholarship, 1994); Sarolta Katalin Gyökér, "Egon Schiele's Self-Portraiture" (MA thesis, Queen's University, 1994); and Dean Zuelsdorf, "Implications of Creativity, Artistic Expression, and Psychological Cohesion: The Self-Portrait as a Reparative Self-Object of Egon Schiele" (PhD diss., The Chicago School of Professional Psychology, 1995).

5 Schorske, *Fin-de-Siècle* Vienna. See also Steven Beller, ed., *Rethinking Vienna 1900*, vol. 3, *Austrian Studies* (New York: Berghahn Books, 2001); Thomas Harrison, *1910: The Emancipation of Dissonance* (Berkeley: University of California Press, 1996); Paul Hofmann, *The Viennese: Splendor, Twilight, and Exile* (New York: Anchor Press, 1988); and Stephen Eric Bronner and F. Peter Wagner, eds., *Vienna: The World of Yesterday, 1889–1914* (Atlantic Highlands: Humanities Press International, 1997).

6 Gemma Blackshaw and Leslie Topp, "Scrutinised Bodies and Lunatic Utopias: Mental Illness, Psychiatry and the Visual Arts in Vienna, 1898–1914," in *Madness and Modernity: Mental Illness and the Visual Arts in Vienna 1900*, eds. Gemma Blackshaw and Leslie Topp (Farnham: Lund Humphries, 2009), 36.

7 Schröder, *Egon Schiele*, 83–88; Steiner, *Egon Schiele*, 48–54; and Patrick Werkner, "The Child-Woman and Hysteria: Images of the Female Body in the Art of Schiele, in Viennese Modernism, and Today," in *Egon Schiele: Art, Sexuality, and Viennese Modernism*, ed.

Patrick Werkner (Palo Alto: The Society for the Promotion of Science and Scholarship, 1994), 51–78. Although it is not explicit in their research, both Schröder and Steiner, like Werkner, only address images of the female body in relation to Schiele's paintings, given that they only examine images in Charcot's *IPS*.

8   Georges Didi-Huberman, *Invention of Hysteria: Charcot and the Photographic Iconography of the Salpêtrière*, trans. Alisa Hartz (Cambridge: The MIT Press, 2003).

9   Regarding *fin-de-siècle* notions of the male hysteric, see Jan Goldstein, "The Uses of Male Hysteria: Medical and Literary Discourse in Nineteenth-Century France," *Representations* 34 (Spring 1991): 134–65; Paul Lerner, *Hysterical Men: War, Psychiatry, and the Politics of Trauma in Germany, 1890–1930* (Ithaca: Cornell University Press, 2003); and Mark Micale, *Hysterical Men: The Hidden History of Male Nervous Illness* (Cambridge, MA: Harvard University Press, 2008).

10 For Wright's analysis of the modern body and its significance in paintings by Matisse, see Alastair Wright, *Matisse and the Subject of Modernism* (Princeton: Princeton University Press, 2005), 55–92.

11 See the epigraph to this chapter, which is taken from Freud's and Breuer's essay "On the Physical Mechanism of Hysterical Phenomena." For the complete essay, see the preparatory remarks in Breuer and Freud, *Studies on Hysteria*, 3–17.

12 See Sigmund Freud, *The Etiology of Hysteria*, ed. James Strachey, trans. James Strachey, vol. 3, *The Standard Edition of the Complete Psychological Works of Sigmund Freud* (1896; London: The Hogarth Press and the Institute of Psycho-Analysis, 1953–74), 189–221.

13 Breuer and Freud, *Studies on Hysteria*, 3–17.

14 Breuer and Freud, *Studies on Hysteria*, 45.

15 Breuer and Freud were responding to Jean-Martin Charcot, *Leçons sur les maladies du système nerveux*, vol. 3 (Paris: 1887).

16 Breuer and Freud, *Studies on Hysteria*, 13.

17 Breuer and Freud, *Studies on Hysteria*, 3–17.

18 The translation of this text is found in Michael Roth, "Falling into History: Freud's Case of Frau Emmy von N.," in *The Psychoanalytic Century: Freud's Legacy for the Future*, ed. David E. Scharff (New York: Other Press, 2001), 10. For the original French version, see Jean-Martin Charcot, "Sur un cas d'amnésie rétro-antérograde: Probablement d'origine hysterique," *Revue de médecine* 12 (1892): 85.

19 Regarding the rise of hypnotism from quackery to a legitimate scientific cure, see Adam Crabtree, *From Mesmer to Freud: Magnetic Sleep and the Roots of Psychological Healing* (New Haven: Yale University Press, 1994), 166–67. Anne Harrington, in her analysis of Charcot's embrace of hypnotism as an effective tool for psychotherapy, suggests that, "Charcot manages, in one fell swoop, both to give an aura of medical respectability to a formerly shunned and suspect subject, and simultaneously to stake a clear claim to the medical profession's exclusive competency to deal with this subject." See Anne Harrington, "Hysteria, Hypnosis, and the Lure of the Invisible: The Rise of Neo-mesmerism in *fin-de-siècle* French psychiatry," in *The Anatomy of Madness: Essays in the History of Psychiatry*, vol. 3, eds. Roy Porter, W. F. Bynum, and Michael Shepherd (London: Routledge, 1988), 277.

20 Michael Roth, for example, has analyzed the historical implications of the belief that hypnotism was an artificial hysteria, which was present in many of Charcot's and Freud's respective writings on the proper use of this technique in treating hysterical attacks. See Roth, "Falling into History," 11.

21 For Charcot's emphasis on forgetting through hypnotism, see Charcot, "Sur un cas d'amnésie rétro-antérograde," 81–96.

22 I am borrowing the term "school of forgetting" from Michael Roth, who suggests that Freud's model of psychoanalysis was in direct opposition to the therapies proposed by Charcot, Janet and others. See Roth, "Falling into History," 7.

23 Didi-Huberman, *Invention of Hysteria*, 77–80.

24 Sigmund Freud, *Letters of Sigmund Freud*, ed. Ernst L. Freud, trans. Tania and James Stern (New York: Basic Books, 1960), 185.

25 Freud, *Letters of Sigmund Freud*, 200.

26 Regarding Freud's mixed feelings toward Charcot, see David Joravsky, "Between Science and Art: Freud versus Schnitzler, Kafka, and Musil," in *The Mind of Modernism: Medicine, Psychology, and the Cultural Arts in Europe and America, 1880–1940*, ed. Mark S. Micale (Stanford: Stanford University Press, 2004), 279; and Didi-Huberman, *Invention of Hysteria*, 80.

27 For the complete collection of photographs, see Jean-Martin Charcot, D. M. Bourneville, and Paul Régnard, *Iconographie photographique de la Salpêtrière*, 3 vols. (Paris: Progrès etrol / V. Adrien Delahaye, 1876–1880).

28 Didi-Huberman, *Invention of Hysteria*, 38.

29 Didi-Huberman, *Invention of Hysteria*, 39, 42.

30 For a theoretical discussion of documentary photography's attempt to record and archive certain "types" of individuals at the turn of the century, see Allan Sekula, "The Body and the Archive," *October* 39 (Winter 1986): 3–64.

31 For Charcot's understanding of the physicality of hysteria, see Charcot, "Sur un cas d'amnésie rétro-antérograde," 81–96; and Charcot, *Leçons sur les maladies du système nerveux*. This latter work is also known as *Leçons sur les maladies du système nerveux faits à la Salpetrière*.

32 See Harold Blum, "Setting Freud and Hysteria in Historical Context," in *The Psychoanalytic Century: Freud's Legacy for the Future*, ed. David E. Scharff (New York: Other Press, 2001), 159–63.

33 See Michel Foucault, *The History of Sexuality: An Introduction*, trans. Robert Hurley, vol. 1 (New York: Vintage Books, 1978), 153. In his earlier work *Madness and Civilization* (1961), Foucault provides a lengthier examination of hysteria that includes seventeenth, eighteenth, and nineteenth-century discourses linking the parallelism, and consequent theorization of, hysteria and hypochondria. Foucault thus analyzes the gendered, psychological, and biological tenets that helped certain individuals—such as Plater, Cullen, Linnaeus, Willis, Blackmore, Raulin, Ferrand, Le Pois, and Pinel—understand these divergent, though analogous, disorders. Like *The History of Sexuality*, Foucault's *Madness and Civilization* does not consider hysteria alongside theories offered by Charcot or Freud, but in contrast to the later work avoids suggesting that it might be conceived of as "the movement of sex." See Michel Foucault, *Madness and Civilization: A History of Insanity in the Age of Reason*, trans. Richard Howard, Second ed. (1961; Oxford: Routledge, 2001), 128–50.

34 Foucault, *The History of Sexuality*, 153.

35 Although this disorder was not called hysteria in the ancient world, the belief that it was caused by uterine movement provided the archetype for early nineteenth-century formulations of hysteria as a physiological affliction caused by a wandering uterus. For a good review of these early theories of hysteria, including Plato's first recorded formulation of it, see Mark J. Adair, "Plato's View of the 'Wandering Uterus'," *The Classical Journal* 91, no. 2 (Dec. 1995–Jan. 1996): 153–63. For other excellent sources on the etiology of hysteria, see Sander L. Gilman, ed., *Hysteria Beyond Freud* (Berkeley: University of California Press, 1993); and John P. Wright, "Hysteria and Mechanical Man," *Journal of the History of Ideas* 40, no. 2 (Apr.–Jun. 1980): 233–47.

36 Regarding Lepois' discoveries, see Wright, "Hysteria and Mechanical Man," 235.

37 Breuer and Freud, *Studies on Hysteria*, 77.

38 Concerning seventeenth-century formulations of hysteria, see Wright, "Hysteria and Mechanical Man," 235–36.

39 Micale, "Discourses of Hysteria in Fin-de-Siècle France," 90.

40 For contemporary (male) responses to the hysterical woman as a femme fatale, see Didi-Huberman, *Invention of Hysteria*.

41 I am here adopting Didi-Huberman's assessment of Charcot's photographs. See Didi-Huberman, *Invention of Hysteria*, 30.

42 See, for example, Didi-Huberman, *Invention of Hysteria*, xi–xii. For a further analysis of Charcot's images, in addition to a review (and criticism) of Didi-Huberman's handling of these photographs and the discourse surrounding hysteria, see Carol Armstrong, "Probing Pictures," *Artforum International* 42, no. 1 (September 2003): 55–56. Klaus Schröder also contends that Charcot's photographs, or "action stills," as he calls them, "acted out"

dramas between male doctors and female patients, in Schröder, *Egon Schiele*, 83–84. Finally, and as previously discussed in this chapter, Mark Micale notes that photographs of Augustine highlight the complex relationship that existed between Charcot, Régnard, and their female muse in Micale, "Discourses of Hysteria in Fin-de-Siècle France," 90.

43 Didi-Huberman, *Invention of Hysteria*, 7, 13.

44 Didi-Huberman, *Invention of Hysteria*, 13.

45 Léon Daudet, quoted in Didi-Huberman, *Invention of Hysteria*, 17.

46 Jean-Martin Charcot, quoted and translated in Didi-Huberman, *Invention of Hysteria*, 87. For the original French, see Charcot et al., *Iconographie Photographique de la Salpêtrière*, vol. 2, 125–28.

47 For literature that discusses the "child-woman" in Viennese expressionism, see Werkner, "The Child-Woman and Hysteria," 68–69. For the appearance of this subject in French painting, particularly the works of Toulouse-Lautrec, see Nichola A. Haxell, "'Ces Dames du Cirque:' A Taxonomy of Male Desire in Nineteenth-Century French Literature and Art," *MLN* 115, no. 4 (2000): 783–800, esp. 793. For this motif in Victorian literature, and thus as a precursor to its use in turn-of-the-century literature and drama, see Claudia Nelson, "The 'Child-Woman' and the Victorian Novel," *Nineteenth Century Studies* 20 (2007): 1–12. And finally, regarding Freud's interest in this subject, see Fritz Wittels, *Freud and the Child Woman: The Memoirs of Fritz Wittels*, ed. Edward Timms (New Haven: Yale University Press, 1996).

48 V. Penelope Pelizzon, "Memoire on the Heliographe," *Fourth Genre: Explorations in Nonfiction* 6, no. 2 (2004): 46.

49 Didi-Huberman, *Invention of Hysteria*, xi.

50 Didi-Huberman, *Invention of Hysteria*, 68.

51 Freud, *Letters of Sigmund Freud*, 185.

52 Micale, "Discourses of Hysteria in Fin-de-Siècle France," 76; and Didi-Huberman, *Invention of Hysteria*, 244.

53 Crabtree, *From Mesmer to Freud*, 166–67.

54 Imre Szecsödy, among others, has questioned the relationship between Freud and Dora, suggesting that the latter was perhaps the invention of the former. For his argument, see Imre Szecsödy, "Dora: Freud's Pygmalion?" in *The Psychoanalytic Century: Freud's Legacy for the Future*, ed. David E. Scharff (New York: Other Press, 2001), 125–38. Freud's and Dora's complicated relationship is also examined by Susan Rubin Suleiman, who argues that Dora's treatment was both a failure and success of psychoanalysis. See Susan Rubin Suleiman, *Subversive Intent: Gender, Politics, and the Avant-Garde* (Cambridge MA: Harvard University Press, 1990), 91–99.

55 Sigmund Freud, *Dora: An Analysis of a Case of Hysteria*, ed. and trans. Philip Rieff (1905; New York: Collier Books, 1963), 2–3.

56 Freud, *Dora*, 2. Regarding Bauer's familial status, see Szecsödy, "Dora: Freud's Pygmalion?" 126.

57 Blum, "Setting Freud and Hysteria in Historical Context," 162.

58 Augustine's true identity is not known for a number of reasons. First of all, Charcot's records do not indicate her name, only her status as a housemaid; and secondly, Augustine eventually escaped the Salpêtrière dressed as a man, never to return to the hospital. See Pelizzon, "Memoire on the Heliographe," 46.

59 Regarding Freud's and Breuer's treatment of male hysteria, see Breuer and Freud, *Studies on Hysteria*, 236.

60 Jean-Martin Charcot, *Oeuvres complètes*, ed. Babinski, Bourneville, Bernard, Féré, Guinon, Marie, Gilles de la Tourette, Brissaud, and Sevestre, vol. 3 (Paris: Progrès médical/Lecrosnier & Babé, 1886–1893), 3.

61 For the first published photographs of male hysteria, see plates I and II in the first volume of Gilles de la Tourette, "L'attitude et la marche dans l'hémiplégie hystérique," in *Nouvelle Iconographie de la Salpêtrière: Clinique des Maladies du Système Nerveux* (Paris: Lescronier et Babbé, 1888).

62 Monique David-Ménard offers an interesting review and analysis of Freud's changing views on hysteria, particularly with regard to the body and mind of the patient. See Monique David-Ménard, *Hysteria from Freud to Lacan: Body and Language in Psychoanalysis*,

trans. Catherine Porter (Ithaca: Cornell University Press, 1989). For a feminist, though positive, analysis of Freud's early theories of hysteria, see Jennifer L. Pierce, "The Relation Between Emotion Work and Hysteria: A Feminist Reinterpretation of Freud's *Studies on Hysteria*," *Women's Studies* 16 (1989): 255–70.

63 It is generally understood that Freud's *Interpretation of Dreams* (1900) signals his independence from the previous theories of neuro-psychopathology offered by Charcot and Breuer. This work is equally significant for its introduction of the notion of repressed desires and dream interpretation to the newly developed theory of psychoanalysis. For Freud's analysis of these concepts, see Sigmund Freud, *The Interpretation of Dreams*, ed. James Strachey, trans. James Strachey, Third revised English ed. (1900; New York: Avon, 1965).

64 Freud, "General Remarks on Hysterical Attacks," 120.

65 Freud, "General Remarks on Hysterical Attacks," 124.

66 For Freud's theory of hysteria in relation to bisexuality, see Sigmund Freud, "Hysterical Fantasies and Their Relation to Bisexuality," in *Dora: An Analysis of a Case of Hysteria*, ed. Philip Rieff (1908; New York: Collier Books, 1963), 113–19.

67 Freud, "General Remarks on Hysterical Attacks," 124.

68 Freud, "Hysterical Fantasies and Their Relation to Bisexuality," 113.

69 See Didi-Huberman, *Invention of Hysteria*, 25.

70 David-Ménard, *Hysteria from Freud to Lacan*, 66.

71 David-Ménard, *Hysteria from Freud to Lacan*, 103.

72 David-Ménard, *Hysteria from Freud to Lacan*, 123.

73 See Leslie Topp, *Architecture and Truth in Fin-de-Siècle Vienna* (Cambridge: Cambridge University Press, 2004).

74 Richard von Krafft-Ebing, *Über gesunde und kranke Nerven*, Fifth revised ed. (Tübingen: H. Laupp'sche Buchhandlung, 1903), 1–15. Although this work would be widely read and was published in multiple editions, Krafft-Ebing's most well-known work was his 1886 book entitled *Psychopathia Sexualis*. See Richard von Krafft-Ebing, *Psychopathia Sexualis: eine klinisch-forensische Studie* (Stuttgart: Ferdinand Enke, 1886).

75 Krafft-Ebing, *Über gesunde und kranke Nerven*, 1–15.

76 Krafft-Ebing, *Über gesunde und kranke Nerven*, 133–73.

77 See Topp, *Architecture and Truth in Fin-de-Siècle Vienna*, 67.

78 For Topp's examination of the Purkersdorf Sanatorium, see Topp, *Architecture and Truth in Fin-de-Siècle Vienna*, 66–69.

79 Krafft-Ebing, *Über gesunde und kranke Nerven*, 1–3, 74–76.

80 Richard von Krafft-Ebing, *Hypnotische Experimente*, second extended ed. (Stuttgart: Ferdinand Enke, 1893).

81 Krafft-Ebing, *Hypnotische Experimente*, 3, 5. The original German reads: "empirisch psychologische Forschung" and "geringfügige Kinderkrankheiten und häufige Anfälle von Kopfweh."

82 Krafft-Ebing, *Über gesunde und kranke Nerven*, 1–15.

83 The idea that a language of theatrical gesture could be translated from the avant-garde theatrical stage to the expressionist canvas corroborates what theater historian W. E. Yates has called the "flowering of modernism" in *fin-de-siècle* Vienna. See W. E. Yates, *Theatre in Vienna: A Critical History, 1776–1995* (Cambridge: Cambridge University Press, 1996), 178.

3 Performing Hysteria

A Vogue for Hystero-Theatrical Gestures

Hysteria is now the fashionable disease.[1]

—Friedrich Brandes, 1905

Sigmund Freud was responsible for providing the literal and theoretical means by which Jean-Martin Charcot's writings and images first entered Viennese society in the mid-1880s, since he not only translated the French physician's texts into German, but also brought copies of the photographic medical journals to Vienna. As previously discussed, it has generally been incorrectly believed that the non-scientific Viennese interest in hysteria was owed entirely to Freud's advances in psychoanalysis, as well as to his personal formulation of hysterical lunacy. In challenging this misconception, this chapter describes an alternative route by which the trope of the clinically hysterical woman became embedded in pre-expressionist cabaret and modern theater performances in Vienna, as well as in *fin-de-siècle* painting, neither of which rely on a psychoanalytic methodology. To establish this historical foundation is to reiterate that the iconography of hysteria had arrived in Vienna prior to the rise of expressionism in the city, and to show that this was a discourse that was already in place, rather than one that developed in tandem with this new artistic style. I am also building on the understanding that the legitimacy of medical experiments was already being called into question at the turn of the century, and that clinical hysteria was understood to be nothing more than a display of modern theatrics. Charcot's Tuesday Lectures offer a prime example to validate this contention, since, from their inception, these "scientific" demonstrations were intended to illustrate how hysteria affected the body of a "mad" woman by first hypnotizing the patient and then having her act out the various gestures and contortions of her illness.[2] Charcot's contemporary, a Parisian physician named Jules Falret, a man who made significant strides in understanding the etiology of both bipolar and obsessive compulsive disorders, was perhaps the first nineteenth-century psychiatrist to note the highly theatrical, and thus artificially constructed, nature of hysteria. Falret wrote:

> These patients are veritable actresses: their greatest pleasure is to deceive everyone with whom they come into contact. The hysterics, who exaggerate their convulsive movements, make corresponding travesties and exaggerations of their feelings, thoughts, and actions. [...] In a word, the lives of hysterics are one long falsehood.[3]

Although it is not explicit, Georges Didi-Huberman's research on Parisian notions of hysteria essentially builds on Falret's historical observations, and consequently concludes that Charcot's interest in his patients' presumed hysterical afflictions did not stem from a purely medical (and thus objective) hypothesis. Instead, Didi-Huberman implies that Charcot, as a male physician, wanted to witness, gaze upon, and consume the spectacle of the hysterical female body *in motion* (see Figures I.6, 2.1–2.3).[4] Once again, the importance of medical observation—or the act of looking at clinical bodies in motion—cannot be overlooked. While Didi-Huberman does not dwell on this issue of bodies in motion, it is clear that mobility develops as a key aspect of the madwoman's performance, because male desire was understood to be agitated by the *active* female body, just as her uterus was historically believed to be agitated within her own body. In opposition to Charcot's claims that the static photographs published in *IPS* (*Iconographie photographique de la Salpêtrière,* or *Photographic Iconography of the Salpêtrière*, 1876–80) revealed the reality of hysteria, the Tuesday Lectures reinforced the formulaic definition of hysteria as a dynamic bodily disorder.[5] But rather than merely being female, the hysterical woman of the Salpêtrière had become a female temptress, whose spastic and erotic movements simultaneously repulsed and excited male physicians. In short, Charcot's concept of the hysterical woman, as embodied by his muse, Augustine, was nothing more than another articulation of the metaphorical femme fatale who could neither escape her guilt, nor her femininity. His was an expression of the trope that was now dressed up in the livery of modern medicine.

In line with this assertion, Didi-Huberman concludes that, "hysteria in the clinic became the spectacle, the invention of hysteria. Indeed, hysteria was covertly identified with something like an art, close to theater or painting."[6] Narrowing this distinction even further, Mark Micale contends that "hysteria proved more adaptable to the theater than any other art," while Rae Beth Gordon similarly argues that the gestures of epilepsy and hysteria, which by the end of the nineteenth century were often conflated into a single disorder, entered the cabaret "well before the form appears in art and literature."[7] With regard to the aesthetic appeal of this "pathological femininity," Klaus Albrecht Schröder suggests that,

> the semiotics of hysteria fitted perfectly into the pathologization of art. The signs made by the female patients had always been a Theater of Hysteria; but until they were documented by photography they were regarded as natural, somatic symptoms.[8]

Schröder's analysis has been augmented by Thérèse Lichtenstein, who refers to this phenomenon as "Charcot's aesthetic-medical model of hysteria," and by Reinhard Steiner, who concludes that "hysteria to some extent became a work of art and the hysterical woman an actress whose repertoire of gestures offered the sheer artistry of nerves."[9]

These recent assessments of hysteria's theatrical nature collectively highlight the historical discourse surrounding the semiotics of pathological gesture and the tension that once existed between the indexical and symbolical signs of hysteria, as revealed in the live spectacles of the Tuesday Lectures, and in their corresponding photographs.[10] Schröder's observations raise questions of origin, insofar as one is left to wonder whether these hysterical women were inherently theatrical because they modeled their antics on those first acted out on the theatrical stage, or whether modern actors and dramatists were first attracted to the theatrics of hysteria when they began to use the clinically hysterical female patient as a muse. In other words, were Charcot's records of his medical experiments nothing more than reformulations, perhaps even copies, of theatrical choreographies? Or were they really the first evidence of the invention of hysteria?

In an attempt to conceptualize the semiotics of theatrical and gestural signs, Marco de Marinis has suggested that the viewer must first of all acknowledge that theatrical performances—more than literature, painting, music, or film—demand immediacy, and consequently establish the pretense of a physical encounter between the actor (the sender) and the audience (the addressee), offering the illusion of normal, everyday life.[11] By reading the Tuesday Lectures through the critical lens of Marinis' findings, it is apparent that these dazzling performances gained popularity in late nineteenth-century medical communities through the immediacy of their impact and the illusion of a reality expressed under the auspices of scientific legitimacy. And what is even more clear is that hysteria became the fashionable disease of *fin-de-siècle* Europe precisely because of its theatrical, artificial, and, most importantly, entertaining qualities. The energetic, gyrating and twisting bodies on view in the Salpêtrière amphitheater were undoubtedly entertaining to their viewers, a homogenous group comprised mainly of white, heterosexual men—not just medical professionals or students, but also actors, artists, journalists, and novelists.[12] In turn, the very presence of these kinds of spectators at the Tuesday Lectures reinforces the theatrical qualities of the menagerie of hysterical patients that Charcot paraded before them, precisely because they (the viewers) were emulating the behaviors of audiences attending an actual theatrical performance. One could therefore argue that, from their very inception, the Tuesday Lectures deliberately sought to blur the line between fiction and reality, and ostensibly did so in order to capitalize on the spectacle of female bodies in motion.

French Spectacles: Sarah Bernhardt and Jane Avril

As noted above, Falret was perhaps the first doctor to observe the theatricality of hysteria as it played out in nineteenth-century Paris, though we should not forget that Freud also spent time in France in the mid-1880s. When Freud first traveled to Paris in 1885 to study neuropathology with Charcot, he regularly found himself discouraged by the neurologist's contemptuous manner, and consequently sought alternative activities in the city. One pastime accessible to the demoralized Austrian was the Parisian stage, which he regularly patronized, attending cabaret and theater performances showcasing the renowned French actress Sarah Bernhardt (née Sarah Marie Henriette Bernard).[13] After seeing Bernhardt in a November 1885 production of *Theodora*, Freud, who was quite taken with her movements, declared that,

> every inch of this little figure was alive and bewitching. As for her caressing and pleading and embracing, the postures she assumes, the way she wraps herself round a man, the way she acts with every limb, every joint—it's incredible. A remarkable creature, and I can well imagine she is no different in life from what she is on the stage.[14]

Freud presumably took notice of the strong similarities between Bernhardt's dramatic portrayals of hysterical women and the real hysterics acting out their pathological symptoms in Charcot's clinic.[15] The Viennese psychiatrist certainly had good reason to note these parallels, as by then both Western and Central European dramatists and actors were utilizing hysterical movements as a modern dramatic language. In line with this assertion, Gordon states further that,

> as early as the 1870s, a number of café-concert and cabaret artists borrowed gestures and movements from asylum inmates. [… As a result,] the enormous popularity of epileptic performers and […] songs about nervous pathologies in the café-concerts contributed to the furor of attention paid to nervous disorders in the 1880s and 1890s.[16]

The iconography of nervous disorders also inspired the use of expressive gestures in modern theater, not simply in café-concerts. By the mid-1880s, Bernhardt had personally studied female patients at the Salpêtrière in order to scrutinize their gesticulations and better understand the aesthetics of hysteria.[17] In an interview published in 1897 in the journal *La Chronique Médicale* (*The Medical Chronicle*), she explained that her visit to the hospital in 1884 was brought about by her desire to perfect the authenticity of a nervous attack suffered by the eponymous character in the play *Adrienne Lecouvreur* (1849) by Ernest Legouvé and Eugène Scribe.[18] Bernhardt stated that in order to truly immerse herself in the role she had even spent time in one of the cells at the Salpêtrière. Her interviewer, S. Veyrac, commented later in the article that Bernhardt's visit to the clinic had also taught her how to act like a somnambulist—for her role as Lady Macbeth—and to convey "frightful agony"—for her role as Marguerite Gautier in the stage adaptation of Alexandre Dumas' *La Dame aux Camélias* (*The Lady of the Camellias*; the novel was written in 1848 and adapted to the stage by 1852).[19] A cabinet card photograph from the late nineteenth century of Bernhardt's performance in *Adrienne Lecouvreur* serves as an effective, though subtle, record of the iconography of theatrical hysteria that the actress had hoped to communicate to her audience, particularly through her clasped hands and exaggerated physiognomy (Figure 3.1).[20] When the photograph is coupled with her personal account of the Salpêtrière published in *The Medical Chronicle*, it is clear that Bernhardt visually incorporated her observational research at Charcot's clinic into her acting style, particularly in her tendency to use histrionic or melodramatic manners and gestures. It is also possible that Bernhardt, apart from actually visiting the Parisian hospital, had also studied the photographs of patients in *IPS* and *NIS* when preparing for her various dramatic roles.

Three years prior to Bernhardt's personal investigation of hysterical symptoms at Charcot's clinic, theater critic Jules Claretie published *Les Amours d'un interne* (*The Loves of an Intern*, 1881), a pseudo-romantic, pseudo-journalistic novel in which a young medical apprentice conducts nocturnal *liaisons amoureuses* and *dangereuses* with his hysterically seductive female patients at the Salpêtrière.[21] One of these patients was another legendary figure of the Parisian stage, Jane Avril, who emerged as the celebrated can-can dancer at the cabaret Moulin Rouge in the 1880s and 1890s. Known largely for her role in the development of avant-garde, expressive dance, Avril was actually a patient at Charcot's clinic during the 1870s.[22] Born Jeanne Beaudon in 1868, Avril left home at the age of thirteen to escape an abusive mother, who had been working as a prostitute in Paris. When authorities collected the young Avril around 1881, she was

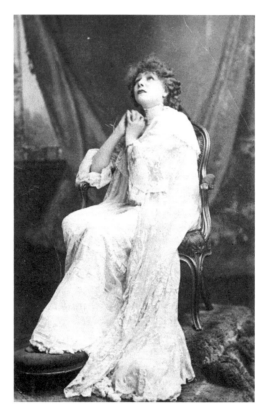

Figure 3.1 W. & D. Downey, Sarah Bernhardt as Adrienne Lecouvreur, 19th century, sepia photograph on paper. Bequeathed by Guy Little. Victoria and Albert Museum, London.
Source: Photo: © Victoria and Albert Museum, London.

deemed clinically insane and sent to the Salpêtrière. During her treatment at the hospital, which lasted eighteen months, Avril was diagnosed—by Charcot—as being afflicted with Sydenham's chorea, also known as Saint Vitus Dance, a disorder that afflicts the limbs and is typically expressed through sporadic and jerky movements. She consequently underwent a rigorous rehabilitation administered by her doctors, after which time Avril was found to be cured of her afflictions and discharged.[23]

The irony is quite apparent, as Avril, who was treated for a pathology she may or may not have actually possessed, adopted her theatrical persona from the very asylum that was said to have cured her of her corporeal afflictions. More amusing still is her paramount role in transferring the hysterical movements commonly exhibited in the clinic to the realm of profitable cabaret entertainment. Her "mad" gesticulations contributed enormously to her notoriety, and are discernible in a number of paintings and posters created by the French post-impressionist artist Henri de Toulouse-Lautrec throughout the 1890s. In Toulouse-Lautrec's painting *Jane Avril dansant* (*Jane Avril Dancing*, c. 1892, Figure 3.2) the modern dancer is depicted with eyelids at half-mast, arms akimbo, and legs jutting unnaturally from her body at almost impossible, yet dynamic and dramatic, angles.

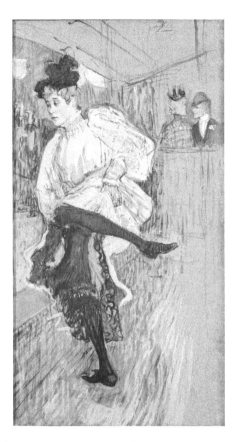

Figure 3.2 Henri de Toulouse-Lautrec, *Jane Avril Dancing*, c. 1892, oil on cardboard. Musée d'Orsay, Paris.
Source: Photo: Gianni Dagli Orti / The Art Archive at Art Resource, NY.

If one recalls Badoureau's drawing (Figure 2.3) of a woman suffering from a hystero-epileptic attack—with her legs crossed and pointed in opposite directions from her body—it would appear, at least in Toulouse-Lautrec's image, that Avril had learned much at the Salpêtrière. Avril's use of hystero-theatrical gestures was also a historical conflation of two different though related turn-of-the-century theatricalities: the movement of Charcot's "madwomen" in the clinic, and the gyrations of avant-garde dancers in Parisian cabarets. In end effect, Bernhardt's historical visit to the Salpêtrière, Toulouse-Lautrec's many depictions of Avril dancing, and Claretie's literary portrayal of melodramatic misconduct at Charcot's hospital collectively highlight the widespread artistic interest in the theatrics of hysteria, be that in literature, theater, or painting, at least in Paris. The proliferation of non-clinical images of hysteria, which included photographs of Bernhardt and paintings of Avril, also recall the typified gestural modes expressed in photographs of Augustine and her fellow hysterics at the Salpêtrière, and therefore visually fortify the idea that "high" theater and "low" cabaret were similarly invested in recreating the "authentic" body language of the institutionalized madwoman.

Hysteria's Mobility: From Paris to the Germanic Stage

It is through Bernhardt that one also discovers an initial, tangible encounter between Parisian explorations of hystero-theatrical gesture, and those enacted in pre-expressionist cabaret and theatrical productions in *fin-de-siècle* Vienna. Bernhardt traveled to Vienna in 1882, 1887, and 1908 to perform a series of plays at the celebrated Theater an der Wien.[24] Although the actress' earliest trip to Austria predates her first known visit to the Salpêtrière in 1884, she had undoubtedly incorporated hystero-theatrical gestures into her 1887 and 1908 performances; and as a result, the Viennese theater seems to have fervently embraced her theatrics. This was also the case with Bernhardt's guest appearances throughout Central Europe, including Germany. According to the *fin-de-siècle* theater critic Franz Hofen, whose reviews often appeared in the celebrated Austro-German journal *Bühne und Welt* (*Stage and World*), Bernhardt's "French" gestures led the actress to be regarded as particularly novel to German-speaking audiences.[25] In spite of Hofen having labeled her as "famously pompous," Bernhardt's celebrity was the envy of most German and Austrian actresses, who reportedly studied her skills in order to better imitate her movements in their own productions.[26]

In a review of Bernhardt's *Figaro* that appeared in the *Wiener Abendpost* (*Vienna Evening Post*) in December 1902, the actress is quoted at length expressing her gratitude for the warm reception the play received following its censorship in France.[27] Irritated by her native country's lack of modern vision, Bernhardt vowed never to return to the French stage: an empty threat that nevertheless indicates just how appealing (and well received) her dramatic experimentations were in Central Europe. A slightly earlier review of her many appearances throughout Germany was published in *The New York Times* in November 1902, which instead claimed that not all Germanic theatergoers were entranced by Bernhardt's modern performances. The critic ridicules both the music in her production of *Hamlet*, as well as her appearance as the lead character, presumably because she was a woman.[28] Whether laudatory or unfavorable, critical reviews of Bernhardt collectively illustrate the changing nature of modern theater in *fin-de-siècle* Europe and her willingness to experiment with the accepted parameters of dramatic gesture, and even gender.

Bernhardt's visits to Austria and Germany are important indicators that Central European dramatists and theater directors were also anticipating and incorporating radical changes in the realm of modern dramaturgy, stage direction, and choreography. In relation to this, W. E. Yates has suggested that "the theatrical life of Vienna was becoming cosmopolitan—flung open not just to popular fashions from Paris, but to the influence of serious modern theatrical experiment."[29] This assertion, which speaks to the widespread processes of cultural exchange under way between Paris, Vienna, Berlin, and Munich, cannot, however, be explained by a single actress' occasional guest performances. Instead, one must examine the multitude of actresses, theater personalities, cabaret owners, and their interlocutors who operated in and around Vienna in the early twentieth century.

Achille Georges d'Ailly-Vaucheret, like Bernhardt, consequently becomes a notable name in the cultural exchange between France and Austria. More commonly known by his pseudonym, "Marc Henry," d'Ailly-Vaucheret was an itinerant French writer and businessman, credited with introducing Parisian cabaret-theater to Vienna, Munich, and Berlin in the late 1890s. As the founder of the bi-monthly, bilingual journal *Revue franco-allemande/Deutsch-französische Rundschau* (*French-German Review/German-French Review*), Henry stimulated interest in French poetry, music, theater and literature in Central Europe, a feat, according to Harold Segel, that helped to narrow "the cultural gap between the French and German peoples."[30] The *Review*, which was published in Munich and distributed in Vienna, Paris, and Brussels, also disseminated French and German essays and poems, as well as literary and theater reviews written by a wide range of literary figures, including well-known personalities like Leo Tolstoy, Émile Zola, Heinrich Heine, and Rainer Maria Rilke. By 1898 the *Review* had become the arbiter of Franco-German theatrical taste in Central Europe, making Henry the authority on cabaret entertainment in all of the aforementioned German-speaking cities.[31] The social prestige that cabaret culture offered Henry also afforded him considerable commercial success outside of Paris.[32] His financial achievements were due in large part to the fact that he had modeled his "new" Franco-German theater on previously established Parisian cabarets and clubs, such as the Moulin Rouge and the Folies-Bergère, which, in turn, served as prototypes for cabarets that opened in Munich and Berlin in the late nineteenth century, and in Vienna in 1901.[33] Before delving into further Viennese theatrical productions, which form the basis of Chapter 4, the remainder of this chapter will focus on hysteria's mobility through the performing arts from Paris to Germany, prior to its arrival on the Austrian stage.

In Germany, Henry's journal reveals how the language of psychology had begun to infiltrate literary and theater reviews published at the turn of the century. In an 1899 review of the play *Kain*, written by the little-known playwright Ernst Prange, and performed at Munich's Schauspielhaus (Playhouse), the critic Leo Greiner argued that the production offered local audiences "a psychologically bungled, insane catastrophe of tragic pathos."[34] Greiner's rather damning critique also claimed that the play revealed a juvenile need for "bombastic" magnitude, in spite of its "dissonant echoes" of plays like *Kollege Crampton* (written by Gerhart Hauptmann in 1892) and *John Gabriel Borkman* (composed by Henrik Ibsen in 1896).[35] Here again, semantics play a significant role in our understanding of how the language of clinical psychology was seeping into the discourse surrounding modern Germanic theater. In his review, Greiner uses the compound word *Wahnsinnskatastrophe* to denote an "insane catastrophe" or "crazy catastrophe," with the German term *Wahnsinn* denoting clinical lunacy, dementia or madness. This seems a rather deliberate maneuver on the part of the writer, given that he chose not to use the adjective *verrückt* commonly used to suggest that something is "crazy" or "loony" in a figurative sense. Griener also states that *Kain* presented a "psychologically bungled" catastrophe, implying that the play itself metaphorically suffered from a pre-existing condition that was only worsened by allusions to modern medicine.

Two years later, Oscar Wilde's controversial play *Salomé* (*Salome*) had its German debut at Munich's Schauspielhaus in May 1901, and not at Berlin's Kleines Theater (Little Theater) on 15 November 1902, as suggested in much of the extant literature.[36] Written by the notorious Irish playwright in 1891, *Salome* was originally composed in French with the expectation that Bernhardt would star in the leading role. The play did not publicly premiere in Paris until 1896, and when it did, Bernhardt was not in the cast.[37] The play then opened a full five years later in Germany, a delay ascribed to the considerable censorship it had been subjected to in France and then Great Britain. Georg Schaumberg, a writer for *Stage and*

World, opened his review of the Munich production of *Salome* with the following statement:

> I owe the strongest impression of this past season to a foreigner, Oscar Wilde, and his fascinating "Salome." Frau Gerhäufer of the Court Theater in Karlsruhe, the wife of our future heroic tenor [Herr Gerhäufer], looked ravishing as Salome.[38] [...] An entire essay would be necessary to elucidate the fascinating effect of this one-act play. But alas, this is not my assignment.[39]

When the play reached Berlin the following year, its transformation from a "fascinating" Bavarian production into an elaborate and modern visual spectacle was the brainchild of the celebrated Viennese director Max Reinhardt. Reinhardt, who worked and traveled between Austria and Germany throughout the first three decades of the twentieth century, eventually immigrated to the United States following the 1938 Anschluss of Austria by Nazi Germany. It is also important to note that Reinhardt, like other *fin-de-siècle* theater personalities and visual artists in German-speaking Europe, was drawn to the cosmopolitan German capital due to the fact that modern, experimental theater was more widely accepted in "Protestant" Berlin, than in "Catholic" Vienna, which was seen as more socially conservative throughout the Austro-Hungarian Empire. One might also recall Franz Ferdinand's conservative attitudes toward Oskar Kokoschka's paintings, as discussed in Chapter 1.

When staging the controversial *Salome*, Reinhardt cast a local actress named Gertrud Eysoldt in the leading role. Reinhardt presumably considered her to be the best choice as the theatrical incarnation of the biblical temptress due to the critical acclaim she had previously received for her portrayal of Trude in the tragic comedy *Ackermann*. Critics had proclaimed that Eysoldt was an actress capable of capturing "haunting character portrayals" through her "truly erotic sensations and demonic fiendishness."[40] Reinhardt's staging of *Salome* ignited an immediate scandal in Berlin, as it had in earlier productions throughout Europe. However, due to the threat of the Berlin censors, who forbade its continued run after the opening night performance, *Salome* was thereafter only presented to private audiences.[41] Such private showings were staged for privileged and discreet viewers, including the likes of Hugo von Hofmannsthal and the German composer Richard Strauss, but only until 29 September 1903 when the public ban was finally lifted.[42]

The controversy surrounding the play was directly linked to the overt sexuality of its characters, and particularly to Eysoldt's erotic and grotesque portrayal of Salome. Tilla Durieux, a well-known, turn-of-the-century Viennese actress, believed that Eysoldt was particularly well suited for the role due to the fact that her body "resembled that of a child and she knew how to accentuate the ambivalence of her child-woman persona without attracting the attention of the censors."[43] Durieux's words recall the *fin-de-siècle* trend of describing theatrically hysterical women as child-women sexually trapped between pre- and post-pubescence. Given that Durieux herself later played the role of Salome in Reinhardt's production, sharing the title role with Eysoldt and Eysoldt's understudies, it is likely that the Viennese actress adopted Eysoldt's child-woman persona in order to make her own performances more compelling.[44] Heinrich Stümcke, the Berlin theater critic for *Stage and World*, and the local reviewer for many of the productions staged at the Kleines Theater, further corroborates Durieux's historical observations. Stümcke notes that, following the Dance of the Seven Veils, Eysoldt exhibited both "the pathological persistence of a spoiled child who immediately nags about the present she is denied, as well as the perverse, erotic, and vengeful lust of a scornful woman."[45] Taken together, these contemporary analyses suggest that Eysoldt's gestural language was historically situated within a discourse centered on the sexualized hysteric or femme fatale, as communicated through her pathological, child-woman persona.

Returning briefly to Prange's *Kain*, it is significant that Griener discusses further plays by Hauptmann and Ibsen in his review, particularly since psychological discord was one of Ibsen's major theatrical leitmotifs.[46] The interest in psychologically driven drama was also evident in Stümcke's review of Hauptmann's *Der arme Heinrich* (*Poor Heinrich*), a reworking of Hartmann von Aue's Middle High German poem that premiered on 6 December 1902 in Berlin.[47] Hauptmann's play was essentially a medieval tragedy cloaked in the psychological turmoil of a lead character suffering from leprosy. In his review, Stümcke once again employed the language of modern medicine to describe the power of Hauptmann's scenes:

> Another question is whether or not the special case of poor Heinrich—who discovers that the miraculous cure for leprosy lies, in fact, in the unconsummated blood sacrifice of a pious female virgin—is appropriate for the stage. The dramatic crux is established here first by the miraculous cure, then by the nauseating disease. Hauptmann does not eliminate the miraculous cure from his dramatic development of the plot, perhaps because he does not want to, even though he otherwise—with all the means of the modern art of the soul—strives for a psychological deepening of the scenes. [...] The first four acts present us with all of the phases of leprosy's corporeal and psychological processes. At the forefront is the deepest melancholy.[48]

Stümcke continues with a description of the actors:

> The male and female lead roles were performed by Rudolf Rittner and Irene Triesch. [...] Triesch is the triumphal incarnation of Salome's sensuality [...] through her scantily clad, girlish form, coy virginity, and ecstatic fervor.[49]

It is notable that throughout his review Stümcke is overwhelmingly interested in the corporeal effects of leprosy, which he describes as *ekelhaft*, meaning "nauseating" or "disgusting." His choice of terminology suggests that Hauptmann may have intended to elicit a visceral reaction from his viewers, hoping they would become transfixed by the "psychological deepening" of the scenes. The plot itself revolves around the rather misogynistic notion that the pious Heinrich must obtain the unspoiled blood of a virgin in order to miraculously cure his disease. Unluckily for poor Heinrich, though in keeping with the vogue for the theatrical child-woman, his would-be virgin is none other than the carnal embodiment of Salome, the ultimate temptress, who, as noted by Stümcke, was expertly portrayed through Triesch's juxtaposition of sensual womanliness and girlish childishness.

Reinhardt and Eysoldt explored the hysterical femme fatale in two further productions staged at the Kleines Theater in the early twentieth century: Frank Wedekind's *Erdgeist* (*Earth Spirit*, 1895) and Hugo von Hofmannsthal's *Elektra* (1903).[50] Originally performed in 1898 as the first of Wedekind's "Lulu" dramas, *Earth Spirit* (sometimes known in English as *Gnome*) is commonly regarded as the work that definitively established Wedekind as the *enfant terrible* of *fin-de-siècle* German literature, a reputation due in large part to the radical and modernist handling of morality and sexual taboos evident in his dramatic works.[51] *Earth Spirit* follows Wedekind's recurring protagonist, Lulu, through her increasingly risqué confrontations with sexual frankness and decadence, allowing the viewer to examine the dialectical nature of his complex heroine. Lulu is thus a patriarchal paradox: she is the ideal embodiment of nature's beauty (*Erdgeist* as the spirit of the earth), as well as a femme fatale (*Erdgeist* as the lustful force of female nature). J. L. Hibberd has asserted that Wedekind intended for Lulu's dialectical nature to be conspicuous throughout *Earth Spirit* and contends that the animal-tamer who acts as the narrator in the play's prologue deliberately highlights Lulu's dualistic nature in an attempt to emphasize the equilibrium of her character.[52] That is to say, in the hands of Wedekind, the character is not simply an incarnation of earthly innocence, nor is she entirely a diabolical femme fatale. Instead, the animal-tamer proclaims:

> Hi, Charlie!—bring our Serpent this way!
> She was created to incite to sin,
> To lure, seduce, poison—yea, murder in
> A manner no man knows.—My pretty beast,
> [...]
> Thou hast no right to spoil the shape most fitting,
> Most true, of woman, with meows and spitting!
> And mind, all foolery and making faces
> The childish simpleness of Vice disgraces.[53]

Despite the animal-tamer referring to Lulu as "our Serpent" (clearly a reference to her complicity in the biblical notion of original sin), he also calls her *süße Unschuld*, or "sweet innocence," a point that allows Hibberd to insist that Wedekind's concept of "childish simpleness" clearly indicates that the character should "be played not as a scheming, sophisticated vamp (as she was by Eysoldt in Reinhardt's 1902 Berlin production), but with the simplicity of a child."[54] Hibberd is convincing in his analysis of the animal-tamer's intentions to reveal Lulu as a binary creation, though it is nevertheless significant that Reinhardt chose to accentuate the sinful side of Lulu (*Erdgesit* as the femme fatale) in his staging of the play. This directorial decision, itself a testament to the play's ability to adapt to avant-garde theater, was also recognized by contemporary critics, with Stümcke once again singling out Eysoldt for her cunning portrayal of the child-woman:

> The Earth Spirit is the ever-eternal embodiment of the demonic side of female nature that bewitches and destroys all men who fall under her spell. Eve, who Wedekind also calls Mignon and Lulu, is an elaborate mixture of childlike naiveté, devotion, depravity, sensuality, and coldness. For a change, Ms. Eve flirts and shows her resplendent limbs for a season in a variety theater. One thinks of Ms. Eysoldt's Salome as a worthy counterpart. Dazzling in a hundred colors, she was wholly the fascinating embodiment of Mignon, Lulu, and Eve, the naughty child, the petulant despot, the perverse illicit lover, and the alluring hedonistic dancer, all in one person.[55]

In describing Lulu throwing her "resplendent limbs" around in "a variety theater," one wonders if Stümcke was envisioning Wedekind's heroine as a dramatized incarnation of Jane Avril, given that they were both cabaret dancers. Irrespective of the inspiration for Stümcke's comment, the parallels between the fictional depiction of Lulu, as a pathological but savvy woman who turns her mental afflictions into an economic asset, and the real-life story of Avril, are surely striking.

To explore this issue further, one must invariably return to the dialectical nature of Lulu's character, since it seems quite deliberate that Lulu constantly walks a metaphorical tightrope between sweet innocence and overt sexuality. Stümcke's analysis of Wedekind's play suggests that a figure like Avril, if not Avril herself, might be regarded as a prototype for Lulu's later exploration of modern dance. Once more, the body of the woman moves, and she stirs the minds and desires of men. As such, Wedekind's conspicuous conflation of Lulu with the symbolic figures of Eve (the original temptress), and Mignon (Lulu as a little girl, since *mignon* means "cute" in French), tellingly echoes the conflation of terms used to describe hysterics at the turn of the century, including interchangeable labels like "theatrical madwoman," "femme fatale," "*bête noire*," or "child-woman." The cult of hysteria, which positioned the disorder as the "fashionable disease" of the *fin de siècle*, must certainly have affected Reinhardt's decision to emphasize Lulu's fallen nature, because, as we learned from the factual example of Avril, the use of hystero-theatrical gestures translated handsomely into profitable entertainment. As such, Lulu, Salome, Trude, and the young maiden in *Poor Heinrich* all can be seen to embody aspects of the hysterical woman on the theatrical stage.

On at least two occasions, the editors of *Stage and World*—which, to repeat, circulated throughout Berlin, Munich and Vienna—invited medical doctors to submit essays describing the role (and toll) of embodying pathologies in dramatic works. One such article, entitled "Schauspieler-Krankheiten" ("Actors' Diseases"), which was penned by Albert Eulenburg, a professor and doctor of medicine, specifically discussed the portrayal of nervous disorders in modern theatrical productions. Given his expertise as a specialist in nervous afflictions, Eulenburg observed that many modern actors and actresses had become "victims of their art, making them martyrs to their nerves."[56] Then, in speaking of "the corporeal and psychological life of actors," he concludes that in pouring themselves into their art, "good" actors develop "a necessary though unfortunate sensitivity to their nerves."[57] Even though Eulenburg's essay preceded the premiere of Reinhardt's production of *Salome*, it is nevertheless telling that the writer cites Ibsen and Hauptmann as two playwrights whose respective works visibly demanded this sensitivity to one's physical health.[58]

In the following year, Dr. L. Fürst, the Berliner Sanitätsrat (Berlin Officer of Health), published an article headlined "Das Pathologische auf der Bühne" ("Pathology on the Stage"), which appeared in *Stage and World* in February 1903. This essay, which discusses plays by Ibsen, is a wealth of information concerning the theatrical interest in modern medical pathologies at the turn of the century.[59] Fürst provides a lengthy and tedious review of observable corporeal and psychological diseases (*Krankheiten*) that had been explored on the modern stage, including disorders like bodily paralysis, the degeneration of the nervous system, hallucinations, visions, deafness, muteness, blindness, depression, melancholy, shaky hands and fingers, and death.[60] While Fürst does not refer to hysteria directly, his discussion of hallucinatory visions, nervous disorders, and the spastic movements of hands and fingers does, nevertheless, utilize the language of the *Modekrankheit* outlined in contemporary medical treatises.

Elektra's Hysteria

The language of hysteria was present moreover in the second major collaboration staged by Reinhardt and Eysoldt at the Kleines Theater: Hofmannsthal's *Elektra*. Alongside Stefan Zweig, Peter Altenberg, and Arthur Schnitzler, Hofmannsthal was one of the most prominent members of Jung Wien, a position that afforded him considerable success and notoriety as a *fin-de-siècle* Viennese poet and playwright associated with cabaret culture, including the Cabaret Fledermaus in Vienna, and theaters throughout Germany. In the early years of the twentieth century, Hofmannsthal became intrigued by the potential to reimagine Sophocles' dramatic works as modernist theater, and thus decided to refashion the tragic figure of Elektra into a hysterical femme fatale. This reincarnation of the ancient Greek play materialized through several conversations on the role of physicality and gestural movements between Reinhardt, Eysoldt, Hermann Bahr and Hofmannsthal, the latter of whom was moving back and forth between Berlin and Vienna during the period.[61] Apart from the new arrangement and staging of the play, the overarching impetus for Elektra's rebirth as a young hysteric seems to lie in Eysoldt's earlier portrayal of Salome, which Hofmannsthal had witnessed at the Kleines Theater.[62] Having written and arranged the role for Eysoldt specifically, both Hofmannsthal and Reinhardt believed that the actress possessed the greatest ability to portray the expressive, hysterical nature of the modernized Elektra.[63]

In her book *Electra After Freud* (2005), Jill Scott analyzes the construction of the *fin-de-siècle* heroine by first charting the etiology of hysteria. Starting with ancient theories of the wandering womb, Scott meanders through Freud's and Breuer's ideas on psychopathology, outlined in *Studies in Hysteria*, before arriving at Hofmannsthal's and Richard Strauss' respective dramatic works, in which Elektra is refigured as a tragic femme fatale.[64] Scott does not, however, propose that Hofmannsthal's *Elektra* had actually become a madwoman. In an attempt to situate the discourse on Elektra within psychoanalytic and feminist criticism, Scott concludes that Elektra should not be perceived as a hysteric, and that any such reading of this sort only "undermines any diagnosis by appropriating and indeed performing the medical discourse and disease as a defensive strategy."[65] Scott thus contends that "Elektra's hysteria is perhaps intrinsic to her femininity" and therefore metaphorically represents "the radical otherness of Elektra as woman" within the context of Hofmannsthal's play.[66] Building on feminist reevaluations of Freudian psychoanalysis offered by Luce Irigaray, Elaine Showalter, Jane Gallop, and Shoshana Felman, as well as on Judith Butler's constructivist theory of sex and gender, Scott employs a postmodern, feminist methodology to elucidate Elektra's sexual difference and the identity politics associated with this gendered character—that is, as a woman who is not actually hysterical, but who acts out hysteria in order to recapture a positive identity for herself.[67]

Although Scott's analysis appropriately scrutinizes the performative nature of hysteria, and thus the inherent theatricality of the disorder, she is largely interested in how this performance occurs within the parameters of *fin-de-siècle* gender biases and historical attitudes toward women. Scott arrives, quite accurately, at the conclusion that being hysterical at the turn of the century was synonymous with being female, as exemplified by Freud's and Breuer's understanding of hysteria in the late nineteenth century, though her analysis ultimately handles the discourse surrounding Elektra as though she were an actual person, like Augustine or Dora. Given that Elektra was of course a fictitious, theatrical character from the start, and all the more so in the hands of Hofmannsthal and Eysoldt, it is somewhat counterintuitive to argue that she gains her autonomy through her performance of hysteria, since Elektra—as a metaphorical character—could only be performed in order to exist. As such, I am more interested in the fact that *fin-de-siècle* theater critics understood Elektra to be a hysteric precisely because of the historical misogyny surrounding the cult of hysteria and hysterical women. Such an understanding has also led Philip Ward to argue that Hofmannsthal deliberately presents Elektra as a hysteric in order to show audiences that hysteria had become a synecdoche for all female movements and behaviors that disturbed the status quo of society.[68]

Prior to his work on *Elektra*, Hofmannsthal consulted with Bahr about Freud's and Breuer's findings on hysteria and repressed memory.[69] It is also known that Hofmannsthal, who possessed a first edition copy of *Studies in Hysteria*, as well as Freud's *Die Traumdeutung* (*Interpretation of Dreams*, 1900), read these works during his development of *Elektra*.[70] Definitive proof that Hofmannsthal literally based Elektra on a historical figure like Anna O. is of course not available, as Hofmannsthal never made such a conclusive claim, at least not in his writings.[71] This notwithstanding, the majority of the critical literature agrees that this connection was undeniably strong, and perhaps even completely convincing in Eysoldt's embodiment of the character. The impetus for Elektra's hysterical movements were derived from Eysoldt's earlier performance as Salome, but Hofmannsthal's initial interest in psychopathology can be linked to his relationship with Bahr, who, by 1902, had begun writing the Freudian-Aristotelian section of his book *Dialog vom Tragischen* (*Dialogue of Tragedies*, 1904), in which he analyzes Freud's theory of hysteria alongside Sophocles' and Euripides' respective versions of *Elektra*. Bahr's personal documents also reveal that he was reading clinical studies by Charcot, Hippolyte Bernheim and Pierre Janet, even though these physicians are not specifically cited in the pages of the *Dialogue*.[72] Lorna Martens has shown, moreover, that Bahr had lent the unpublished section on Freud and *Elektra* to Hofmannsthal and asked for his editorial comments prior to July 1903, so Hofmannsthal was unequivocally aware of the connections that Bahr was drawing between clinical hysteria and ancient Greek tragedy.[73]

It should therefore come as no surprise that Bahr was the first *fin-de-siècle* critic to specifically identify the main character in Hofmannsthal's play as a hysterical woman, stating in a 1904 letter that the playwright "wonderfully brought out the hysteric, via Eysoldt, in Elektra."[74] Within the play, one is made aware of Elektra's role as a hysterical femme fatale when one sees that the vengeance that she seeks for her father's death is only satisfied after she convinces her brother, Orestes, to kill their mother, Klytaemnestra.[75] At this point, we realize that the femme fatale is not only a conduit for hysterical fits and a demonic lust for vengeance, but that she also transfers this need for revenge onto her brother, thus corrupting a man in the process. It thus stands to reason that Klytaemnestra, the woman who premeditates the murder of Agamemnon (her husband and Elektra's father), can also be identified as a theatrical incarnation of the destructive femme fatale. If one agrees with Heinz Politzer's observation that the character of Klytaemnestra is also a hysteric, then Hofmannsthal's *Elektra* presented audiences with not just one, but two hysterical madwomen.[76]

As previously mentioned, Bahr, a Viennese critic, was a fan of *Elektra*, yet a number of German critics had mixed opinions of Hofmannsthal's play. Alfred Kerr, a Berlin theater critic for the *Neue Deutsche Rundschau* (*New German Review*), argued that all of Hofmannsthal's plays seemed to develop as "internalized, stylized forms of art, from the first moment to the next with penetrating force."[77] Although this review seems favorable, Kerr nevertheless states that in *Elektra*, "Hofmannsthal is a reveler; often a subtle reveler; here a reveler of blood."[78] Another Berlin critic, writing for the *Neue Preußische Zeitung* (*New Prussian Newspaper*), criticized *Elektra*, claiming that Hofmannsthal had eradicated lyrical drama from the play by abandoning character development in favor of atmosphere.[79] By contrast, a third critic, Alfred Klaar, endorsed Hofmannsthal's efforts and praised the "sensual images" created by the play's novel handling of theatrical atmosphere, immediacy, and forcefulness.[80]

Despite their varied reviews, it is clear that all of these German critics were responding to Hofmannsthal's new style of writing and Reinhardt's modern direction, rather than to the main character or the play's allusions to modern medicine. This is telling for a number of reasons. First, Kerr and the theater critic for the *New Prussian Newspaper* were both writing for conservative German audiences who, beyond a reasonable doubt, were principally accustomed to traditional forms of theater. Second, we know that Kerr detested Reinhardt and his ideas on avant-garde theater and modern stage direction, things that Hofmannsthal wholly embraced.[81] What is more, Kerr was only concerned with how the use of disquieting, atmospheric lighting created discord between the characters and the audience.[82] Klaar, by contrast, noted that these unconventional lighting techniques communicated Elektra's psychological turmoil and her need for revenge to the audience. In summary, Klaar argued that Elektra was "an uncanny, wild, flickering, vengeful little flame that, at the whiff of victory and fulfillment, is extinguished."[83] His critique is also the first instance in which the language of psychopathology appears in *fin-de-siècle* reviews of *Elektra*. In describing the stage design, the critic noted that the murderous atmosphere was rife with "the tyranny of insanity."[84] Here, Klaar employs the word *Wahnsinn*—again, a word that either denotes insanity, lunacy, or clinical madness. This historical observation seemingly dispels any doubt that Elektra's pathology was lost on contemporary audiences. Instead, it appears that Hofmannsthal effectively brought clinical hysteria to the German stage prior to transferring the semblance of hystero-theatrical gestures to his native Vienna.

Conclusion

Turning to the epigraph of this chapter, I want to go back to the notion that hysteria had become the *Modekrankheit* of the *fin de siècle*, particularly in the realm of modern theater. The use of the term "fashionable disease" in relation to clinical hysteria was initially employed by the theater critic Friedrich Brandes who, after seeing Richard Strauss' opera *Salome* at the Dresden Opera in December 1905, suggested that the lead character's portrayal of pathological symptoms was indicative of the popular trend for avant-garde playwrights and theater directors to capitalize on the expressive potential of the hysterical madwoman.[85] In light of the previously reviewed critical literature discussing the fashion for corporeal and psychological disorders, and considering also their corresponding movements and gestures in *fin-de-siècle* drama, Brandes' review could easily be applied to any one of the modernist productions staged by Reinhardt in Berlin in the early twentieth century. That is to say, Brandes manages—in a single phrase—to surmise what his contemporaries were stating with less brevity: that hysteria had not only become the fashionable disease of the turn of the century, but had transformed itself into the favorite disease of modernity, particularly in the realm of the performing arts.

In the following chapter, I build on Brandes' observation and subsequently explore the Viennese interpretation of hystero-theatrical gestures in modern dramatic productions, and in symbolist and expressionist paintings created in *fin-de-siècle* Vienna. As a way of bridging these two realms, I turn to a series of photographs taken during the Viennese premiere of Strauss' opera *Elektra* (1909). Understood as "modern" due to its novel musical composition, which explored dissonance and avant-garde tonalities, Strauss' *Elektra* also incorporated expressive gestural movements choreographed for its singers. Parroting the theatricality of Eysoldt in her roles as Salome and Elektra in Reinhardt's earlier productions, a number of photographs housed in the archive of the Austrian Theater Museum show the hystero-theatrical gestures enacted by the immensely popular Viennese soprano Anna Bahr-Mildenburg (née Anna Bellschan von Mildenburg).

The wife of Hermann Bahr, Bahr-Mildenburg was one Austrian performer who conspicuously adopted the language and typology of hysteria in her portrayal of psychopathology on the stage. As analyzed by Nicholas Baragwanath, Bahr-Mildenburg's success as a commanding lead soprano at the Vienna Opera (and elsewhere) can be credited to her immense stage presence and use of expressive gestures.[86] Basing his findings on Bahr-Mildenburg's own writings on avant-garde performance, including her musings on the importance of mimicking various psychological states, Baragwanath argues that she was instrumental in developing a semiotics of pathological movements on the Austrian stage.[87] Photographs housed in the Austrian Theater Museum can therefore be said to serve as physical and visual evidence of these gesticulations, allowing scholars to gain greater insight into the use (and re-use) of hystero-theatrical gestures in modern performances, in this instance opera. These images, which serve as some of the initial case studies discussed in Chapter 4, allow us to journey from the Parisian and Berlin theater scenes of the late nineteenth- and early twentieth-centuries, to the world of *fin-de-siècle* Viennese theater and its similar embrace of hysteria as the *Modekrankheit*. Importantly, charting such a path draws us into the cultural milieu that the Viennese expressionists encountered in 1909–10, when their activities ultimately came to fruition.

Notes

1 Friedrich Brandes, "Dresdener Uraufführung der Salome von Wilde-Strauss," *Deutsche Tageszeitung*, December 11, 1905, n.p.

2 Mark S. Micale, "Discourses of Hysteria in Fin-de-Siècle France," in *The Mind of Modernism: Medicine, Psychology, and the Cultural Arts in Europe and America, 1880–1940*, ed. Mark S. Micale (Stanford: Stanford University Press, 2004), 76. See also Georges Didi-Huberman, *Invention of Hysteria: Charcot and the Photographic Iconography of the Salpêtrière*, trans. Alisa Hartz (Cambridge, MA: MIT Press, 2003), 244.

3 Jules Falret, quoted in Manfred Schneider, "Hysterie als Gesamtkunstwerk," in *Ornament und Askese: Im Zeitgeist des Wien der Jahrhundertwende*, ed. Alfred Pfabigan (Vienna: C. Brandstätter, 1985), 223n15. For Falret's early research on hysteria and epilepsy, see Jules Falret and Brierre de Boismont, *Über gefährliche Geisteskranke und die Special-Asyle für die sogenannten verbrecherischen Irren: Zwei psychiatrische Abhandlungen*, trans. Carl Stark (Stuttgart: H. Lindemann, 1871), 18.

4 Didi-Huberman, *Invention of Hysteria*, xi. In a somewhat related vein, Susan Rubin Suleiman and David Lomas have both examined Charcot's theatrical images of hysteria

in relation to surrealism's interest in psychoanalysis and the sexually commodified female body. See Suleiman, *Subversive Intent: Gender, Politics, and the Avant-Garde*, 99–109; and David Lomas, *The Haunted Self: Surrealism, Psychoanalysis, Subjectivity* (New Haven: Yale University Press, 1999), 53–93.

5 Didi-Huberman, *Invention of Hysteria*, 68.

6 Didi-Huberman, *Invention of Hysteria*, xi. In addition to Didi-Huberman's examination of Charcot and the theatrics of the Salpêtrière, Sarah J. Rudolph and Ellen W. Kaplan have analyzed the popularity and spectacle of the gestures of "lunatic" patients in London's Bethlehem Hospital. Robert Whitaker has likewise examined a similar trend in the Pennsylvania Hospital, which offered ward visits as a form of entertainment for the public. See Ellen W. Kaplan and Sarah J. Rudolph, ed., *Images of Mental Illness Through Text and Performance*, vol. 33, *Studies in Theatre Arts* (Lewiston: The Edwin Mellen Press, 2005), 7–8.

7 For Micale's analysis, see Micale, "Discourses of Hysteria in Fin-de-Siècle France," 76. For Gordon's analysis, see Rae Beth Gordon, "From Charcot to Charlot: Unconscious Imitation and Spectatorship in French Cabaret and Early Cinema," in *The Mind of Modernism: Medicine, Psychology, and The Cultural Arts in Europe and America, 1880–1940*, ed. Mark S. Micale (Stanford: Stanford University Press, 2004), 100, 104.

8 Klaus Albrecht Schröder, *Egon Schiele: Eros and Passion*, trans. David Britt (Munich: Prestel, 1989), 84. Rae Beth Gordon's research essentially contradicts Schröder's assertion that hysterical gestures first appear in paintings and therefore precede Charcot's photographs as well as the appearance of these gestures in theater and literature. Moreover, Schröder does not analyze the appearance of these gestures in theater but only in painting. See Gordon, "From Charcot to Charlot," 100–04.

9 For Lichtenstein's analysis concerning the misogynistic foundation of Charcot's model, see Thérèse Lichtenstein, *Behind Closed Doors: The Art of Hans Bellmer* (Los Angeles: University of California Press, 2001), 202n10. For Steiner's comments, see Reinhard Steiner, *Egon Schiele, 1890–1918*, trans. Michael Hulse (Cologne: Taschen Verlag, 2000), 50.

10 For a well-formulated discussion on the semiotics of gestural signs in theater, see Erika Fischer-Lichte, *The Semiotics of Theater*, trans. Jeremy Gaines and Doris L. Jones (1983; Bloomington: Indiana University Press, 1992), 39–58. For a discussion of theatrical gesture, see Fernando de Toro, *Theatre Semiotics: Text and Staging in Modern Theatre*, ed. Carole Hubbard, trans. John Lewis (Toronto: University of Toronto Press, 1995), 76–82.

11 Marco de Marinis, *The Semiotics of Performance*, trans. Áine O'Healy (1982; Bloomington: Indiana University Press, 1993), 53–54.

12 Christopher G. Goetz, Michel Bonduelle, and Toby Gelfand, *Charcot: Constructing Neurology* (New York: Oxford University Press, 1995), 238–39.

13 Didi-Huberman, *Invention of Hysteria*, 77–79; Steiner, *Egon Schiele*, 50; and Thomas Medicus, "Das Theater der Nervosität. Freud, Charcot, Sarah Bernhardt und die Salpêtrière," *Freibeuter* 41 (1989): 93–103.

14 Freud, *Letters of Sigmund Freud*, 181.

15 Thomas Medicus suggests that Freud was aware of this relationship. See Medicus, "Das Theater der Nervosität," 93–103.

16 Gordon, "From Charcot to Charlot," 94.

17 S. Veyrac, "Nos Interviews: Une heure chez Sarah Bernhardt," in *La Chronique Médicale: Revue bi-mensuelle de médecine, historique, littéraire et anecdotique* 4, no. 19 (October 1, 1897): 614.

18 Veyrac, "Nos Interviews," 614. This anecdote has also been repeated widely in the current scholarship on Bernhardt. See, for example, Gordon, "From Charcot to Charlot," 105; Rae Beth Gordon, *Why the French Love Jerry Lewis: From Cabaret to Early Cinema* (Stanford: Stanford University Press, 2001), 29; Asti Hustvedt, *Medical Muses: Hysteria in Nineteenth-Century Paris* (New York: W. W. Norton, 2011), 93; and Micale, "Discourses of Hysteria in Fin-de-Siècle France," 76.

19 Veyrac, "Nos Interviews," 616.

20 Thomas Medicus was the first and, to my knowledge, the only scholar to date to analyze Charcot's images of hysteria alongside photographs of Bernhardt's theatrical personas. See Medicus, "Das Theater der Nervosität," 93–103.

21 Jules Claretie, *Les amours d'un interne* (Paris: Dentu, 1881). In addition to this novel, Claretie would also publish the novel *Hypnotisme* in 1892, which dealt with scientific experiments at the Salpêtrière and its hysterical women. For further analyses of Claretie's novel in relation to clinical hysteria, see Janet Beizer, *Ventriloquized Bodies: Narratives of Hysteria in Nineteenth-Century France* (Ithaca: Cornell University Press, 1994), 15–29; and Micale, "Discourses of Hysteria in Fin-de-Siècle France," 75.

22 Gordon, "From Charcot to Charlot," 94; and Hustvedt, *Medical Muses*, 94–97.

23 For Avril's biography, see François Caradec, *Jane Avril: Au Moulin Rouge avec Toulouse-Lautrec* (Paris: Fayard, 2001).

24 W. E. Yates, *Theatre in Vienna: A Critical History, 1776–1995* (Cambridge: Cambridge University Press, 1996), 178.

25 Franz Hofen, "Sarah Bernhardt in Deutschland," *Bühne und Welt: Zeitschrift für Theaterwesen, Litteratur und Musik* 5, no. 3 (November 1902): 89–93. See also Heinrich Stümcke, "Von den Berliner Theatern 1902/03," *Bühne und Welt: Zeitschrift für Theaterwesen, Litteratur und Musik* 5, no. 4 (November 1902): 167. The journal *Bühne und Welt* was founded in 1898 by Stümcke as the official publication of the *Deutscher Bühnenverein* (German Theater and Orchestra Association).

26 Hofen, "Sarah Bernhardt in Deutschland," 92–93. Regarding Bernhardt's popularity with German-speaking actors, see Heinrich Stümcke, "Von Den Berliner Theatern 1902/03," *Bühne und Welt: Zeitschrift für Theaterwesen, Litteratur und Musik* 5, no. 3 (November 1902): 167–70.

27 "Theater und Kunst," *Wiener Abendpost: Beilage zur Wiener Zeitung*, no. 263, December 14, 1902, 8. The *Wiener Abendpost* was the official newspaper of the Austrian government, and even though it would occasionally adopt a non-monarchist viewpoint, it was generally understood to take an illiberal stance on basic issues. For a history of Viennese newspapers and their political affiliations, see Kurt Paupié, *Handbuch der Österreichischen Pressegeschichte, 1848–1959*, vol. 1 (Vienna: Wilhelm Braumüller, 1960).

28 "Dramatic and Musical Events in Germany. Sarah Bernhardt Criticised – Recitals from the Bible – An American Pianist," *The New York Times*, November 2, 1902, 5.

29 Yates, *Theatre in Vienna*, 178–79.

30 Harold B. Segel, *Turn-of-the-Century Cabaret: Paris, Barcelona, Berlin, Munich, Vienna, Cracow, Moscow, St. Petersburg, Zurich* (New York: Columbia University Press, 1987), 143–44.

31 Segel, *Turn-of-the-Century Cabaret*, 144–45.

32 Segel, *Turn-of-the-Century Cabaret*, 145.

33 Segel, *Turn-of-the-Century Cabaret*, 184.

34 Leo Greiner, "Münchener Theater," *Revue franco-allemande/Deutsch-französische Rundschau* 2, no. 21 (November 1899): 295. The entire review reads as follows: "Prange's 'Kain' ersetzt durch die Unmöglichkeit der Voraussetzungen die Glaubwürdigkeit der Vorgänge, durch misstönende Anklänge an 'Kollege Krampton' und 'John Gabriel Borkmann' eigene Gestaltungskraft, durch eine psychologisch verpfuschte Wahnsinnskatastrophe das tragische Pathos. Ich will nicht sagen, dass der Verfasser ohne Talent ist. Aber sein Werk zeigt all' das Streben nach bombastischer Grösse und toller Ungeheuerlichkeit der Motive, wie es gewissen Jugendarbeiten anhaftet, welche vorsichtigere Dichter weise im Schreibpult verschliessen."

35 Greiner, "Münchener Theater," 295.

36 See Georg Schaumberg, "Münchener Brief," *Bühne und Welt: Zeitschrift für Theaterwesen, Litteratur und Musik* 3, no. 16 (May 1901): 700. Each of the following scholars incorrectly states that the Berlin premiere was also the German premiere of Wilde's *Salome*, even though the play was first staged in Munich in 1901. See Horst Uhr, *Lovis Corinth* (Berkeley: University of California Press, 1990), 166; Peter Jelavich, *Berlin Cabaret* (Cambridge, MA: Harvard University Press, 1993), 62; and Segel, *Turn-of-the-Century Cabaret*, 142.

37 Despite having written the play in French, Wilde intended to premiere *Salome* in London, but the censors immediately banned all public performances in 1892. It is unclear whether Bernhardt ever appeared in any private performances staged in London, though she was not performing in the lead role when it premiered in Paris in 1896. Toni Bentley argues that Wilde did not write the play for Bernhardt, though he could imagine no one other than the

forty-seven-year-old actress to play Salome. See Toni Bentley, *Sisters of Salome* (Lincoln: Bison Books, 2005), 27–28.

38　Schaumberg, "Münchener Brief," 696. The original German reads: "Den stärksten Eindruck der verflossenen Saison verdanke ich einem Ausländer, Oskar Wilde, und seiner faszinierenden 'Salome'. Frau Gerhäufer von Karlsruher Hoftheater, die Gattin unseres zukünftigen Heldentenors, sah als Salome entzückend aus."

39　Schaumberg, "Münchener Brief," 700. The original German reads: "Eine eigene Abhandlung wäre nötig, um die faszinierende Wirkung dieses Einakters klar zu machen. Das ist aber nicht meine Aufgabe."

40　Stümcke, "Von den Berliner Theater 1902/03," vol. 5, no. 4, 168–69.

41　Steven Price and William Tydeman, *Wilde: Salome* (Cambridge: Cambridge University Press, 1996), 31.

42　Segel, *Turn-of-the-Century Cabaret*, 142. Segel only discusses Strauss' attendance at this private performance, though it is known that Hofmannsthal also attended the production. See Price and Tydeman, *Wilde*, 33.

43　Tilla Durieux quoted in Uhr, *Lovis Corinth*, 167.

44　Regarding Durieux's performances as Salome, see Price and Tydeman, *Wilde*, 34.

45　Heinrich Stümcke, "Von den Berliner Theatern 1902/03," *Bühne und Welt: Zeitschrift für Theaterwesen, Litteratur und Musik* 5, no. 5 (December 1902): 215. In speaking of a painting by Lovis Corinth depicting Eysoldt in her role as Salome, which has since been destroyed, Horst Uhr argues that Corinth's canvas presented an "image of depravity, partly, perhaps, in response to the then current vogue for pictures of the prototypical *femme fatale*." See Uhr, *Lovis Corinth*, 167.

46　Although this point is stressed in much of the current scholarship on Ibsen's work, I would call the reader's attention to a contemporary German review/essay that stressed the playwright's interest in the psychological turmoil of his characters. See Philipp Stein, "Ibsen auf den Berliner Bühnen 1876/1900," *Bühne und Welt: Zeitschrift für Theaterwesen, Litteratur und Musik* 3, no. 12 (March 1901): 489–504.

47　Regarding the play's Berlin premiere, see Heinrich Stümcke, "Von Den Berliner Theatern 1902/03," *Bühne und Welt: Zeitschrift für Theaterwesen, Litteratur und Musik* 5, no. 6 (December 1902): 254. For a somewhat contemporary analysis of Hauptmann's work within expressionist drama, as well as his overwhelming interest in psychological and pathological disease, see Manfred Schneider, *Der Expressionismus im Drama* (Stuttgart: Julius Hoffmann, 1920), 13–18.

48　Stümcke, "Von Den Berliner Theatern 1902/03," vol. 5, no. 6, 254–55. The original German reads: "Eine andere Frage ist es, ob der Spezialfall des armen Heinrich, die wunderbare Heilung des Aussätzigen durch das freilich nicht vollzogene Blutopfer der frommen Jungfrau, sich für die Bühne eignet. Die dramatische crux bilden hier einmal das Wunder, dann die ekelhafte Krankheit. Hauptmann hat das Wunder aus seiner dramatischen Entwicklung des Falles nicht beseitigt, vielleicht auch nicht beseitigen wollen, obgleich er sonst mit allen Mitteln moderner Seelenkunst sich um die psychologische Vertiefung der Vorgänge bemüht. [...] Die vier ersten Akte zeigen uns alle Phasen des leiblichen und seelischen Krankheitsprozesses. Zuerst die tiefe Melancholie."

49　Stümcke, "Von Den Berliner Theatern 1902/03," vol. 5, no. 6, 256. The original German reads: "Die männliche und weibliche Hauptrolle waren mit Rudolf Rittner und Irene Triesch besetzt. [...] Irene Triesch, die in Inkarnationen der Sinnlichkeit wie Salome, Anisja, Rahel sonst triumphiert, schuf mit kluger Kunst eine glaubwürdige Ottogebe von mädchenhafter Dürftigkeit der Formen, schämiger Jungfräulichkeit und der ekstatischen Inbrunst."

50　Uhr, *Lovis Corinth*, 167.

51　For critical responses to Wedekind's play, including discussions of its importance to the development of the modern theater, see Jeannine Schuler-Will, "Wedekind's Lulu: Pandora and Pierrot, the Visual Experience of Myth," *German Studies Review* 7, no. 1 (February 1984): 27–38; and J. L. Hibberd, "The Spirit of the Flesh: Wedekind's Lulu," *The Modern Language Review* 79, no. 2 (April 1984): 336–55. Harold Segel discusses Wedekind's notoriety in Segel, *Turn-of-the-Century Cabaret*, 143.

52　See Hibberd, "The Spirit of the Flesh," 338.

53 Frank Wedekind, *Erdgeist (Earth-Spirit)*, trans. Jr. Samuel A. Eliot (1895; New York: Albert and Charles Boni, 1914), 9. The original German reads: "He, Aujust! Bring mir unsre *Schlange* her! Sie ward geschaffen, Unheil anzustiften, Zu locken, zu verführen, zu vergiften - Zu morden, ohne daß es einer spürt. [...] Du hast kein Recht, uns durch Miaun und Fauchen, Die *Urgestalt* des *Weibes* zu verstauchen, Durch Faxenmachen uns und Fratzenschneiden, Des *Lasters Kindereinfalt* zu verleiden!"

54 Hibberd, "The Spirit of the Flesh," 338.

55 Heinrich Stümcke, "Von den Berliner Theatern 1902/03," *Bühne und Welt: Zeitschrift für Theaterwesen, Litteratur und Musik* 5, no. 7 (January 1903): 300. The original German reads: "Der Erdgeist ist die urewige Verkörperung der dämonischen Weibsnatur, die alle Männer, die in ihren Bannkreis geraten, bethört und zernichtet. Eva, die bei Wedekind auch Mignon und Lulu heißt, eine raffinierte Mischung von kindlicher Naivität, Hingebung, Verdorbenheit, Sinnlichkeit und Kälte. Frau Eva flirtet und zeigt ihre Gliederpracht zur Abwechslung jetzt ein Weilchen in einem Variété-Theater. Frau Eysoldt hat ihrer Salome ein würdiges Gegenstück zugesellt. Sie war, in hundert Farben schillernd, ganz die faszinierende Verkörperung der Mignon, Lulu und Eva, das ungezogene Kind, die launische Despotin, die perverse Buhlerin und die lockende Tanzmänade in einer Person."

56 Albert Eulenburg, "Schauspieler-Krankheiten," *Bühne und Welt: Zeitschrift für Theaterwesen, Litteratur und Musik* 4, no. 9 (February 1902): 388. The original German reads: "die ausgezeichnetsten Bühnenkünstler zugleich zu Opfern ihrer Kunst, zu 'Nervenmärtyrern' machen."

57 Eulenburg, "Schauspieler-Krankheiten," 388. The original German reads: "das körperliche und seelische Leben des Schauspielers" and "notwendigen aber unglücklichen Empfindsamkeit ihrer Nerven."

58 Eulenburg, "Schauspieler-Krankheiten," 389.

59 L. Fürst, "Das Pathologische auf der Bühne," *Bühne und Welt: Zeitschrift für Theaterwesen, Litteratur und Musik* 5, no. 9 (February 1903): 375–79.

60 See Fürst, "Das Pathologische auf der Bühne," 375–79.

61 Jelavich, *Berlin Cabaret*, 82; and Sally McMullen, "From the Armchair to the Stage: Hofmannsthal's 'Elektra' in its Theatrical Context," *The Modern Language Review* 80, no. 3 (July 1985): 638.

62 Jelavich, *Berlin Cabaret*, 82. Jelavich bases this information on Hofmannsthal correspondence, which is reproduced in Hugo von Hofmannsthal, *Briefe 1900–1909* (Vienna: Bermann-Fischer Verlag, 1937). See also Gertrud Eysoldt, *Der Sturm Elektra: Gertrud Eysoldt, Hugo von Hofmannsthal Briefe* (Salzburg: Residenz Verlag, 1996).

63 Jelavich, *Berlin Cabaret*, 82.

64 Jill Scott, *Electra after Freud: Myth and Culture* (Ithaca: Cornell University Press, 2005), 25–43, 57–80. Graham Wheeler has also explored notions of gender within the construction of Elektra, though only within Sophocles' play. See Graham Wheeler, "Gender and Transgression in Sophocles' 'Electra'," *The Classical Quarterly* 53, no. 2 (November 2003): 377–88.

65 Scott, *Electra after Freud*, 58.

66 Scott, *Electra after Freud*, 58.

67 Scott, *Electra after Freud*, 58.

68 See Philip Marshall Ward, "Hofmannsthal, *Elektra* and the Representation of Women's Behaviour Through Myth," *German Life and Letters* 53, no. 1 (2003): 37–55. In line with Scott's research, however, Ward also concludes that Hofmannsthal does not literally represent Elektra as a hysteric.

69 Hofmannsthal, *Briefe 1900–1909*, 142.

70 See Michael Hamburger, "Hofmannsthals Bibliothek," *Euphorion* 55 (1955): 27; and Hofmannsthal, *Briefe 1900–1909*, 384. Thanks to Bernd Urban's 1978 study *Hofmannsthal, Freud und die Psychoanalyse*, scholars know the specific passages Hofmannsthal demarcated in Freud's texts, though it is unclear whether these notations were made prior to, or following, the years 1902 and 1903 when Hofmannsthal was composing the play. See Bernd Urban, *Hofmannsthal, Freud und die Psychoanalyse* (Frankfurt: Lang, 1978). For a sampling of the scholarship connecting Hofmannsthal's play to Freud's writings on psychoanalysis and hysteria, see McMullen, "From the Armchair to the Stage," 637–51;

Lorna Martens, "The Theme of the Repressed Memory in Hofmannsthal's *Elektra*," *The German Quarterly* 60, no. 1 (Winter 1987): 38–51; Heinz Politzer, "Hugo von Hofmannsthal's 'Elektra': Geburt der Tragödie aus dem Geiste der Psychopathologie," *Deutsche Vierteljahrschrift* 47 (1973): 95–119; Michael Worps, *Nervenkunst* (Frankfurt: Europäische Verlagsanstalt, 1983), 259–95; and E. M. Butler, "Hoffmannsthal's [sic] 'Elektra'. A Graeco-Freudian Myth," *Journal of the Warburg Institute* 2, no. 2 (October 1938): 164–75.

71   Even though their conclusions are speculative, both Worps and Martens find that Hofmannsthal's *Elektra* was a kind of modernization of Breuer's case study of Anna O. See Martens, "The Theme of the Repressed Memory in Hofmannsthal's *Elektra*," 40; and Worps, *Nervenkunst*, 280–87. By contrast, Scott asserts: "My own concern is not whether it can be proved without doubt that Anna O. served as the model for Hofmannsthal's heroine. Rather it is my aim to compare the manifestation of hysteria in each case and examine their separate attempts to manipulate the imposed pathologies into a performance, be it theatrical, somatic, or psychological," in *Electra after Freud*, 63.

72   See Hermann Bahr, *Dialog vom Tragischen* (Berlin: S. Fischer, 1904), 9–78. Unpublished documents written by Bahr (known as "Merkbuch" and "Notizbuch," and which document his collection of psychological texts by Freud, Breuer, Janet, Charcot and Bernheim) can be found in the Theatersammlung of the Österreichische Nationalbibliothek in Vienna.

73   See Lorna Martens, *Shadow Lines: Austrian Literature from Freud to Kafka* (Lincoln: University of Nebraska Press, 1996), 62–63.

74   This statement is found in an unpublished document, by Bahr, in the Theatersammlung of the Österreichische Nationalbibliothek in Vienna. Portions of this letter have also been reproduced in Martens, "The Theme of the Repressed Memory in Hofmannsthal's *Elektra*," 40. The original German reads: "Ihren einen Ton, den Hysterischen, haben Sie ihr in der Elektra wunderbar gebracht."

75   Regarding the plot of the play, see Hugo von Hofmannsthal, *Elektra* (Stuttgart: Schauspiel Staatstheater, 2003).

76   For Politzer's analysis of Klytaemnestra, see Politzer, "Hugo von Hofmannsthal's 'Elektra,'" 108.

77   Alfred Kerr, "Rose Bernd und Elektra," *Neue Deutsche Rundschau* 14 (1903): 1316. The original German reads: "Alle Hofmannsthalische Kunst ist verinnerlichte Stilkunst, zum ersten Male jetzt mit durchbrechender Gewalt."

78   Kerr, "Rose Bernd und Elektra," 1315. The original German reads: "Hofmannsthal ist ein Schwelger; oft ein zarter Schwelger; hier ein Blutschwelger."

79   "Feuilleton," *Neue Preußische Zeitung*, no. 512, October 31, 1903, n.p. The *Neue Preußische Zeitung* was politically affiliated with the Prussian Conservative Party, whose conservative members had opposed Bismarck's plans to unite Germany.

80   For Klaar's review of *Elektra*, see Alfred Klaar, ["Elektra,"] *Vossische Zeitung*, no. 511, October 31, 1903, n.p. The original German reads: "sinnliche Bilder." The *Vossische Zeitung* was a liberal newspaper, considered by many to be the German national newspaper of record at the turn of the century.

81   Regarding Kerr's hostility towards Reinhardt, see G. J. Carr, "'Organic' Contradictions in Alfred Kerr's Theatre Criticism," *Oxford German Studies* 14 (1983): 111–24. For an analysis of Hofmannsthal's interest in Reinhardt's direction, see McMullen, "From the Armchair to the Stage," 641, 43.

82   See Alfred Kerr, *Die Welt im Drama*, 5 vols., vol. 2 (Berlin: S. Fischer, 1917), 325.

83   Klaar, *Vossische Zeitung*. The original German reads: "ein unheimliches, wild flackerndes Flämmchen, Rache, übrig geblieben ist, das im Hauche des Sieges, der Befriedigung, erlischt."

84   Klaar, *Vossische Zeitung*. The original German reads: "die Tyrannei sich in Wahnsinn."

85   Brandes, "Dresdener Uraufführung der Salome von Wilde-Strauss."

86   See Nicholas Baragwanath, "Anna Bahr-Mildenburg, gesture, and the Bayreuth style," *Musical Times* 148, no. 1901 (Winter 2007): 63–74.

87   Baragwanath, "Anna Bahr-Mildenburg, gesture, and the Bayreuth style," 63–74.

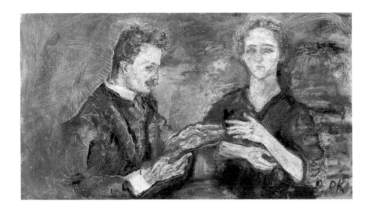

Plate 1 Oskar Kokoschka, *Hans Tietze and Erica Tietze-Conrat*, 1909, oil on canvas. Abby Aldrich Rockefeller Fund, The Museum of Modern Art, New York.

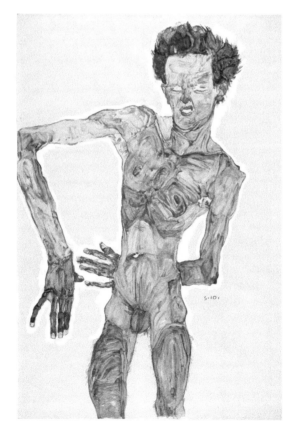

Plate 2 Egon Schiele, *Nude Self-Portrait*, 1910, gouache, watercolor and white heightening. Graphische Sammlung Albertina, Vienna, Austria.

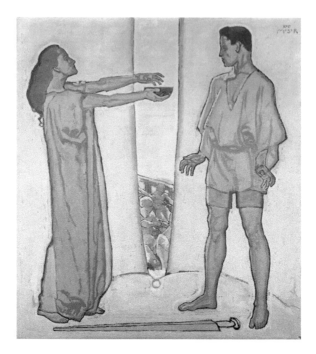

Plate 3 Koloman Moser, *The Love Potion—Tristan and Isolde*, 1915, oil on canvas. Leopold Museum, Private Collection, Vienna.
Source: Photo: Leopold Museum.

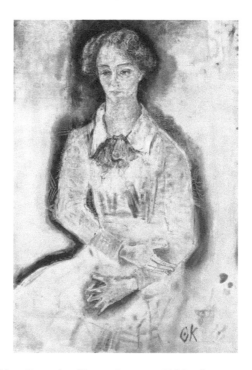

Plate 4 Oskar Kokoschka, *Portrait of Lotte Franzos*, 1909, oil on canvas. The Phillips Collection, Washington, D.C., USA. Acquired 1941.
Source: © 2016 Fondation Oskar Kokoschka / Artists Rights Society (ARS), New York / ProLitteris, Zürich. Photo: Bridgeman Images.

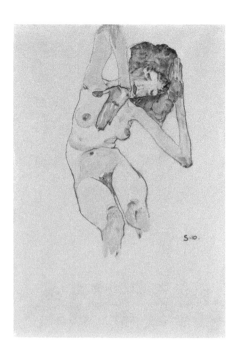

Plate 5 Egon Schiele, *Seated Female Nude with Tilted Head and Raised Arms*, 1910, gouache,
    watercolor and black ink on paper. Private Collection.
Source: Photo: © Sotheby's / akg-images.

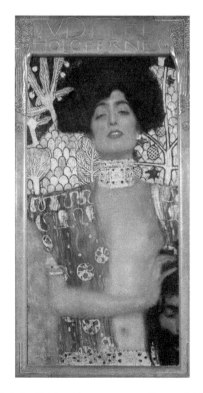

Plate 6 Gustav Klimt, *Judith I*, 1901, oil on canvas. Österreichische Galerie im Belvedere,
    Vienna.
Source: Photo: Erich Lessing / Art Resource, NY.

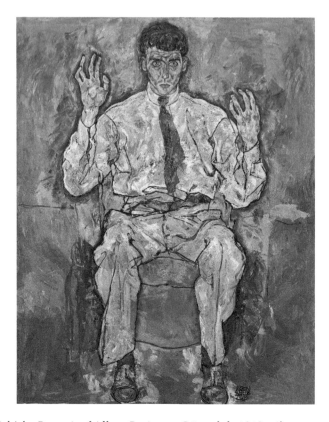

Plate 7 Egon Schiele, *Portrait of Albert Paris von Gütersloh*, 1918, oil on canvas. Minneapolis
Institute of Art, Minneapolis, USA. Gift of the P. D. McMillan Land Company.
Source: Photo: Bridgeman Images.

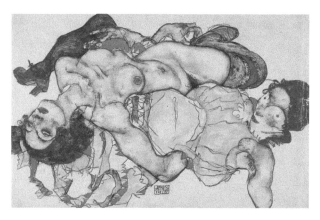

Plate 8 Egon Schiele, *Two Girls, Lying in an Entwined Position*, 1915, gouache and pencil
on paper. Graphische Sammlung Albertina, Vienna, Austria.
Source: Photo: HIP / Art Resource, NY.

4   A Tale of Three Hysterics
Elektra, Isolde, and Salome

> We [psychoanalysts] have the right to analyze a poet's work, but it is not right for the poet to make poetry out of our analyses.[1]
> —Sigmund Freud, addressing the Vienna Psychoanalytic Society, 1909

As in *fin-de-siècle* Paris and Berlin, hystero-theatrical gestures carried the ability to communicate a language of the modern body to Viennese audiences. Viennese theater directors like Hermann Bahr and Max Reinhardt, and numerous female stage performers (some Austrian, some not), including Maud Allan, Anna Bahr-Mildenburg, Gertrude Barrison, Isadora Duncan, Tilla Durieux, Gertrud Eysoldt, and Ruth St. Denis, together participated in theatrical productions across the city that probed the potential for expressive movements to embody the female hysteric on the page, and on the stage. Just as Parisian cabaret had utilized hystero-theatrical gestures as an emotive art form, Viennese playwrights like Hugo von Hofmannsthal made use of these gesticulations in operas and plays centered on pathological themes and characters. Accordingly, Hofmannsthal's and Richard Strauss' collaborative opera *Elektra* (1909), Gustav Mahler and Alfred Roller's production of Richard Wagner's *Tristan and Isolde* (1903), Hofmannsthal's and Reinhardt's experimental staging of Hofmannsthal's *Oedipus Rex* (1906), and Maud Allan's production of *The Vision of Salomé* (1906) all serve as examples of "mad" performances in this chapter's exploration of modern theater in *fin-de-siècle* Vienna.

During this period, hystero-theatrical gestures in theatrical productions seemingly received more critical attention than those appearing in symbolist, Secessionist, and expressionist works of art. This is a further indication that expressionists were themselves more interested in the physical and visceral manifestation of avant-garde corporeal movements enacted in theater than in the static gestures recorded in photographic medical journals that they may or may not have studied. A number of young expressionist artists were active in the city's most notable cabaret—Die Fledermaus (The Bat)—and the use of expressive movements on the stage there points to an interest in, and collaborative exploration of, hystero-theatrical gesture among artists working in a range of disciplines in this particular Viennese setting. Many of the artists affiliated with the Wiener Werkstätte participated in the shared effort to decorate the Cabaret Fledermaus and make it the foremost example of the *Gesamtkunstwerk* (or "total work of art"), while others designed stage sets or composed and directed cabaret productions in its theater. The Fledermaus was only one of many theater spaces devoted to artistic activities, though it was the center of arguably the most avant-garde scene in Vienna, and one of the few stages that hosted expressionist theatrical productions, which were not common in the city. The dramatic works discussed in this chapter, however, almost all predate such productions, and therefore now appear to have been prototypes for the appearance of the pathological body in later expressionist drama.

W. E. Yates has recently observed that the "flowering of modernism" in *fin-de-siècle* Vienna cannot be viewed solely in terms of the literature, architecture, or fine arts produced by artists and poets associated with the Vienna Secession, the Wiener Werkstätte, and the expressionist movement.[2] Instead, Yates advocates a sort of *Gesamtkunstwerk* vision of Viennese modernism by insisting that the radical changes unfolding in avant-garde theater went hand-in-hand with the flourishing of the visual arts. In line with Yates' contention, this chapter begins by briefly charting the movement of hystero-theatrical gestures from Strauss' premiere of *Salome* in Dresden, to the later staging of *Elektra* in Dresden and then Vienna. This examination is based on the appearance of these expressive gestures in French and German theater, as outlined in the previous chapter, and also explores the twentieth-century Viennese interest in bringing aspects of modern medicine—particularly the discourse surrounding hysteria—into theatrical performance. The appearance and reappearance of theatrical madwomen made familiar by characters like Salome and Elektra, and Klytaemnestra and Isolde, provide a fascinating look into the role that hystero-theatrical gestures played in the Austrian capital. This chapter not only discusses these important examples of theatrical hysterics, but also establishes their legacy in *fin-de-siècle* Viennese painting, which includes works by Gustav Klimt, Koloman Moser, and Egon Schiele.

Like Mother, Like Daughter: Elektra and Klytaemnestra

As with the performances involving the hysterical femme fatale in Reinhardt's productions at Berlin's Kleines Theater, the trope of the hysterical madwoman resurfaced in Strauss' operatic versions of *Salome* (1905) and *Elektra* (1909). Adapted from Oscar Wilde's and Hofmannsthal's respective plays, Strauss' operas are today regarded as the composer's most modernist works. Sander Gilman and Lawrence Kramer have both tackled the theme of disease and culture in these operas, arguing that the works supported patriarchal, misogynistic, anti-Semitic, gendered, and disease-ridden notions.[3] Intrigued by the idea that contemporary audiences believed the lead character in *Salome* to be diseased, Gilman concludes that,

> Strauss discovered the avant-garde opera and was in turn discovered by the avant-garde. It is this avant-garde, understood by Strauss (and, indeed, by much of fin-de-siècle culture) as "Jewish," which sets the stage for the selection of *Salome* as his first "modern" opera.[4]

Building upon Gilman's assessment of *Salome* as a model of "theatrical and political anti-Semitism," Kramer similarly claims that Strauss treated

> Salome not as a monstrous sexual icon but as a focal point for the representation of a bundle of instabilities produced by the *fin-de-siècle* gender system. Questions of sexuality, both male and female, are certainly involved, but so are questions of gender, writing and cultural authority.[5]

In her essay, "The Taste of Love: Salome's Transfiguration" (2006), Anne Seshadri concludes that Kramer's analysis fails to consider racial differences, while Gilman's approach places too much weight on the notions of avant-gardism, homosexuality, degeneracy, and Orientalism.[6] In attempting to correct this, Seshadri argues that Strauss' *Salome* can more accurately be understood as a *Judenoper*, or "Jewish opera," since audiences of the period would themselves have interpreted it as such, given its exploration of the "subjective and collective meanings of Jewishness as a category of racial and national identity."[7] She further argues that contemporary viewers would have understood Salome's death at the conclusion of Strauss' opera as wholly unrelated to the one that unfolds in Wilde's play, since "the Jewish princess Salome, through the music of Strauss, transcended her Jewishness and was transfigured."[8] On one level, Seshadri seems to echo Jill Scott's formulation of the character Elektra as a gendered construct acting out female pathologies in order to be transformed into an autonomous woman. Nevertheless, Seshadri's argument abandons the reclamation of gender in favor of the redemptive power of racial and social transfiguration. The correlation between Harold Blum's comments regarding the conflation of cultural signifiers like "diseased" and "Jewishness," as discussed in Chapter 2 in relation to Ida Bauer (Freud's "Dora"), is therefore most striking when compared to Gilman's and Kramer's respective analyses of Strauss' turn-of-the-century femme fatale.

Strauss unveiled his other modernist opera, *Elektra*, on 25 January 1909 at the Dresden Semperoper (Dresden Opera), where *Salome* had debuted four years earlier. *Elektra* was the first major collaboration between Strauss and Hofmannsthal, the latter of whom adapted the libretto from his own 1903 play. As such, a very deliberate and distinct connection exists between Hofmannsthal's lyrical Elektra and the subsequent incarnation of the singing madwoman in Strauss' opera. The music correspondent for the *Neues Wiener Journal* (*New Viennese Journal*) commented on this relationship in a review published on 26 January 1909, stating that Strauss' *Elektra* owed much to Reinhardt's and Hofmannsthal's production in Berlin, including Eysoldt's portrayal of the crazed protagonist.[9] Equally telling is the fact that the unnamed critic used as many words to discuss Strauss' *Salome* as he or she did commenting on *Elektra*, concluding that the latter opera was essentially an extension of the former opera's musical experimentations.[10]

When *Elektra* opened on 23 March 1909 at the Wiener Hofoper (Vienna Court Opera, now the Wiener Staatsoper/Vienna Opera), Anna Bahr-Mildenburg (who was not yet married to Hermann Bahr) appeared as Klytaemnestra, Elektra's murderous mother.[11] Contemporary accounts unvaryingly suggest that the soprano's commanding stage presence, distinct body gestures, and undeniable talent enraptured audiences during her debut in the role.[12] One such observer was Erwin Stein, an Austrian writer, musician, and pupil of the expressionist composer Arnold Schoenberg, who recalled that Bahr-Mildenburg was not only regarded by critics as a talented singer, but also as a great tragic actress, given the emphasis she placed on the grandeur of her movements.[13] In this sense, Bahr-Mildenburg might be regarded as the Austrian Sarah Bernhardt, given the propensity for both actresses to rely on the histrionics of the *Modekrankheit* to enhance their performances.

Examples of Bahr-Mildenburg's expressive body language and physiognomy can be found in numerous photographs of the actress housed in the collection of the

Austrian Theater Museum (see, for example, Figures 4.1 and 4.2). In one image (Figure 4.1), taken during the Vienna Court Opera's 1909 production, Bahr-Mildenburg is shown with her eyes shut and hands draped over her staff, suggesting that she is either lost in thought, caught in a trancelike state, or reminiscing about the nefarious plot she pursues to kill her late husband, Agamemnon.

In a second photograph (Figure 4.2), captured during the London premiere of *Elektra* at Covent Garden in 1910, Bahr-Mildenburg (now married to Bahr) appears in the same costume that she wore in the earlier Viennese production, but this time is shown with a wide-eyed stare, outstretched arms, and twisted "hysterical" fingers (as in Figure 2.3). Taken together, her eyes, arms, and fingers, as recorded in the second photograph, seem like a more explicit set of physical symbols of Klytaemnestra's crazed, murderous intent. It is worth remembering that audiences who had attended Hofmannsthal's and Reinhardt's *Elektra* in Berlin in 1903 regarded the character of Klytaemnestra as a dangerous femme fatale. And since Hofmannsthal had provided the libretto for the opera, it is generally understood that the modernist aspects of Reinhardt's staging at the Kleines Theater were also liberally, if not literally, applied to the presentation of Strauss' opera in Dresden, Vienna, and London. Strauss' monumental task, however, was to convey the language of hysteria through music, rather

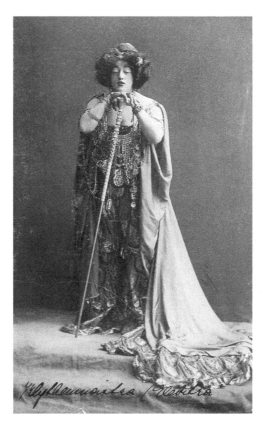

Figure 4.1 Anna Bahr-Mildenburg as Klytaemnestra in Richard Strauss' *Elektra*, 1909, photograph. Theatermuseum, Vienna.
Source: Photo: KHM-Museumsverband, Theatermuseum Vienna.

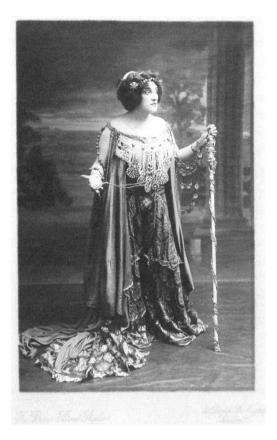

Figure 4.2 Anna Bahr-Mildenburg as Klytaemnestra in Richard Strauss' *Elektra*, 1910, photograph. Theatermuseum, Vienna.
Source: Photo: KHM-Museumsverband, Theatermuseum Vienna.

than the spoken word. To this end, the dissonant chromaticity of the bitonal "Elektra chord" and the iconography of the opera's costumes and set designs were orchestrated to capture the various psychological states of the opera's characters.

With the exception of Heinz Politzer, who has argued that Klytaemnestra can be read as a second hysteric in Hofmannsthal's play (and, by extension, Strauss' opera) this character does not seem to conspicuously embody the overtly hysterical mad-woman, at least not in Hofmannsthal's portrayal of Klytaemnestra. It is clear, however, that Klytaemnestra is a second femme fatale in the play/opera, due to the fact that she conspires to murder her husband Agamemnon in order to marry her para-mour Aegisth (or Aegisthus) and rule the kingdom of Mycenae. This discord suggests that Bahr-Mildenburg may have adopted gestures that were previously codified as hysterical in order to express the inner nature of her character, but without the inten-tion of portraying Klytaemnestra as a woman suffering from a clinical disorder. Such an interpretation suggests that hystero-theatrical gestures, at least by 1909 in Vienna, had begun to be transmuted into a more generalized psychological or pathological language of movements capable of communicating to the audience the connection between an actor's dramatic gestures and modern medicine. It is equally conceivable that Bahr-Mildenburg's movements, as Stein observed in 1909, were designed to compete visually with the gestures used by the opera's lead protagonist and the actual hysteric: Elektra.

In a production photograph taken during the 1909 premiere of the opera in Dresden, the physiognomy and corporeal gestures of Annie Krull, who debuted the operatic role of Elektra, visually communicate that the character is frightened and crazed, perhaps even driven wild by anxiety (Figure 4.3). After seeing the production in Germany, the critic Otto Sonne wrote on 29 January 1909 in the *Illustrirte Zeitung* (*Illustrated Newspaper*, published in Leipzig and Berlin): "One example of talent worth mentioning is the impressive achievement of Frau Krull as Elektra; in terms of acting, elocution and music, she exhausted—to the point of authenticity—the pathological nature of this character."[14] Given that Krull later revived her role as Elektra at the Vienna Court Opera on 9 November 1909, the "Dresden" photograph effectively provides (in the absence of any similar photographs from Vienna) a record of the dramatics that Sonne witnessed in Dresden, and those that viewers would have observed when Krull appeared in the Austrian capital playing opposite Bahr-Mildenburg.[15] Viewers of the

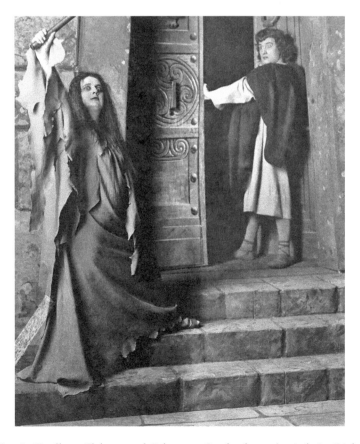

Figure 4.3 Annie Krull as Elektra and Johannes Sembach as Aegisth in Richard Strauss'
          Elektra, 1909, photograph.
Source: Photo: © SZ Photo/Scherl/Bridgeman Images.

photograph will notice the heavy, thickly applied black make-up surrounding the actress' eyes, as well as the telltale physicality of the clinically hysterical woman: her head is thrown back and her eyes are frozen in a wide, feral stare. Were Krull's body language not enough to convey the appearance of hysteria, any doubt is dispelled through the look of fright that is registered on the face of Johannes Sembach, here playing the role of Aegisth.

Viewers will also note that the photograph shows Krull with long, black disheveled hair, and wearing a tattered, witch-like garment. Her costume may have been envisioned as a further theatrical device intended to convey Elektra's "demonic" nature, but might also have been designed to conspicuously recall the ragged, burlap sack costume worn by Eysoldt in the earlier 1903 play.[16] This probable correlation is significant for a number of reasons, primarily because it implies that the popularity and novelty of the madwoman motif in Hofmannsthal's play had been solidified in Strauss' opera. This was certainly the case when another Austrian singer, Maria Gärtner, performed the role of Elektra at the Vienna Court Opera in August and September 1909.[17] Adorned in a costume by the artist Alfred Roller, a co-founder of the Vienna Secession and later chief set designer at the Vienna Court Opera, Gärtner was photographed with a wide-eyed stare, wild hair and hand gestures, and nearly identical garment as that worn by Krull in the "Dresden" image (Figure 4.4).

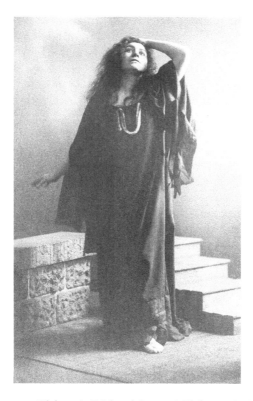

Figure 4.4 Maria Gärtner as Elektra in Richard Strauss' *Elektra*, 1909, photograph. Theatermuseum, Vienna.
Source: Photo: KHM-Museumsverband, Theatermuseum Vienna.

The importance of costuming Elektra as a hysteric in Strauss' opera, so that her outer appearance might reflect her inner turmoil, also suggests that the operatic Elektra was essentially a singing version of Hofmannsthal's original, lyrical hysteric. If this is indeed the case, then Austrians who were familiar with or had seen the play in Berlin, may have already recognized Strauss' Elektra as a hysterical character when Gärtner, Krull, and others performed the role at the Vienna Court Opera throughout the early twentieth century. The transferal of the *Modekrankheit* from one theatrical venue to another seems to have therefore served as a particularly fruitful device when staging *Elektra* in *fin-de-siècle* Vienna. Elektra and Klytaemnestra were not, however, the earliest incarnations of the Viennese modern body in the dramatic arts, since this role was first occupied by another crazed character: Isolde.

Isolde, the Hypnotic Sleepwalker

The stylized movements recorded in photographs from various productions of *Elektra* resemble expressive gestures that appear in Viennese expressionist paintings, particularly those incorporated into Koloman Moser's *The Love Potion—Tristan and Isolde* (1915, Plate 3). The title of Moser's painting suggests nevertheless that the artist was more interested in providing material form to the tragic heroes of Richard Wagner's opera *Tristan and Isolde* (1859), rather than the characters in Hofmannsthal's and Strauss' works. During its run in the nineteenth-century, German-speaking theater world, *Tristan and Isolde* generally received favorable reviews and was famously praised by Friedrich Nietzsche, who admired the opera's ecstatic music.[18] Wagner's overall influence on Viennese art was just as profound as his impact on its musical heritage: Bahr-Mildenburg, who was under contract with the Vienna Court Opera from 1898 until 1917,[19] is today remembered primarily as a Wagnerian soprano, and Wagner's concept of the *Gesamtkunstwerk* greatly inspired collaborative activities between the Vienna Secession and the Wiener Werkstätte, which Moser had co-founded in 1903.[20] *Tristan and Isolde* also represented the principal avenue by which Gottfried von Strassburg's Middle High German chivalric tale *Tristan* reached modern audiences. To clarify, the medieval Germanic-Norse legend was not a popular theme amongst German or Austrian visual artists until the early twentieth century, but it was known to the Pre-Raphaelite Brotherhood in England during the previous century. The subject matter of Moser's canvas, with its theatrical staging of modern bodies, was therefore particularly novel in late Secessionist and expressionist artworks.

Wagner's tragic opera, which premiered in Munich in 1865, opens with Isolde, an Irish princess who possesses magical healing powers, standing aboard a ship bound for southwest England, where she will marry King Marke of Cornwall. A young Breton nobleman named Tristan, who Isolde despises, has been given the task of transporting her safely to Cornwall, since he is Marke's nephew and adopted heir. Isolde loathes the knight, firstly because he is taking her to Marke, who she does not wish to marry, but principally because Tristan was responsible for killing Morold, her previous fiancé. Isolde recounts to her handmaid, by means of a flashback, how she had previously, though unknowingly, healed Tristan when she found him mortally wounded. When his true identity was finally revealed, she attempted to kill him, but was ultimately moved to pity and allowed him to live, making him swear never to return to her lands. Now aboard the ship to Cornwall, it is clear that Tristan has knowingly broken his oath, and Isolde therefore conspires to punish him by asking him to drink what she says is a special potion that will enable him to atone for his transgressions, but which, in reality, is a deadly poison. When Isolde's handmaid learns of her mistress' treacherous plot, she secretly replaces the poison with a love potion. At the close of Act One, Isolde offers Tristan the poison/love potion and drinks half herself, believing their lives will end before they reach Cornwall. Instead, the two fall madly in love. However, since Isolde is still promised to Marke, her handmaid's deviousness guarantees that Tristan and Isolde will remain star-crossed lovers until their deaths at the end of Act Three.

Moser's painting focuses on the moment in Act One when Isolde offers Tristan the love potion disguised as poison that will forever change their lives. While the depiction of Tristan's hands is certainly expressive in itself, Isolde's unconcealed use of hystero-theatrical gestures are, in fact, much more visually arresting. With eyes closed, arms outstretched from her torso, Isolde emerges as a painted somnambulist. Symbolically, the iconography of Moser's sleepwalker suggests that her inner visions, her dreams, and perhaps even her nightmares or fantasies are guiding her across the surface of the canvas toward her ill-fated lover. It is also worth noting that Moser's Isolde is adorned in a sack-like garment that strongly resembles the costumes worn by Krull and Gärtner in their roles as Elektra in Dresden and Vienna. *The Love Potion* therefore seemingly confirms that the trope of the theatrically hysterical femme fatale, as popularized in various theater productions at the *fin de siècle*, was also being explored in the visual arts produced by Secession/Werkstätte artists.

In 1882 Charcot concluded that somnambulism was in fact one of the three stages of hypnosis, which was, in turn, believed to be applicable to (and thus an effective treatment for) hysterics alone.[21] One of Charcot's former pupils at the Salpêtrière, the French neuropathologist Gilles de la Tourette, thus concluded: "As natural somnambulism is a precursor of hysteria, so hypnotic somnambulism is only a further manifestation of hysteria."[22] Early theorists of hypnotism and sleepwalking surmised that these phenomena were not simply induced states, but psychological conditions innate in the hysterical patient. Freud also wrote about sleepwalking, beginning as early as 1895 in his *Studies on Hysteria*, and then in his notes on Frau Emmy von N., in which he said that her memories were at their most lucid during her somnambulist episodes.[23] Hypnotic sleepwalking thus became synonymous with clinical hysteria at the turn of the century, both in Paris and Vienna. A review of *fin-de-siècle* medical journals and writings reveals, however, that Charcot had seemingly never published photographs of somnambulists in his various publications, and neither did Freud in *Studies on Hysteria* or in his later studies on hysterical attacks. In other words, the discourse surrounding somnambulism directly connected this phenomenon to hysteria, even though photographic or printed images of clinical patients "afflicted" with sleepwalking were not publicized during the period.

Rather than arguing that Moser was studying medical photographs of somnambulism, which do not seem to have existed, I am proposing that the painter was instead observing representations of the Viennese modern body shown on the theatrical stage, in particular, the body of Bahr-Mildenburg. As with her performance as Klytaemnestra in *Elektra*, the soprano had previously made a great impact on Austrian theatergoers when she appeared as Isolde in Wagner's *Tristan and Isolde* at the Vienna Court Opera in February 1900.[24] She reprised the role in February 1903, this time in a new staging of the opera organized by Alfred Roller and the celebrated Austrian conductor and composer Gustav Mahler. Mahler had become director of the Vienna Court Opera in 1897 and brought Bahr-Mildenburg back to Vienna (from Germany)

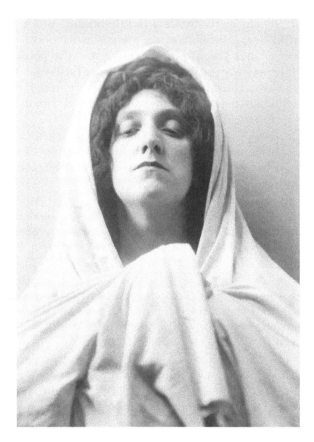

Figure 4.5 Anna Bahr-Mildenburg as Isolde in Richard Wagner's *Tristan and Isolde*, c. 1900, photograph. Theatermuseum, Vienna.

Source: Photo: KHM-Museumsverband, Theatermuseum Vienna.

in 1898.[25] In a portrait photograph from circa 1900 (Figure 4.5), Bahr-Mildenburg is depicted wrapped in the ample folds of a voluminous white costume reminiscent of a shroud. The lids of her eyes are nearly closed as she gazes down on the viewer, suggesting any number of possibilities: that she, as Isolde, is casting a magic spell, is falling asleep, is about to fall madly in love with Tristan, or is about to die.

Similarly, in Roller's design for Bahr-Mildenburg's costume for the later 1903 Viennese production of *Tristan and Isolde* (Figure 4.6), the artist depicts the actress with her eyes shut and her right hand extended as if to support her body since she cannot use her corporeal sight for guidance. Roller's Isolde wears a much more elaborate, beaded robe than the simpler, peplos-like garment worn by Moser's female figure, yet closed eyes are a feature common to both of the painted Isoldes. This artistic device is particularly intriguing in Roller's image, since the work was arguably only meant to serve as an illustration for the finished costume, but it nevertheless captures the very essence of Isolde's character and reinforces her persona as a somnambulist in a *fin-de-siècle* Viennese opera production. Given that Bahr-Mildenburg is depicted as a modern sleepwalker in Roller's costume design, the iconography and semiology of the expressive female body in Moser's later painting becomes somewhat clearer.

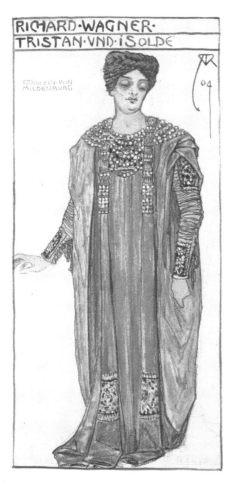

Figure 4.6 Alfred Roller, costume design for Anna Bahr-Mildenburg as Isolde in Richard Wagner's *Tristan and Isolde* (1903), dated 1904, mixed media on paper. Theatermuseum, Vienna.

Source: Photo: KHM-Museumsverband, Theatermuseum Vienna.

Returning to Brandes' observation from 1905 that hysteria had become the *Modekrankheit*, it is significant that the term *Mode* in German denotes a commercial style, or clothing that is fashionable or trendy.[26] If one were to separate this compound noun into its two distinctive units: *Mode* and *Krankheit*, or to hyphenate the word to form *Mode-Krankheit*, the result suggests that the modern actress could literally wear this disease, as one might don a modish outfit like Roller's costume for Isolde. It is therefore plausible that actresses appearing on the Viennese stage were seen by viewers as figuratively and literally wearing their hysteria. This notion of a "portable" disease allows me to return to the notion that hysteria was *the* disease of the turn of the century, signifying that it was both fashionable and modern to adopt this particular disorder when attempting to represent the sexualized woman through the mediums of art or drama.[27] It is also important to remember that theatrical photographs, including those of Bahr-Mildenburg as Isolde, were as carefully orchestrated as Moser's painting, revealing that the director, composer, photographer, and actress were all involved in spreading the idea that the theatrical femme fatale was draped in hysteria.

Somewhat paradoxically, another strong parallel between theatrical photographs and Moser's stylized Isolde can be seen in the image of the physically ruined male body, as opposed to the female form. In this instance, commonalities are found between Moser's Isolde and the main character in Reinhardt's and Hofmannsthal's second collaborative production: Hofmannsthal's *Oedipus Rex* (1906). In many ways, *Oedipus Rex* represented Reinhardt's and Hofmannsthal's return to, and continued interest in, adapting classical theater to the modern stage. As with their earlier work on the play *Elektra*, the two men transformed Sophocles' *Oedipus the King* into an expressive exploration of corporeal, psychological, and emotional decrepitude. The experimental, arena-style play was first performed in Munich in 1910, then later in 1910 at Berlin's Zirkus Schumann, with actors from the Deutsches Theater (German Theater).[28] Reinhardt's troupe eventually traveled to Vienna in May 1911 and transformed the city's Zirkus Busch into a modern theater.[29] During its run in the Austrian capital, the Italian-born Albanian actor Alexander Moissi (born Aleksandër Moisiu), who starred in the title role, performed a pseudo-somnambulist walk for enthusiastic audiences, which included Freud. Freud wrote about the spectacle, calling it a "tragedy of the 'arranged libido'" in a letter dated 12 May 1911 to his Swiss colleague, the equally famous psychiatrist and analytic psychologist Carl Jung.[30]

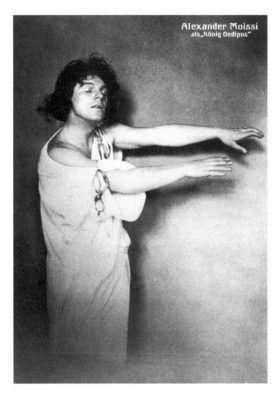

Figure 4.7 Alexander Moissi as King Oedipus in Hugo von Hofmannsthal's and Max Reinhardt's *Oedipus Rex*, c. 1910, photograph.

Source: Photo: bpk, Berlin / Art Resource, NY.

A cabinet card photograph from the play documents Moissi's performance as the "sleepwalking" Oedipus (Figure 4.7). With arms outstretched in front of his torso, Moissi's tragic character shares striking iconographic affinities with Moser's hysterical somnambulist: both characters exhibit closed eyes, grasping arms, and costumes that resemble ancient tunics. With this in mind, we might suppose that the Oedipus of the Reinhardt-Hofmannsthal production served as a male counterpart to female archetypes like Salome and Elektra. This conclusion also presumes that Reinhardt and Hofmannsthal transplanted the aesthetics of Elektra's hysterical persona onto the body of the actor, so that Oedipus could also be transformed into—and thus become "readable" as—a male character suffering from psychological afflictions. It is certainly true that Moissi's gestures could simply have been intended to convey the blindness of his character as he wandered precariously around the theatrical arena. A more nuanced reading, however, might conceive that Moissi's Oedipus should theoretically be viewed as a synecdoche for all of the psycho-physiological pathology present in early twentieth-century theater, or alternatively, as a dramatic example of a *fin-de-siècle* male hysteric.

Hysterical men were uncommon in medical studies of the period, yet they do exist in theories published by Charcot, and Breuer and Freud, as briefly discussed in Chapter 2.[31] As recently analyzed by Janet Beizer, if a man were diagnosed with hysteria at the turn of the century, particularly at the Salpêtrière, then he would often be considered an inadequate male since this disorder was stereotypically associated with "inferior" genders, races, and classes at the hospital; in Charcot's writings, this label was often applied to women and Jews.[32] More common in the case of male patients was the diagnosis of neurasthenia, and even Freud was said to have self-identified as a neurasthenic.[33] One wonders, however, if—as a Jew—Freud had adopted this diagnosis in order to restore a sense of "dignity" to his masculinity, or, perhaps more probably, because he wanted to distance himself from Charcot's latent anti-Semitism. I will address this issue of the link between hysteria and anti-Semitism later in the chapter, but in returning to the photograph of Moissi, one might ultimately conclude that hysterical female actresses like Bahr-Mildenburg, Krull, and Gärtner had metaphorically "infected" the neurasthenic male actor with *her* theatrical disorder, not his.

In either case, the use and reuse of hystero-theatrical gestures by actors suggests that the explicit language of the dramatic body was continually responding to changes in the meaning bestowed onto its constituent movements during performances in Germanic theater. Take, for example, another photograph of Bahr-Mildenburg from the late 1920s (Figure 4.8) and the little-known watercolor drawing by Egon Schiele entitled *Frau mit blauem Haar* (*Woman with Blue Hair*, 1908, Figure 4.9). In the photograph, the actress' costume is strikingly similar to the garment Bahr-Mildenburg wore in the 1900 production of *Tristan and Isolde* (Figure 4.5), but in the later image her eyes are wide open, her head thrown back, and her arms raised. Similarly, in Schiele's *Woman with Blue Hair*, the subject is depicted wearing a peplos-like dress, with her head thrown back, eyes open, and her arms extended in front of her body as she stares directly out at the viewer. Schiele's blue-haired woman seems menacing, as though a supernatural spirit possesses her, or, more appropriately, as though she is overcome with a hysterical fit of sleepwalking, except with her eyes open. Her body language is completely theatrical, just as Bahr-Mildenburg's gestures suggest that she is revealing a strange combination of the wild ferocity of Elektra, the arm movements

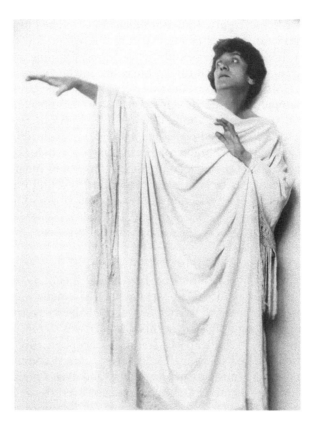

Figure 4.8 Anna Bahr-Mildenburg, c. 1928/30, photograph. Theatermuseum, Vienna.
Source: Photo: KHM-Museumsverband, Theatermuseum Vienna.

and costuming of Moissi's Oedipus, Moser's Isolde, and Schiele's entranced woman. Is this, then, an example of life (Bahr-Mildenburg) imitating art (*The Love Potion*, or *Woman with Blue Hair*)? Perhaps so, given the striking similarities between all of the images. More importantly, all of these artistic subjects reinforce my contention that hystero-theatrical gestures were a language of the Viennese modern body that, by the turn of the century, had circulated throughout the city. In support of this theory, Moser's *The Love Potion* and Schiele's *Woman with Blue Hair* are prime historical examples of the rich dialogue that developed between the visual and performing arts when it came to an exploration of identifiably pathological characters.

But why paint Isolde as a hysteric at all, when Salome or Elektra would appear to be more fitting artistic subjects? Novelty could certainly account for Moser's selection of this lesser-known character in modern Germanic painting. When one considers that Wagner's Tristan is responsible for murdering Isolde's fiancé Morold, it stands to reason that when she offers him the love potion (again, believed to be poison by both Tristan and Isolde) audiences would have understood that Wagner's femme fatale was attempting to lure the young man to his death by using her feminine wiles. The fact that Isolde also drinks the poison in the opera therefore becomes irrelevant, since in Moser's painting the hypnotized madwoman thrusts the toxic elixir toward the male

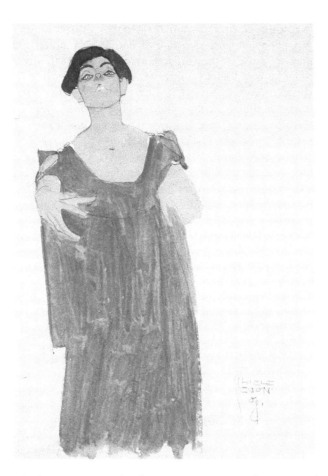

Figure 4.9 Egon Schiele, *Woman with Blue Hair*, 1908, gouache, watercolor and pencil on paper. Private Collection.
Source: Photo: © Christie's Images/Bridgeman Images.

protagonist alone. Moser's Tristan observes this potentially mortal threat with surprise, which can be seen in his body language. The dramatic division of the canvas between male and female forces supports this interpretation visually since Moser places the two characters on opposite sides of the ship's tent, which is left slightly open in the middle of the composition. As a result, and unlike theatrical photographs, *The Love Potion* does not simply document the Isolde of Wagner's opera, but instead presents the femme fatale as a hypnotized hysteric. Moser's Isolde is thus the madwoman reborn on the canvas, rather than the stage.

Salome's Deadly Dance

Unveiled during the height of expressionist activity in Vienna, *The Love Potion* is a rather mature example of the litany of hysterical women that appeared in symbolist, Secessionist, and expressionist paintings throughout the long nineteenth century. As in modernist theater, early painted images of anti-heroines often focused on the consummate femme fatale of the *fin de siècle*: Salome, who was now symbolically interpreted as the epitome of the carnal madwoman.[34] Even though painters throughout the sixteenth and seventeenth centuries treated the biblical narrative of Salome as a popular religious subject matter, it was the pathological nature of Salome's body that captured the imagination of nineteenth-century artists like no other historical woman throughout the period.[35] The French novelist Joris-Karl Huysmans was arguably the first modern author to discuss hysteria in direct relation to Salome. In Huysmans' writings, the artistic femme fatale emerges unambiguously alongside descriptions of Salome in his book *À rebours* (*Against Nature*, or *Against the Grain*, 1884), which is often considered his most definitively avant-garde, decadent work of fiction.[36] Huysmans' novel follows its main protagonist, Jean Des Esseintes, as he retreats from the confines of nineteenth-century bourgeois Parisian society into a more pastoral environment, where he enjoys the inner contemplation of art, literature, and humanistic thought. At one particularly memorable moment in the narrative, Des Esseintes stands in front of two paintings by Gustave Moreau, including his *L'Apparition* (*The Apparition*, 1874–76, Figure 4.10), which Des Esseintes purchased for his private collection due to the ecstatic feelings that the dancing girl evoked in him.[37]

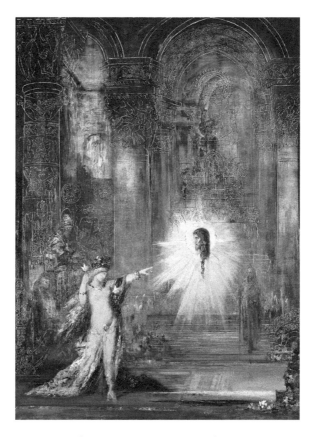

Figure 4.10 Gustave Moreau, *The Apparition*, 1874–76, oil on canvas. Musée Gustave Moreau, Paris, France.
Source: Photo: Erich Lessing / Art Resource, NY.

Although passages from Huysmans' book have found their way into the critical literature examining *fin-de-siècle* notions of the femme fatale, Des Esseintes' personal musings on the corporeal nature of Salome bear repeating in the context of this chapter. This reiteration is largely justified by the fact that Huysmans' prose echoes a language of pathology extracted from late nineteenth-century medical discourses describing the physical mechanisms of hysterical attacks. When read through this lens, it is clear that Huysmans' description of Moreau's paintings provides a further account of the seductive qualities of the hysterical female body in both the visual and literary arts. Huysmans writes:

> Amid the heady odor of these perfumes, in the overheated atmosphere of the basilica, Salome slowly glides forward on the points of her toes, *her left arm stretched out in a commanding gesture.* [...] Her eyes fixed in the *concentrated gaze of a sleepwalker*, she sees neither the Tetrarch, who sits there quivering, nor her mother, the ferocious Herodias.[38] (Emphasis mine)

And then,

> In Gustave Moreau's work, which in conception went far beyond the data supplied by the New Testament, Des Esseintes saw realized at long last the weird and superhuman Salome of his dreams. Here she was no longer just the dancing-girl who extorts a cry of lust and lechery from an old man by the *lascivious movements of her loins*; who saps the morale and breaks the will of a king with the heaving of her breasts, the twitching of her belly, the quivering of her thighs. She had become, as it were, the symbolic incarnation of undying Lust, the Goddess of immortal *Hysteria*, the accursed Beauty exalted above all other beauties by the *catalepsy that hardens her flesh and steels her muscles*, the monstrous Beast, indifferent, irresponsible, insensible, poisoning, like the Helen of ancient myth, everything that approaches her, everything that sees her, everything that she touches.[39] (Emphasis mine)

Huysmans' description of Salome evokes the iconography of hysterical symptoms supplanted onto the body of the femme fatale. This interest in the sensual qualities of the pathological body signaled the dualistic nature of Salome as a woman who corrupts man through her female sensuality while having a body that is itself physically compromised by disease. Huysmans' acknowledgment that Moreau has altered the biblical account of Salome—something that was also noted by critics writing about Oscar Wilde's *Salome*—is important because it permits him to view her not as a strictly religious figure, but as an alluring woman who uses the sensuality and theatrical movements of her body to evoke voyeuristic pleasure in the male viewer as she dances.[40] As the term femme fatale implies, there is the ever-present and explicit danger that mere proximity to such a woman can lead to a man's death, as exemplified by the decapitation of John the Baptist in both the biblical and theatrical versions of the story. What is more, Moreau and Wilde each focused on Salome's necrophilic lust for the dead prophet in their respective works. In this regard, both the visual and dramatic arts reveal that Salome is by nature a destructive force, even though her impetus to bring about the ruin of her male victim may, in turn, be the cause of her own body's "quivering" and "twitching" spasms, as if she were under the influence of cataleptic hysteria.

So is hysteria actually to blame for Salome's simultaneously alluring and destructive power? Or does she seek to destroy men not because of her own innate and corrupt nature, but because she is the vulnerable puppet of her own body, whose hysterical madness drives her to perform her sexualized dance? The fact that Huysmans mentions both sleepwalking and catalepsy—again, understood in late nineteenth-century neurological medicine as symptoms of hysteria—suggests that the novelist was astutely aware of the contemporary clinical language used to describe this highly expressive female disorder. In his particular French formulation of hysteria, we might presume that the disease—which, historically, had been created by men to subjugate women in the clinic—was meant to ensnare the body of the femme fatale, just as she had ensnared the body of men with her sexuality.

Like Moreau, a number of European symbolist and art nouveau artists famously claimed Salome as their muse, including Aubrey Beardsley, Gustav Klimt, Max Klinger, Edvard Munch, Max Oppenheimer, and Franz von Stuck. Stuck, a German Symbolist artist and co-founder of the Munich Secession, completed a number of expressive canvases in 1906 with Salome as their subject, two of which conspicuously feature hystero-theatrical gestures being performed by the femme fatale (see Figures 4.11 and 4.12). When comparing Stuck's conceptualization of Salome to Moreau's representation, the viewer is confronted in all three works with a scantily clad, sensuous dancing girl, although Stuck's femme fatale is not the cool, statuesque character that materializes in *The Apparition*. Instead, Stuck depicts Salome's body in a three-quarter view, with head thrown back, lips parted, and arms frozen in a deliberately theatrical gesture. These paintings suggest visually that Stuck's subjects—with their bejeweled bodies and discernible expressions of pleasure—were designed to highlight hysteria as the *Modekrankheit*. As with images of Elektra and Isolde, the female body in Stuck's *Salome* paintings can be seen to be involved in a theater of exaggerated movements, now codified as hysterical ecstasy in order to represent Salome's pathology.[41]

Given that Stuck was a Bavarian rather than Austrian painter, it may not be readily apparent that his *Salome* paintings had, in fact, been inspired by a theatrical body he observed in Vienna. Much like Richard Strauss, who had attended a private performance of Reinhardt's staging of *Salome* in Berlin and subsequently constructed his operatic libretto based on the play, Stuck attended a performance of Maud Allan's *The Vision of Salomé*, which was loosely based on Wilde's original one-act tragedy and Reinhardt's subsequent production at the Kleines Theater.[42] Allan, an English-speaking Canadian actress and dancer, began her career at the Hochschule für Musik in Berlin (now the Berlin University of the Arts), where she studied classical piano between 1895 and 1898. Abandoning the instrument in 1898, she turned to expressive dance as a creative and professional outlet. In 1906 she famously unveiled—in Vienna, rather than Berlin or Munich—her new theatrical production, *The Vision of Salomé*, which included a risqué version of the Dance of the Seven Veils that led her to being billed across Europe as the "Salomé Dancer" (see Figure 4.13).[43] Stuck, an avid supporter of modern theater, saw Allan perform in Vienna and then helped to arrange the Munich debut of her play.[44] He reportedly became incensed when the Bavarian censors prohibited additional public performances after the opening night in Munich on the basis that too much of the actress' body was exposed to the audience. Stuck petitioned the censors, though Allan continued to perform *The Vision of Salomé* in the Bavarian capital at private venues.

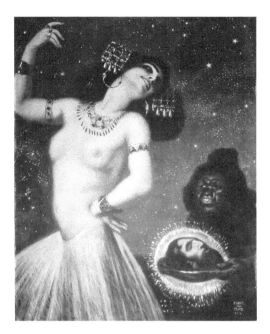

Figure 4.11 Franz von Stuck, *Salome*, 1906, distemper on canvas. Städtische Galerie im Lenbachhaus, Munich.
Source: Photo: bpk, Berlin / Städtische Galerie im Lenbachhaus / Lutz Braun / Art Resource, NY.

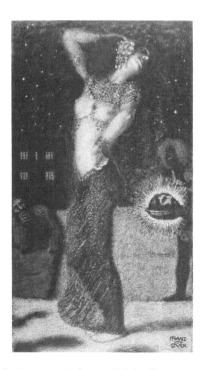

Figure 4.12 Franz von Stuck, *Dancing Salome*, 1906, oil on wood panel. Private Collection.
Source: Photo: bpk, Berlin / Art Resource, NY.

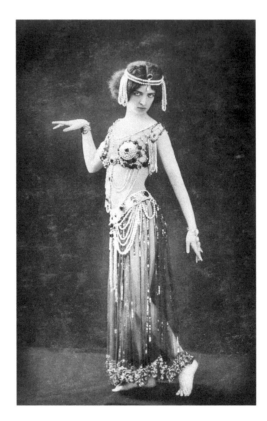

Figure 4.13 Maud Allan as Salome in *The Vision of Salomé*, c. 1908, photograph. Private
      Collection.
Source: Photo: Prismatic Pictures/Bridgeman Images.

In her personal memoirs, Allan describes her lexicon of corporeal gestures and
dramatic movements. She writes:

> In the mad whirl of childish joy she [Salome] is drawn again to dance—dance
> around this strange silent presence [the head of Jokanaan].[45] [...] What passes in
> those few moments through this excited, half-terror-stricken, half-stubborn brain
> makes of little Salomé a woman! Now, instead of wanting to conquer, she wants
> to be conquered [...]. A sudden wild grief overmasters her, and the fair young Prin-
> cess, bereft of all her pride, her childish gaiety, and her womanly desire, falls, her
> hands grasping high above her for her lost redemption, a quivering huddled mass.[46]

In speaking of Salome, Allan (like Charcot, Freud, and Frank Wedekind), describes
the allure of the femme fatale by utilizing words that recall images of the young,
hysterical child-woman, whose body and gestures are controlled by her developing
sexuality.[47] In keeping with this notion, Felicia McCarren has astutely observed
that the relationship between hysteria and the hypnotic movements performed by
the American dancer Loïe Fuller provide a further parallel to the processes at work
in the execution and reception of Allan's Dance of the Seven Veils.[48] McCarren has

argued that meaning was created when *fin-de-siècle* French viewers (mostly male) saw Fuller perform, or saw photographs of her dances, and attempted to read her body through Stéphane Mallarmé's poetic gaze, which McCarren suggests is at the root of Mallarmé's linguistic descriptions of Fuller's corporeal form, as well as in the medical gaze popularized by Charcot in the Tuesday Lectures. McCarren suggests that Fuller's "mesmerizing" dances were thus a direct confrontation between the "medical stereotypes of the hysterical body and the cultural conception of femininity" that each of these gazes—one literary, the other scientific, but both constructed around the notion of male voyeuristic pleasure—created and sustained.[49]

As with McCarren's analysis of Fuller's body, Allan's terminology brings to mind the iconography of female bodies in motion for male pleasure. To promote the show, Allan produced photographs of herself in the role, many of which capture the actress' expressive hand movements, her bejeweled diaphanous skirt, and scantily clad breasts (Figure 4.13). Comparing the photograph to Stuck's paintings, the three images share startling affinities, particularly with regard to costuming and corporeal gestures. Considering that Stuck knew Allan personally and had seen *The Vision of Salomé* in Vienna and Munich, and given that the play and Stuck's images were produced at similar times and share similar aesthetics, it seems clear that Allan's Salome served as the inspiration for Stuck's paintings.[50] Coupled with Allan's sensuous physiognomy, and the language she employed to evoke images of the child-woman finding sexual maturity through expressive dance, Stuck's canvases appear to be two further examples of the "Viennese" modern body in painted form, and speak to the historical interest paid to hysteria as an artistic *Modekrankheit*. The two *Salome* paintings thus definitively communicate the power that a real-life, theatrical "femme fatale" had over a modern visual artist.

Perhaps the most infamous Salome of the *fin-de-siècle* Germanic art world was a painting of an entirely different subject altogether: Klimt's *Judith I* (1901, Plate 6). Routinely and purposefully mislabeled "Salome" in contemporary reviews and exhibitions, *Judith I* was repeatedly interpreted by turn-of-the-century viewers as the seductive New Testament femme fatale, even though Klimt's original frame bears the title *Judith und Holofernes*.[51] In an exhibition review published in 1901 in the Munich-based journal *Die Kunst* (*Art*), Fritz von Ostini said: "Klimt shows his rich decorative taste in [...] a 'Judith,' which would actually be better identified as 'Salome'."[52] Nadine Sine has more recently explored this relationship, demonstrating that *fin-de-siècle* critics like Ostini actually favored the incorrect *Salome* title.[53] Her research also highlights that the desire to conflate Judith with Salome was somewhat strange, given that the visual depictions of the two women share only one common iconographic feature: a decapitated male head. Biblically speaking, both women are Jewish, and each is credited with the death of a powerful man, though the similarities end there. Tellingly, the connection between Judith—who saves the Israelites from imminent annihilation by the Assyrians—and Salome—the dancing seductress of Judea during the time of Christ—parallels the Judeo-Christian tradition of treating female nature as one of two extremes: the pious virgin, or the corrupt harlot. Like Sine, Jane Kallir and Susanne Kelley have both analyzed the historical attitudes surrounding Klimt's painting, as well as the discourse focused on cultural identity and representations of the female Jewish body in turn-of-the-century Vienna. By focusing their scholarship on the critical literature of the period, Kallir's and Kelley's research demonstrates that Klimt's *Judith I* confronted non-Jewish male viewers with a powerful female sexuality that unsettled their misogynist and largely anti-Semitic prejudices, which, according to Kallir and Kelley, were typical of the cultural *milieu* of Vienna circa 1900.[54]

Alessandra Comini has further argued that the golden, cloisonné choker worn by the female figure in Klimt's painting visually, symbolically, and paradoxically separates her head from her body, thereby suggesting that the Austrian artist deliberately painted two decapitated heads: that of Judith (or Salome), and the other of Holofernes (or John the Baptist).[55] Comini's astute analysis expresses the idea that Klimt's femme fatale is not only savage in her desire to ravage flesh, but is reciprocally (and ironically) fragmented and destroyed through her own sexual lust and desires. Often construed as exhibiting a look of sexual gratification or elation, Judith's facial physiognomy, with her disembodied head tilted slightly upward, her lips parted, and her eyes partially closed, offered Viennese viewers a glimpse into the aesthetics of the dangerous femme fatale. This point notwithstanding, historical and contemporary scholars alike have tended to neglect the manner in which Klimt chose to paint his hybrid Judith/Salome as a physically and psychologically diseased woman. *Judith I* is cleverly rendered in such a way that pathological taxonomies are subverted through the presumed sexual ecstasy experienced by Klimt's partially nude subject. Attentive viewers may have therefore noted that the figure's left front tooth is not only more clearly outlined than her other teeth, but has been rendered in a brighter shade of white paint. By highlighting this tooth, Klimt draws the viewer's eye down towards the parted mouth and to the symbolic moment when Judith/Salome lets go a breath of sexual gratification. By isolating the tooth, however, Klimt also illustrates a misaligned maxillary incisor, a defect known as dental malocclusion, or even fluorosis, which manifests as a permanent discoloring of the tooth's enamel. This may seem too nuanced a reading of such a small detail in a painting of a biblical figure, but an important artistic metaphor is nonetheless created through Judith/Salome's condition: Klimt has given the woman a fang.

Symbolically, this reading proposes that Klimt's subject is most probably Salome, the ravenous and carnal seductress, or, according to Robin Lenman, a prime example of the fashionable "vampire-*femme fatale*" that was popular among artists of the period.[56] In this sense, *Judith I* shares allegorical rather than iconographic affinities with Josef von Divéky's theatrical poster titled *Kabarett Fledermaus* (*Cabaret Bat*, 1907, Figure 4.14). As with Klimt's painting, Divéky's graphic work presents an image of the predatory femme-fatale, though here Divéky's creation materializes as a half-woman, half-animal hybrid in the form of a giant vampire bat—the symbol for the Fledermaus—whose curly locks of hair become horns, and whose spiked talons and deadly grin convey an impending threat to the (male) viewer. Divéky's femme fatale is thus a vampire woman capable of enticing the viewer into the cabaret only to ensnare him with the club's trappings. In line with this notion, I believe Klimt's *Judith I* can also be read as a female subject that symbolically personifies the trope of the bloodthirsty murderess, which in turn reveals her destructive nature, as well as her psychological complexities.

The most convincing evidence that *Judith I* embodies corporeal maladies can be seen in her eyes, which are intriguing primarily because they are visually dissimilar from one another. In particular, her right eye is noticeably more closed than her left. Klimt's decision to paint her in such a manner may suggest that Judith/Salome is casting sensual eyes of seduction toward the male viewer, who then symbolically

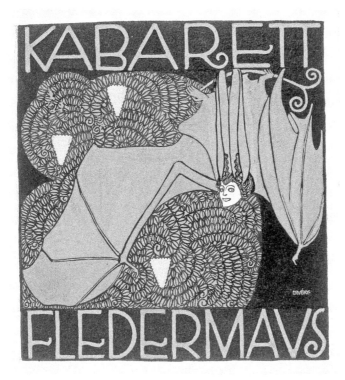

Figure 4.14 Josef von Divéky, *Poster for the Cabaret Fledermaus*, 1907, color lithograph. Sammlungen der Universität für angewandte Kunst Wien, Vienna.
Source: Photo: akg-images / Imagno / Josef von Divéky.

becomes her victim. But this incongruous feature might also suggest that the depravity of Judith/Salome's erotic nature has physically corrupted her body, causing her to suffer from an actual physio-pathological condition, perhaps ptosis or Horner's syndrome, also known colloquially as a "drooping eye," in which the skin of the eyelid collapses abnormally over the eyeball. If this is the case, then her sensual stare fails to be purely seductive, and instead communicates a subtle grotesqueness mapped onto her otherwise comely face. It also suggests that the features of her head—and not just the "decapitated" head itself—have become deformed.

The validity of this argument rests largely in my reading of the image as a representation of the modern pathological body, since it is undeniable that her left eyelid is more stricken by ptosis than the right one. If Klimt simply wanted to convey orgasmic rapture on Judith/Salome's face, then why paint the eyelids at different levels, given that the asymmetry creates an arresting though unsettling affect that, once noticed by the viewer, is not easily ignored? What is more, if Klimt's painting is of a female Jewish body suffering a pathology, then this painting may have unintentionally been seen to coincide with *fin-de-siècle* notions of the diseased body that were being linked with anti-Semitic beliefs about the "grotesque" Jewish body in Vienna. It is therefore plausible that a misogynistic, anti-Semitic male viewer may have concluded that Klimt's femme fatale suffered from two pathological disorders—"Jewishness" and hysterical lust—which, according to the period literature, were "conditions" routinely conflated by the Austro-German public, as previously highlighted by the reception of Strauss' "Jewish" operas.[57] This is not to say that Klimt himself was anti-Semitic or interested in promulgating the notion that Jewish bodies were inherently diseased. On the contrary, in conceiving of the pathological body as a semblance of Viennese modernism, and in choosing the female Jewish body to do so, Klimt's painting attempts to elevate the Jewish body to a high stature, while simultaneously (and ironically) falling in line with historical attitudes concerning Jewish individuals in *fin-de-siècle* Vienna.[58] To support my claim that *Judith I* could have been read as a pathological femme fatale at the turn of the century, it is important to recall that antagonistic critics writing in Vienna's anti-Semitic newspaper, the *Deutsches Volksblatt* (*German People's Paper*), were voicing the same concerns about the "diseased" bodies in Klimt's *Philosophy* and *Medicine* (Figures I.4 and I.5), which the artist so vehemently defended.[59]

The controversial Austrian philosopher Otto Weininger, whose cultural theories relied heavily on his own anti-Semitic and misogynistic beliefs, historically promulgated the association between hysteria and Judaism. Although by no means a part of mainstream turn-of-the-century philosophical or sociological thought, Weininger's writings blatantly reveal some of the more disturbing ideas and fears concerning European Jews and the pathological body. Among other things, Weininger's infamous *Geschlecht und Charakter* (*Sex and Character*, 1903) analyzes the erroneous claim that women, Jews, and hysterics were, by nature, all corrupt. Weininger writes:

> Women are incapable of overcoming their sexuality, which will always enslave them. Hysteria was a powerless defense against sexuality. If their struggle against their own desire were honest and authentic, if they *sincerely wished* to defeat desire, it would be possible for women to do so. Hysteria, however, is itself that which hysterics desire; they do not really seek to recover from it.[60] (Weininger's emphasis)

Certainly deplorable for its gender-based prejudices, Weininger's investigation nevertheless reveals, however unintentionally, the artificial nature of the disease of hysteria. By suggesting that the affliction was a "powerless defense" against female sexuality, Weininger concludes that women who wished to remain slaves to their corrupted sexual nature *willingly* adopted the disorder. In drawing this prejudiced conclusion, he argues that hysteria was a sort of voluntary disease that women could shroud themselves in when attempting, in vain, to defeat men through their sexualized bodies. A parallel therefore seems to emerge between hysteria as a constructed and superficial disorder, as a *Modekrankheit* or "wearable disease," and the modern artist's attempt to recreate the appearance of corporeal pathologies through the artifice of a painting's surface. In light of the unfavorable reception that Klimt's *Faculty Paintings* received, *Judith I* seems only to confirm that the artist continued to explore corporeal pathology as a key feature of the Viennese modern body, even in the face of anti-Semitic detractors.

This point is corroborated by the fact that Klimt submitted *Judith II (Salome)* (Figure 1.1) to the 1909 Kunstschau in Vienna following the controversy of the *Faculty Paintings*. Since the artist himself gave the painting the subtitle "Salome," there can be no doubt that this later work deliberately re-examines the Judith/Salome duality that he previously explored in the first *Judith* painting. In *Judith II (Salome)*, the body of the femme fatale is partially concealed beneath the decorative wrappings of a mosaic-like dress, or perhaps under an ornate background, since it is difficult to discern where her body resides in the claustrophobic space of the canvas. This second Judith/Salome exhibits a drooping eyelid similar to the figure in *Judith I*, although any semblance of ptosis is not easily discernible here, given that only one eye is visible to the viewer. Her breasts are exposed, her body hunched, and her fingers twist into claws that grab at the fabric of her dress, as well as at the long brown tresses of her male victim. The white curvilinear shapes that coil around her body add to the menacing quality of the composition, since these quizzical arabesques resemble giant, animal-like pincers or tusks, or even large scythes, all of which were possibly used to sever the Baptist's head from his body. As with *Judith I*, the visual language of *Judith II (Salome)* reveals that the carnal vixen has ensnared her prey and is proudly displaying his head as her trophy. Klimt's temptress thus makes clear to her viewers that death is her desire—a yearning that was shared by other murderous madwomen who appeared on the turn-of-the-century stage or canvas, namely Klytaemnestra, Elektra, Isolde, and Judith. For better or for worse, Salome had captured the mind of man at the *fin de siècle*, and like the Baptist's head, she did not let go. It is within this *milieu* that Klimt's "Salome" paintings persist as steadfast examples of the Viennese modern body in painted form.

Conclusion

Within the historical parameters of *fin-de-siècle* Vienna, individuals in both the visual and performing arts were recognizing the potential for the body of the femme fatale to be moved, not simply out of her own perverse *Lustmord*, or "love-death," but by the uncontrollable convulsions of her own diseased body, itself a victim of her inescapable gender. In this conceptualization of hysteria, the relationship between victim and perpetrator is somewhat inverted, though this operation takes place on a lateral rather than hierarchical axis, given that the male victim does not suddenly become the instigator of the femme fatale's actions. Instead, the female body—as a third and external agent—metaphorically acts as the Grand Executioner, bringing forth a reign of terror on the opposite sex. The complexities and nuanced interpretations of turn-of-the-century constructions of the femme fatale subsequently allowed composers, playwrights, directors, actors and actresses to transfer this "scientific" construction into the realm of the performing arts, precisely because these complicated readings of the sensual woman as both victim and perpetrator lent themselves so well to the medium of acting, particularly in tragic dramas. In turn, visual artists who attended these dramatic performances, or who were otherwise aware of the power of the hysterically theatrical madwoman, incorporated her image into their respective artworks.

Freud recognized this phenomenon in the early twentieth century, and commented on the fact that the arts had begun to adopt the discourse surrounding psychopathology and psychoanalysis as an expressive language. In one fiery statement made in May 1909 at a meeting of the Vienna Psychoanalytic Society, Freud called for the deliberate separation of the visual and literary arts from the realm of modern medicine. He warned that,

> the art of the poet does not consist of finding and dealing with problems. That he should leave to the psychologists. [...] What is unconscious ought not, without

more ado, be rendered conscious. [...] We [psychoanalysts] have the right to analyze a poet's work, but it is not right for the poet to make poetry out of our
analyses.[61]

With regard to this conflation of the arts and psychology in his native Vienna, Freud
also chastised colleagues who favored an entertaining, rather than scientific, reading
of hysteria. In his opening essay for *Dora*, Freud wrote:

> I am aware that—in this town, at least—there are many physicians who (revolting
> though it may seem) choose to read a case history of this kind not as a contribu-
> tion to the psychopathology of neuroses, but as a *roman à clef* designed for their
> private delectation.[62]

In his essay "Freud and the Poet's Eye," Norman Holland suggests that Freud's
inward hostility towards the arts—which Freud outwardly conveyed as ambivalence
toward poets, playwrights, and painters—was driven by the physician's envy towards
artists and their ability to assess a person's psychological state more easily than a neurologist.[63] Holland's interpretation reinforces the previously held belief that expressionists working in *fin-de-siècle* Vienna were more attuned to their inner visions and
emotions than their optical observations when seeking artistic truths. In Chapter 1,
I problematized this limited reading of expressionism alongside Kokoschka's vision
dialectic, but the truth remains that countless contemporary art critics and historians
have worked to reinforce the idea that expressionism was a deeply emotional and
internal way of making art. Freud's objection to the artistic uses of psychoanalysis inadvertently suggests that the modern doctor invariably used his optical sight to "see"
and diagnose, while the modern artist "felt" and "interpreted" pathological neuroses
for his or her own "private delectation." It is not too extreme to imagine that Freud's
comments might also have extended to the highly entertaining realm of *fin-de-siècle*
drama. If this were the case, then those other physicians who were reading Freud's
Dora as a *roman à clef*, might also have imagined the modern psychiatrist as a man
who manipulated his hysterical female patients as though they were malleable puppets or dolls on a theatrical stage.

The metaphor of the turn-of-the-century artist or physician as a puppet master
tellingly developed as an additional motif throughout the period literature, in marionette theater, and in paintings produced in Austria that linked *fin-de-siècle* medicine
with the modern artistic body. Like the corporeal gestures used by living actors in
cabaret and theater performances, movements expressed by inanimate objects like
marionettes underscored the idea that the aesthetics of human pathology had become
amenable to the puppet stage: either as puppet plays, or as dramas involving human
actors in the guise of marionettes. In turn, these objects served as additional metaphors for the modern body, since puppets and puppet-inspired dramas mimicked the
simultaneous interest in the inaudible language of expressive, pathological gestures.

Although the marionette motif has been explored in the secondary literature on
avant-garde theater, no scholar has thus far fully examined the influence of this trope
within the visual arts of *fin-de-siècle* Vienna, and neither have scholars discussed this
metaphorical construct alongside contemporary discourses on corporeal pathology in
modern Viennese theater or painting.[64] This is a lacuna worth resolving since (as early
as 1908) Wilhelm Worringer, though not a Viennese scholar, had identified a symbolic

connection between (Germanic) puppets, expressive gestures, and a modern pathos. In speaking of modern art and the puppet, Worringer surmised that one mode of artistic expression could be seen to develop through the viewer's emotional response to suffering, communicable through the movements of the marionette.[65] Worringer specifically states: "It is from the same rising pathos that exists in all mechanical emulations of organic functions, for example, in marionettes, that expression develops."[66] Although Worringer did not provide an actual analysis of the viewer's response to these movements, and even though he was not actively writing in the Austrian capital at the turn of the century, his claim nevertheless serves as a fruitful springboard in the following chapter for my exploration of critical responses that conflated the modern body with the language of the metaphorical puppet in *fin-de-siècle* Vienna.

Notes

1 Sigmund Freud, during a weekly meeting of the Vienna Psychoanalytic Society on 31 May, 1909, quoted and translated in Herman Nunberg and Ernst Federn, eds., *The Minutes of the Vienna Psychoanalytic Society*, vol. 2 (New York: International Universities Press, 1967), 189.

2 W. E. Yates, *Theatre in Vienna: A Critical History, 1776–1995* (Cambridge: Cambridge University Press, 1996), 178.

3 See Sander L. Gilman, "Strauss, the Pervert, and Avant Garde Opera of the Fin de Siècle," *New German Critique* no. 43, Special Issue on Austria (Winter 1988): 35–68; Sander L. Gilman, "The Image of the Hysteric," in *Hysteria Beyond Freud*, ed. Sander L. Gilman (Berkeley: University of California Press, 1993), 345–452; Sander L. Gilman, "Salome, Syphilis, Sarah Bernhardt and the 'Modern Jewess'," *The German Quarterly* 66, no. 2 (Spring 1993): 195–211; Lawrence Kramer, "Culture and Musical Hermeneutics: The Salome Complex," *Cambridge Opera Journal* 2, no. 3 (November 1990): 269–94; and Lawrence Kramer, "*Fin-de-siècle* Fantasies: *Elektra*, Degeneration and Sexual Science," *Cambridge Opera Journal* 5, no. 2 (July 1993): 141–65.

4 Gilman, "Strauss, the Pervert, and Avant Garde Opera of the Fin de Siècle," 37.

5 Kramer, "Culture and Musical Hermeneutics," 271. Kramer's understanding of Strauss' *Elektra* also builds on his own ideas concerning the instabilities of gender at the turn-of-the-century, as outlined in his essay on Salome, but also pays tribute to Gilman's analysis of Salome by refiguring Elektra as a diseased and degenerate Jewess. See Kramer, "*Fin-de-siècle* Fantasies," 141–65.

6 See Anne L. Seshadri, "The Taste of Love: Salome's Transfiguration," *Women & Music: A Journal of Gender and Culture* 10 (2006): 24–44.

7 Seshadri, "The Taste of Love," 24.

8 Seshadri, "The Taste of Love," 25. In addition to Seshadri, W. Eugene Davis has also analyzed contemporary responses to Strauss' *Salome* published in the German press between 1902 and 1905. For his essay, see W. Eugene Davis, "Oscar Wilde, Salome, and the German Press 1902–1905," *English Literature in Transition, 1880–1920* 44, no. 2 (2001): 149–80.

9 "Feuilleton. Richard Straußens 'Elektra'," *Neues Wiener Journal* 17, no. 5483 (January 26, 1909): 1.

10 "Feuilleton. Richard Straußens 'Elektra'," 1–3.

11 Bryan Gilliam, *Richard Strauss's Elektra* (Oxford: Oxford University Press, 1996), 139. The role of Elektra was performed by Lucie Marcel at the Vienna premiere. See the digitized archive record of the Wiener Staatsoper, available at: https://db-staatsoper.die-antwort.eu/performances/27596.

12 For a review of the contemporary criticism surrounding Bahr-Mildenburg's performance as Klytaemnestra, see Gilliam, *Richard Strauss's Elektra*.

13 Stein's reminiscences are recounted in Erwin Stein, "Mahler and the Vienna Opera," in *The Opera Bedside Book*, ed. Harold Rosenthal (London: V. Gollancz, 1965), 296–317.

14 Otto Sonne, "Strauss–Hofmannsthal *Elektra*," *Illustrirte Zeitung*, January 28, 1909, n.p. The original German reads: "Eine Talentprobe von imponierender Vollendung ist die Elektra der Frau Krull zu nennen: in darstellerischer, deklamatorischer und musikalischer Hinsicht erschöpfte sie das krankhafte Wesen dieses Charakters bis zur Glaubwürdigkeit."

15 Joy H. Calico, "Staging Scandal with Salome and Elektra," in *The Arts of the Prima Donna in the Long Nineteenth Century*, eds. Rachel Cowgill and Hilary Poriss (New York and Oxford: Oxford University Press, 2012), 71. See also the following digitized archive record of the Wiener Staatsoper, available at: https://db-staatsoper.die-antwort.eu/performances/27964.

16 Calico, "Staging Scandal with Salome and Elektra," 68–69.

17 See the following digitized archive record of the Wiener Staatsoper, available at: https://db-staatsoper.die-antwort.eu/search/person/8685.

18 For Nietzsche's interest in Wagner, see Dietrich Fisher-Dieskau, *Wagner and Nietzsche*, trans. Joachim Neugroschel (New York: The Seabury Press, 1976).

19 For Bahr-Mildenburg's biographical information, see Karin Martensen, "Anna Bahr-Mildenburg," in *MUGI. Musikvermittlung und Genderforschung: Lexikon und multimediale Präsentationen*, eds. Beatrix Borchard und Nina Noeske (Hamburg: Hochschule für Musik und Theater Hamburg, 2003). Also available at: http://mugi.hfmt-hamburg.de/Artikel/Anna_Bahr-Mildenburg.

20 For Wagner's influence on Viennese modernism, see Kevin C. Karnes, *A Kingdom Not of This World: Wagner, the Arts, and Utopian Visions in Fin-de-Siècle Vienna* (New York: Oxford University Press, 2013).

21 Charcot did not publish any work on hypnotism and somnambulism until 1882. He did, however, begin to conduct studies as early as 1878 on hypnotism, lethargy and catalepsy, and their relationship to hysteria. For his extant work on hypnotism, see Jean-Martin Charcot, *Oeuvres complètes*, ed. Babinski, Bourneville, Bernard, Féré, Guinon, Marie, Gilles de la Tourette, Brissaud, and Sevestre, vol. 3 (Paris: Progrès médical/Lecrosnier & Babé, 1886–1893), 16. It is believed that Charles Richet's 1875 essay on hypnotism was the impetus for Charcot's exploration of this technique. For Richet's essay see Charles Richet, "Le somnambulisme provoqué," *Journal d'Anatomie et de Physiologie Normale et Pathologique* 11 (1875): 348–78. For a more recent examination of this discourse, see Adam Crabtree, *From Mesmer to Freud: Magnetic Sleep and the Roots of Psychological Healing* (New Haven: Yale University Press, 1994).

22 Gilles de la Tourette, *L'hypnotisme et les états analogues au point de vue médico-légal* (Paris: 1887), 174. Tourette also discusses lethargy, catalepsy, and somnambulism on pages 81–112.

23 Josef Breuer and Sigmund Freud, *Studies on Hysteria*, trans. and ed. James Strachey (1895; New York: Basic Books, 2000), 97–101.

24 Martensen, "Anna Bahr-Mildenburg."

25 Oswald Georg Baker, "…'daß der Ausdruck Eindruck werde.' Gustav Mahler und Alfred Roller: Die Reform der Wiener Wagner-Szene," *Bayerische Akademie der Schönen Künste Jahrbuch* 11 (1996/97): 55–95; Paul Stefan, *Anna Bahr-Mildenburg* (Vienna: Wiener Literar. Anst., 1922), 26–27; and Manfred Wagner, *Alfred Roller in seiner Zeit* (Salzburg: Residenz Verlag, 1996), 73–74.

26 Brandes, "Dresdener Uraufführung der Salome von Wilde-Strauss."

27 I want to thank Kimberly Smith for her nuanced reading of my analysis of *Modekrankheit*, and particularly for her observation that the term *Mode* (or "fashion") in German and Austrian *fin-de-siècle* discourses on modern design and manufactured goods differs significantly from *Stil* (or "style"). For Smith's research in this area, see Kimberly A. Smith, "The Tactics of Fashion: Jewish Women in Fin-de-Siècle Vienna," *Aurora: the Journal of the History of Art* 4 (2003): 135–54.

28 Hugo von Hofmannsthal, *Briefe 1890–1909*, vol. 2 (Berlin: S. Fischer Verlag, 1937), 384n95. See also Richard H. Armstrong, "Oedipus as Evidence: The Theatrical Background to Freud's Oedipus Complex," *PsyArt: An Online Journal for the Psychological Study of the Arts* 2, no. 6a (January 1999): n.p. Available at: http://www.psyartjournal.com/article/show/armstrong-oedipus_as_evidence_the_theatrical_backg; and Judith Beniston, *Welttheater: Hofmannsthal, Richard von Kralik, and the Revival of Catholic Drama in Austria, 1800–1934*, vol. 46, *MHRA Texts and Dissertations* (London: W. S. Maney & Sons, 1998), 138, 141.

29 Armstrong, "Oedipus as Evidence."
30 William McGuire, ed. *The Freud/Jung Letters: The Correspondence Between Sigmund Freud and C. G. Jung*, trans. Ralph Manheim and R. F. C. Hull, vol. 94, *Bollingen Series* (Princeton: Princeton University Press, 1974), 184.
31 Jean-Martin Charcot, *Leçons sur l'hystérie virile*, ed. Michèle Ouerd (Paris: 1984); and Breuer and Freud, *Studies on Hysteria*, 236. For a more recent analysis of historical discourses on male hysteria, particularly in Charcot's research, see Ouerd's introduction in Charcot, *Leçons sur l'hystérie virile*, esp. 27–28; Mark S. Micale, "Charcot and the Idea of Hysteria in the Male: Gender, Mental Science, and Medical Diagnosis in Late Nineteenth-century France," *Medical History* 34, no. 4 (October 1990): 363–411; and Jan Goldstein, "The Uses of Male Hysteria: Medical and Literary Discourse in Nineteenth-Century France," *Representations* 34 (Spring 1991): 134–65.
32 Janet L. Beizer, *Ventriloquized Bodies: Narratives of Hysteria in Nineteenth-Century France* (Ithaca: Cornell University Press, 1994), 50.
33 Michael S. Myslobodsky, *The Fallacy of Mother's Wisdom: A Critical Perspective on Health Psychology* (Hackensack: World Scientific Publishing Co., 2004), 92.
34 Judith Ryan equally asserts that, "the figure of the femme fatale, frequently represented by Salomé, proliferated in literature and the visual arts. Both women, Judith and Salomé, were regarded as motivated by perverse eroticism and teetering on the brink of insanity." See Judith Ryan, *Rilke, Modernism and Poetic Tradition* (Cambridge: Cambridge University Press, 2004), 103.
35 For readers interested in sixteenth-century images of Salome as a popular religious subject in Renaissance painting, see, for example, works by the German artists Lucas Cranach the Elder and Lucas Cranach the Younger, the German-Swiss painter Joseph Heintz the Elder, and the Italian painters Bernardino Luini, Titian, Veronese, Donatello, Andrea Solario, Cesare da Sesto, and Luciani. With regard to baroque painting of the seventeenth-century, see works by the Dutch artist Matthias Stromer, the Flemish painter David Teniers the Younger, and the Italian artists Bernardo Strozzi, Guido Reni, Onorio Marinari, Giacomo Zoboli, and Caravaggio.
36 For Huysmans' discussion of Moreau's paintings of Salome, see Joris-Karl Huysmans, *Against Nature (À rebours)*, trans. Robert Baldick and Patrick McGuinness (London: Penguin Books, 2003), 50–57.
37 Huysmans, *Against Nature*, 50.
38 Huysmans, *Against Nature*, 51.
39 Huysmans, *Against Nature*, 52–53.
40 Within the critical literature on Wilde's play, one essay in particular, by the English writer and preacher F. W. Farrar, stands as a good example of the overall criticism Wilde received for *Salomé*. See Frederic W. Farrar, "The Bible on the Stage," *The New Review* 8 (January–June 1893): 185.
41 To my knowledge, turn-of-the-century reviews of Stuck's images of Salome only refer to this figure as a femme fatale, and not as a hysteric, or a woman whose movements might be understood as hystero-theatrical gestures.
42 Harold B. Segel, *Turn-of-the-Century Cabaret: Paris, Barcelona, Berlin, Munich, Vienna, Cracow, Moscow, St. Petersburg, Zurich* (New York: Columbia University Press, 1987), 142.
43 Maud Allan, *My Life and Dancing* (London: Everett & Co., 1908).
44 Allan, *My Life and Dancing*, 84.
45 Allan, *My Life and Dancing*, 126.
46 Allan, *My Life and Dancing*, 127.
47 Allan, *My Life and Dancing*, 84.
48 Felicia McCarren, "The 'Symptomatic Act' circa 1900: Hysteria, Hypnosis, Electricity, Dance," *Critical Inquiry* 21, no. 4 (Summer 1995): 748–74.
49 McCarren, "The 'Symptomatic Act' circa 1900," 751–52.
50 Udo Kultermann has previously suggested that Maud Allan actually posed nude for Stuck's paintings, even though he does not substantiate his confident claim with historical sources. See Udo Kultermann, "The 'Dance of the Seven Veils': Salome and Erotic Culture around 1900," *Artibus et Historiae* 27, no. 53 (2006): 200.
51 For a discussion centered on *fin-de-siècle* reviews of Klimt's painting, see Nadine Sine, "Cases of Mistaken Identity: Salome and Judith at the Turn of the Century," *German Studies Review* 11, no. 1 (February 1988): 9–29.

52 Fritz von Ostini, "Die VIII. Internationale Kunstausstellung im KGL Glaspalast zu München," *Die Kunst* 3 (1900–1901): 542. The original German reads: "Seinen reichen dekorativen Geschmack...zeigt Klimt noch in...einer 'Judith,' die eigentlich besser in 'Salome' umgetauft würde."

53 Nadine Sine, "Cases of Mistaken Identity: Salome and Judith at the Turn of the Century," *German Studies Review* 11, no. 1 (February 1988): 9–29.

54 Jane Kallir, *Gustav Klimt: 25 Masterworks* (New York: Harry N. Abrams, 1995), 16; and Susanne Kelley, "Perceptions of Jewish Female Bodies Through Gustav Klimt and Peter Altenberg," *Imaginations* 3, no. 1 (May 2012): 109–22.

55 Alessandra Comini, *Gustav Klimt* (New York: George Braziller, 1975), 22.

56 Robin Lenman, *Artists and Society in Germany, 1850–1914* (Manchester: Manchester University Press, 1997), 89–90. In speaking of these biblical figures, Lenman refers to them as "fashionable vampire-females," and states that Stuck, in particular, continually explored the "vampire/*femme fatale* theme" in his paintings.

57 For a review of various historical attitudes held by the general public regarding this erroneous claim, see the sources listed in note 3.

58 Jane Kallir discusses these prevalent anti-Semitic attitudes in Kallir, *Gustav Klimt*, 16.

59 See Hermann Bahr, ed., *Gegen Klimt: Historisches, Philosophie, Medizin, Goldfische, Fries* (Vienna: Eisenstein & Co., 1903), 35.

60 Otto Weininger, *Geschlecht und Charakter: Eine prinzipielle Untersuchung* (Vienna: Wilhelm Braumüller, 1904), 378. A good English translation of this passage can be found in Ryan, *Rilke, Modernism and Poetic Tradition*, 103–4.

61 Sigmund Freud, during a weekly meeting of the Vienna Psychoanalytic Society on May 31, 1909, quoted and translated in Nunberg and Federn, eds., *The Minutes of the Vienna Psychoanalytic Society*, 189.

62 Sigmund Freud, "General Remarks on Hysterical Attacks," in *Dora: An Analysis of a Case of Hysteria*, ed. Philip Rieff (1909; New York: Collier Books, 1963), 3.

63 Norman N. Holland, "Freud and the Poet's Eye: His Ambivalence Toward the Artist," *PsyArt: An Online Journal for the Psychological Study of the Arts* 2 (1998). Available at: http://www.psyartjournal.com/article/show/n_holland-freud_and_the_poets_eye_his_ambivalence_.

64 See Segel, *Turn-of-the-Century Cabaret*; Harold B. Segel, *Pinocchio's Progeny: Puppets, Marionettes, Automatons, and Robots in Modernist and Avant-Garde Drama* (Baltimore: The Johns Hopkins University Press, 1995); Peter Jelavich, *Munich and Theatrical Modernism: Politics, Playwriting, and Performance, 1890–1914* (Cambridge, MA: Harvard University Press, 1985); Peter Jelavich, *Berlin Cabaret* (Cambridge, MA: Harvard University Press, 1993); Scott Cutler Shershow, *Puppets and "Popular" Culture* (Ithaca: Cornell University Press, 1995); John Bell, ed., *Puppets, Masks, and Performing Objects* (Cambridge, MA: The MIT Press, 2001); and Steve Tillis, *Toward an Aesthetics of the Puppet: Puppetry as a Theatrical Art* (Westport: Greenwood Press, 1992).

65 Wilhelm Worringer, *Abstraktion und Einfühlung: Ein Beitrag zur Stilpsychologie*, Third edn (1908; Munich: R. Piper & Co., 1911), 117.

66 Worringer, *Abstraktion und Einfühlung*, 117. The original German reads: "Es ist dasselbe gesteigerte Pathos, das in aller mechanischen Nachahmung organischer Funktionen, so z. B. in den Marionetten, zum Ausdruck kommt."

5   The Inanimate Body Speaks
The Language of the Marionette Theater

My situation, in short, is this: I have utterly lost my ability to think or speak coherently about anything at all. [...] To me, then, it is as though my body is made up of nothing but ciphers that give me the key to everything.[1]

—Hugo von Hofmannsthal, 1902

We presently have a theater that actors and artists should visit, for all could learn something there. This is the theater of marionettes.[2]

—Hermann Bahr, 1913

As already demonstrated, the assimilation of the aesthetics of clinically hysterical female bodies and their movements into the choreography and iconography of the modern theater, and into symbolist and expressionist paintings, was unmistakable in *fin-de-siècle* Vienna. My investigation has thus far looked at representations of hystero-theatrical gestures in a number of cultural forms. These include late nineteenth-century photographs of clinical patients orchestrated by the French neuropathologist Jean-Martin Charcot, as well as turn-of-the-century photographs documenting expressive movements performed by French, German, and Austrian actors and actresses in modern theatrical productions. The same corporeal movements also feature in the visual and dramatic representation of puppet bodies and the metaphorical implications involved in utilizing these inanimate objects as appropriate surrogates, or doppelgängers, for the modern pathological body in Vienna. As such, artists and playwrights like Oskar Kokoschka and his contemporaries began writing for a different stage—the puppet theater—and thus adapted these expressive gestures to pursue the dramatic and metaphorical aims of this alternative avenue within the performing arts.

The present chapter explores this avenue of expression in order to demonstrate how the use of hystero-theatrical gestures enacted by inanimate bodies served as an additional mode of communication that visual artists in *fin-de-siècle* Vienna found more fruitful than words. The "language crisis" that befell the dramatic and literary arts during this period also parallels this new tension between written words and painted or performed gestures. Austrian expressionist artists, as well as Viennese playwrights and writers like Hugo von Hofmannsthal, together explored the idea that traditional forms of verbal communication—that is, written or spoken language—had to answer to their ability to represent meaning at this particular juncture in history.[3] It is my contention that hystero-theatrical gestures therefore served as an idiom capable of communicating a nonverbal (or inaudible) language of modernism that could be expressed through the aesthetics of the modern body and its gesticulations. The language of these gestures thus permitted bodies to "speak" the language of pathology and, by extension, allowed viewers to understand that hystero-theatrical bodies—whether represented in painted or dramatic form—communicated modernity more effectively than the spoken or written word.

In turn-of-the-century Vienna, this language crisis manifested itself in the belief that words could no longer be seen to embody the concepts and semiotics that they were meant to represent. Somewhat ironically, this distrust in the written word was promulgated by Austrian literary figures, including Hofmannsthal, Rainer Maria Rilke, and Arthur Schnitzler, whose avant-garde prose attempted to conceal or complicate meaning. The crisis of language is also at the very root of my earlier theorization of Kokoschka's dialectic of vision, given that the artist and his interlocutors were critically analyzing the hermeneutics of words signifying "vision" in the German language. One should here recall that Kokoschka utilized the term *Gesichte* ("faces") to imply both inner visions and optical sight. Hermann Bahr similarly asserted during this period that a conundrum of modern vision developed when one attempted to decipher what "vision" and "seeing" meant to different expressionist artists. Furthermore, in his essay "Der Brief des Lord Chandos" ("The Letter of Lord Chandos," 1902), Hofmannsthal indirectly suggests that this crisis of vision does not arise from a disagreement over the *meanings* of the word, but rather, through the understanding that any coherent articulation of what vision *is* cannot be articulated by verbal or written language.[4] Instead, Hofmannsthal suggests that the body and its non-verbal language—as a codified proxy for one's emotions, feelings, and visions—provide the key to understanding the world. In this sense, the reader observes that the human body and its encrypted parts must be decoded in order for meaning to be created.

Andreas Huyssen is perhaps the most recent scholar to address this historical conundrum, arguing that the problem arose from a "crisis of vision as related to the problematic relation of language and narrative in Vienna modernism."[5] Huyssen's assessment resolves any tension that may have existed between modern visual culture and literature, insofar as he argues that a crisis of language ultimately developed when writers attempted to deploy visual metaphors—extracted from paintings, design, and architecture—in their literary works.[6] As a complement to Huyssen's study, which assesses this crisis in Viennese literature alone, I examine the original visual metaphors in paintings that Huyssen views as the precursors, purveyors, or even instigators of the crisis of language and vision. As a means of further investigating the modern body, this chapter, along with Chapter 6, examines these visual metaphors in marionette theater and in expressionist paintings that combine hystero-theatrical gestures with elements of the puppet body. As previously stated, these expressive bodies and their codified gestures offered *fin-de-siècle* viewers a language of the modern body envisioned by artists, but filtered through the language of modern medicine and theater. It is in this sense that hystero-theatrical gestures participated in the crisis of language that was part and parcel of the intellectual *milieu* of Vienna circa 1900. In doing so, expressionists presented viewers with a language of the artistic body that could be read on the stage or canvas, and not just the pages of a book.

That Viennese modernists sought a new language with which to express their avant-garde approach to vision, life, and art is indisputable. In her analysis of corporeal gestures appearing in Viennese expressionist art, Gemma Blackshaw argues that this particular sign system was given meaning when Kokoschka, Max Oppenheimer, and Egon Schiele incorporated and advanced the iconography of diseased and patho-logical bodies that Gustav Klimt had first developed in his much-scrutinized *Faculty Paintings*.[7] As previously discussed, Blackshaw formulates a strong argument con-cerning these iconographies and their relation to photographs of medical pathologies, particularly those published by Charcot. Itzhak Goldberg has similarly argued that a "new body language" played an "incomprehensible role" in Viennese expressionist paintings, and suggests that Charcot's photographs articulate "a new corporeal typo-logy," which Goldberg believes was utilized by a number of visual artists at the turn of the century.[8] In an idea that is similar to my conceptualization of hystero-theatrical gestures, Goldberg argues that this new body language was not exclusive to the realm of painting, since he observes that it can also be witnessed in modern dance, particu-larly in performances staged at the Cabaret Fledermaus.[9] Rather than simultaneously turning to an examination of theatrical gestures in modern theater, he instead roots Schiele's *oeuvre* in Klimt's earlier aesthetic, and concludes that hand gestures in both Schiele's and Kokoschka's respective paintings are rooted in a language of Freudian erotic desire. Goldberg's analysis is therefore an indirect extension of Michael Huter's 1994 study of the crisis of language in relation to Schiele's pictorial idiom, but is nevertheless one filtered through a psychoanalytic methodology.[10]

Building on this literature, I believe that the strange and enigmatic gestures that feature in expressionist artworks were literally (that is, visibly) and figuratively un-derstood to express a language of modernity filtered through the modern and the-atrical pathological body. The importance of the hand to the artist or writer as the instrument of his or her profession, and the tool through which he or she expresses meaning, is incontestable. This contention is made clear in a number of essays writ-ten by Viennese artists, critics, and poets, and by individuals associated with the Vienna Secession, all of whom were quick to discuss the importance of expressive hands and bodies in works by foreign artists, including the French sculptor Auguste Rodin, and the English illustrator Aubrey Beardsley.[11] The discussion that follows subsequently advances the theory that Viennese modern artists were using a language of signs and visual metaphors based on myriad gestures extracted from the world of hysterical patients, modern theatrical performances, and finally, of marionettes. As genderless, androgynous, or sexless "things," marionettes, dolls, and puppets (again, collectively known as *Puppen* in German) were successful in challenging the viewer's preconceived notions about the language of the sexualized body. Puppet-like bodies in expressionist artworks were also capable of disturbing the medical and dramatic visions that previously codified the hysteric patient as a victim of her gender. All of these factors communicated to *fin-de-siècle* Viennese viewers that what they were seeing was the new and modern body.

On the Marionette Theater

From the outset, I want to assert that the Viennese modern body in the visual arts was historically "read" as one might read words, texts, or images on a page. Huys-sen's analysis of the crisis of vision in Viennese modern literature is therefore sup-portive of my conceptualization of corporeal gesture in modernist painting. He appropriately opens the second section of his essay "The Disturbance of Vision in Vienna Modernism" (1998), with an examination of disrupted vision and the threat of blindness in Sigmund Freud's handling of E. T. A. Hoffmann's German romantic story "Der Sandmann" ("The Sandman," 1816), and the role that vision plays in Freud's subsequent theory of the uncanny, as outlined in "Das Unheimliche," ("The Uncanny," 1919).[12] Hoffmann's tale reveals to its reader that the body of the automaton Olympia—the lifeless femme fatale—is responsible for the crisis of vision experienced by the protagonist, Nathaniel, who is deceived by what he sees, believing Olympia to be alive. Freud argues, however, that the life-sized doll in "The Sandman" cannot be regarded as an uncanny object, since it is a known object and therefore not capable of inducing or eliciting fear in the viewer. Instead, Freud posits that the loss of one's eyes—representing, for Freud, the fear of castration—is at the root of Hoffmann's psychological fable.[13] In short, Hoffmann toys with the idea that the uncanny is linked to the body of a non-living automaton that appears to be human, whereas Freud is focused on the corruption of biological functions, particularly the loss of one's sight or genitalia.

In his introductory remarks to "The Uncanny," Freud interestingly highlights the dearth of literature (and we can assume that Freud meant medical literature, as opposed to dramatic or fictional literature) examining the concept of the uncanny in relation to the arts. Although Huyssen does not analyze this particular aspect of Freud's work, Freud's desire to subsume "visual metaphors" into his theory invariably draws us back to Huyssen's contention concerning the relationship between visual and written texts in modern Vienna. An awareness of the crisis befalling both vision and language in Freud's writings also serves as the foundation for Peter Brooks' slightly earlier analysis of Freud's treatment of Dora's hysteria. In his book *Body Work* (1993), Brooks argues that Freud was literally attempting to read the symptomology of Dora's disease, as though her pathological gesticulations could articulate a specific language or discernible typology of the hysterical body.[14] Freud also believed, according to Brooks, that he alone could interpret this language. If Brooks' examination of Freud holds true, then Dora—the diseased female patient—essentially became the puppet of her doctor's ulterior aspirations: to translate the semiotics of hysteria for his professional and intellectual gain.

Freud was not, however, the first physician in the early twentieth century to analyze the uncanny within the literary arts. The earliest known examination of the *Unheimliche* appeared instead in a 1906 essay titled "Zur Psychologie des Unheimlichen" ("On the Psychology of the Uncanny") penned by the German psychologist Ernst Jentsch.[15] In this essay, which "The Uncanny" was largely a response to, Jentsch argues that in the realm of literature, the use of humanlike and life-sized automatons is the most reliable device an author can employ to leave the reader with a feeling of unease or uncertainty.[16] Jentsch does not specifically discuss "The Sandman," nor the automaton named Olympia in Hoffmann's story, though he does argue that Hoffmann "repeatedly made use of this psychological artifice [automatons] with success."[17] Jentsch is quick to note, however, that dolls or small automatic toys cannot convey a sense of the uncanny to the viewer or reader since they are "very familiar" objects.[18] When, in "The Uncanny," Freud subsequently criticizes Jentsch for arguing that children's dolls might function as uncanny objects and thus elicit fear in adulthood, he surprisingly reveals his bias against, and inattentive reading of, Jentsch's text. In choosing to dismiss the idea that small dolls and life-sized automatons could be objects imbued with a notion of the uncanny, Freud puts forward the idea that the truly uncanny device in Hoffmann's romantic tale is the Sandman—the sinister robber of children's eyes—who is, after all, a human character. As a result, Freud steers his theory of the *Unheimliche* away from threatening, inanimate objects like wax figures, and instead insists that this psycho-physiological fear is enacted by a living, albeit fictional, man.

This brief account of Hoffmann's "The Sandman," as situated in Freud's theory and Jentsch's essay, moreover reveals that it was Jentsch, not Freud, who argued that life-sized dolls were capable of eliciting an uncanny response in the minds of their human counterparts, precisely because such doppelgängers belie their lifelessness as objects. The "humanness" of the inanimate doll was likewise discussed by another German romantic writer, Heinrich von Kleist, whose well-known essay "Über das Marionettentheater" ("On the Marionette Theater") was serialized in the *Berliner Abendblätter* (*Berlin Evening Paper*) in December 1810.[19] Although Kleist's text was written nearly a century before Vienna's modernist period, it is known that Kleist's essay greatly inspired Bahr's musings on modernist theater, as well as Rilke's poetry, particularly his *Duino Elegies*, which I discuss later in this chapter. In fact, as early as 1898, Rilke was responding to Kleist's literary *oeuvre*, a fact that ostensibly situates "On the Marionette Theater" as the earliest example of Germanic literature to indicate the crisis of language and the puppet body that eventually dominated the intellectual and creative output of Kleist's successors in *fin-de-siècle* Vienna.[20] Although Kleist conceived of the essay (sometimes considered a novella) as a complex exegesis of consciousness and its role in shaping notions of self-identity and human redemption, the content of his narrative allows one to turn to a theorization of the marionette as a symbol for the modern body and its pathological movements.

In the opening of Kleist's modern parable of human nature, the author makes clear that the animated marionette is more expressive than a human body and its emotive gestures. Speaking in first-person, the narrator—that is, the "Ich" of the essay, who is also enigmatically referred to as "Herr K"—begins his story by recalling a lengthy conversation he had with his friend ("Herr C"), who was then the lead dancer in the local opera company. The encounter between the two men takes place when the narrator serendipitously runs into Herr C at a puppet theater in Munich. In recounting his tale, Herr K states:

> I told him that I was astounded to find him on more than one occasion at a marionette theater erected in the market square to amuse the plebs with short dramatic burlesques interwoven with song and dance. He assured me that the pantomime of these puppets brought him much pleasure, and he let it be known that a dancer hoping to cultivate his art could learn something from these marionettes.[21]

Herr K is quick, however, to question whether the mechanical gestures of the marionette can actually be understood as more expressive and refined movements than those enacted by the body of a skilled dancer, given that Herr K unstintingly advocates the supremacy of conscious bodies over inanimate objects. What is more, by suggesting that the marionette theater exists for "the plebs," Herr K draws a distinction between "low" and "high" art forms: between popular amusements, and cultural entertainment appealing to a more sophisticated or bourgeois sensibility. As a German romantic like Hoffmann, Kleist utilizes the conversation between Herr C and Herr K to discuss the symbolic role of the marionette or puppet as a metaphor for the expressive human body, and not simply within the art of dance or the performing arts, but also in the visual arts, drawing allusions to paintings by the seventeenth-century Flemish painter David Teniers the Younger and sculptures by the Italian baroque artist Gian Lorenzo Bernini. At a pivotal moment in the conversation, the narrator offers a plea for the superiority of man:

> I replied that although he [Herr C] handled his paradoxes with skill, he would never convince me that in a mechanical figure there could be more grace than in the structure of the human body. He replied that it would be almost impossible for a man to attain even an approximation of a mechanical being.[22]

The theoretical conclusion of this final line sees Kleist—through the words of Herr C—arguing that the puppet might offer a way for mankind to find redemption, should man attempt to return to the state of the marionette, whose unconscious grace, Kleist argues, acts as a foil to man's consciousness, or "fall from grace." In terms of artistic inspiration, Kleist's conclusion is important since it suggests that the puppet or marionette not only has the potential to serve as an expressive muse for the artist, but is also an artistic object that can operate on a deeper, internal level untainted by the inescapably corrupt nature of man. Here, Kleist establishes an interesting dichotomy between living flesh and bone, and inanimate wood and paint, or rather, between consciousness and unconsciousness. In end effect, the puppet, according to Kleist, becomes the double of man and, somewhat ironically, man's superior through the "infinite consciousness" of the god-like puppet.[23]

According to Paul de Man, Rilke and his German contemporary, Thomas Mann, were both drawn to the enigmatic and metaphorical language of Kleist's "On the Marionette Theater" for its proto-modernist observations on the semiotics of language.[24] At the root of this language crisis and the modernist aesthetic that it created—consider Huyssen's assertions that modern Viennese literature underwent a crisis due to its attempts to come to terms with, and subsequently incorporate, the language of visual metaphors—de Man argues that the disarticulated and mechanized (and thus, inanimate) body of the marionette, as well as the dismembered human body supported by prosthetics, convey a dehumanized language to the reader. In this sense, Kleist's work highlights the crisis of language through the metaphor of the marionette, suggesting that the body of the puppet is akin to the pathological or defiled body of modern man. This is evident in a later conversation between Herr K and Herr C, who discuss the gracefulness of dismembered bodies augmented by artificial, and in Herr C's opinion, superior prostheses.[25]

One of the more immediate and telling examples of this language crisis, and one that echoes Herr C's notion that the disarticulated human body might be more advanced than a completely natural, non-augmented body, is seen in the problem that arises when one attempts to understand the characters' identities through their ambiguous names. Given the truncated forms of the signifiers, the direct relationship between signifier and signified is destroyed, effectively allowing Kleist to communicate to his readers that knowing a person's name is not the same as knowing his or her identity. Although we might assume that Herr K (the narrator) is an abbreviated form of "Herr Heinrich von Kleist"—thus positioning the author as the narrator of the work—we cannot know for certain that this character is actually meant to represent Kleist. What is more, the remaining character, Herr C, is completely unknowable to the reader, since Kleist fails to provide any additional clues to the man's identity. Perhaps this desire to identify the specificity of these characters is irrelevant, given that their words, rather than their identities, are the catalyst for the story's narrative. However, by hiding the characters' identities in the course of their discussion of inanimate bodies, Kleist paints a picture of a physiologically incoherent view of humanity, and one that is psychologically severed from names, identities, and body parts. In other words, not only is humanity likened to marionettes in Kleist's tale, but so are the characters themselves: the "living" humans in the story have also become disarticulated puppets.

Neither Huyssen nor de Man discuss Bahr in relation to Kleist's text, though it is clear that there is a strong relationship between Bahr's understanding of marionettes and the primacy of these objects in the writings of his romantic predecessor. When working as a theater director and critic in *fin-de-siècle* Vienna, Bahr became intrigued by the role of the modern puppet, so much so that he penned an essay in 1913 titled "Marionetten" ("Marionettes") on the importance of these inanimate figures to the theater. As stated in the epigraph to this chapter, Bahr argued in "Marionettes" that, "we presently have a theater that actors and artists should visit, for all could learn something there. This is the theater of marionettes."[26] Here, Bahr's statement is largely prescriptive, given that he suggests that human actors and artists should study the gesticulations of marionettes in order to learn how to describe the body, either through choreography or iconography, in a more meaningful way. This sentiment therefore replicates, almost verbatim, Kleist's words (as spoken by Herr C) when he states that the success of any modern dancer lies in his or her ability to replicate the puppets' expressive movements. Although Bahr does not specifically mention Kleist in his essay, the latter's proto-modernist view of the puppet as an appropriate didactic instrument for man, or his metaphorical doppelgänger, resonates in the former's work.

For Bahr, this need to identify the puppet as an expressive tool for the visual or performing artist seems to position the marionette as a sort of illustrative reference, like an artist's dummy. This conceptualization of the puppet or marionette as a doll manipulated by strings, or the puppeteer's hands, leads us back to the semantics of the German word *Puppe*, which denotes any one of three things: a puppet, a marionette, or a doll. I therefore want to suggest that despite the slight differences between these objects, puppets, dolls and marionettes were nonetheless blurred together when they became the object of discussion in the critical literature of the long nineteenth century. For example, Olympia in Hoffmann's "The Sandman" is an automaton, but the author nevertheless refers to it as a doll, as did Freud in "The Uncanny." Furthermore, the marionette in Kleist's work becomes a sort of Nietzschean *Übermensch* (superman), while in Bahr's essay it serves as a surrogate "master instructor" for visual and performing artists who wish to learn an expressive body language.[27] In Bahr's formulation, then, one also observes that the body of the marionette may be symbolic and entertaining, but it is also "good for business" as a pedagogical tool, just as the hysterical femme fatale was being used as an instrument with which to create profitable theatrical productions at the turn of the century.

Rilke and the Modern Puppet

As with Bahr's "Marionettes," but unlike Hoffmann's "The Sandman" and Kleist's "On the Marionette Theater," Rilke's writings on the metaphorical marionette, namely his poems titled *Duineser Elegien* (*The Duino Elegies*, 1911–22) and his essay "Puppen" ("Puppets," 1914), were published when expressionist activities were on the rise in turn-of-the-century Vienna. Begun in September 1911 during Rilke's stay at Duino Castle (in the Trieste province of Italy) as a guest of Princess Marie von Thurn und Taxis-Hohenlohe, his *Elegies* were left incomplete until February 1922, owing to Rilke's struggle with compositional concerns, the outbreak and aftermath of World War I, and the poet's personal battle with depression throughout the period.[28] Rilke composed ten elegies in total, though I will focus solely on the fourth due to its pertinence as an examination of the symbolic nature of the puppet and the theatrical stage. Unlike later poems in the cycle, the *Fourth Elegy* was completed in Munich in either 1914 or 1915.[29] In the poem, Rilke, like Bahr, calls attention to two principal elements that captivated the artistic mind at the turn of the century: the theater and the puppet. In the second stanza of the elegy, Rilke writes:

> Who has not sat expectant
> before the curtain of the heart's theater?
> And up it went. A scenery of farewells.
> Easy to picture. The remembered garden,
> the backdrop faintly stirred. Then came the dancer.
> Not *him*. I've had enough. For all his footwork,
> he is a fraud, a bourgeois in disguise,
> and passes through the kitchen to his dwelling.
> I cannot take these half-invested masks.
> Better the puppet. That is full, and honest.
> Out with pretense. I can accept the wires,
> the stuffing and integuments, that face
> of mere appearance. On with the show. I'm here.[30]

Much like Kleist's Herr C in "On the Marionette Theater," the narrator of the elegy (presumably Rilke himself) is the witness of a play, and not just any play, but the spectacle of his life, his love, and his emotions, as indicated by the poet's insistence that he is speaking of the theater of the heart. Although the narrator later refers to this theater as the *Puppenbühne*, or puppet stage, it is unclear whether he is referring to a drama with living actors—who he symbolically relates to animated puppets—or whether he is watching a marionette play, like those discussed in Kleist's and Bahr's respective essays.[31] Rilke's inclusion of the dancer in his *Fourth Elegy* also finds a parallel in Kleist's and Bahr's works, insofar as the dancer/artist is seen as secondary to the expressive qualities and authenticity of the puppet. Rilke subsequently suggests that the puppet stands naked before the viewer, stripped of all pretense, unmasked, pure, and in utter contrast to the "half-invested" human actor (or dancer) that Rilke refers to as a bourgeois *poseur* hiding his identity behind the façade of modernism— or the curtain of a burlesque skit—in order to be regarded as a bohemian, avant-garde performer. Whereas Kleist and Bahr hope to educate their readers by stressing the importance of the marionette's expressive movements, Rilke's dancer is instead a reminder that the figure's art form is merely an act similar to the daily "charade" per-formed by man in order to conceal his true self or identity. In end effect, the body of the puppet and its physicality is of prime importance to Rilke, in spite of its artificial stuffing and its conspicuous strings.

   On this point, de Man has suggested that Rilke's fetishistic desire for the pup-pet is meant to echo Herr C's voyeuristic pleasure in viewing puppet burlesques, arguing that the inanimate body becomes a sexualized object when it comes under the voyeur's gaze.[32] Rilke's abandonment of the half-invested (or half-filled) masks in favor of the wholeness of the puppet further suggests that there is a shared humanity between the onlooker (Rilke) and his doppelgänger (the puppet). He therefore accepts the mechanical elements of the puppet in order to connect with the artificial gaze that meets his own. Like Herr C, the narrator in Rilke's elegy is ultimately consumed by the spectacle of the puppet stage and the "objecthood" of the puppets, to which he longs to feel connected.

Working in the 1930s, the Czech linguist and theorist Otkar Zich explored viewer responses (like those appearing in Rilke's *Fourth Elegy*) to puppet dramas staged at the turn of the twentieth century in Central Europe. In his work, Zich argues that modern puppets give rise to a dialectic because they were viewed either as "lifeless material" or "living beings."[33] Zich's analysis of the overall *fin-de-siècle* fascination with what Jentsch called the uncanny aspects of life-sized dolls offers a third interpretation of these objects as living things in relation to *their* doppelgänger, the human actor. In this sense, the viewer might assume that all bodies, living or lifeless, are nothing more than shells or costumes that human actors imbue with life and meaning, whether this be corporeal bodies, or the wooden bodies of the puppets/ marionettes they manipulate.

Inherent in Zich's examination of the dialectic of the puppet, is a recognition of this inverted doppelgänger motif. His theorization, however, is not without its complications, as more recently highlighted by Scott Shershow in his book *Puppets and "Popular" Culture* (1995), which, among other things, examines Zich's failure to properly conceptualize the viewer–object relationship that emerges in puppet theater.[34] Zich's study nevertheless contends that as viewers, we perceive the puppet as both a lifeless form and as an actual living being, and if we believe the puppet to be inanimate, then we conclude that its lifeless movements are simply "grotesque"—an interpretation that was often voiced in relation to the figures in Klimt's *Faculty Paintings* or Schiele's and Kokoschka's portraits (see, for example, Figures I.4 and I.5 and Plates 1, 2, 4 and 5).[35] If, on the other hand, we view the puppet as a living being, an automaton, or a doll-come-to-life, then we must re-evaluate its grotesqueness, rigidity, and awkwardness as metaphorical manifestations of the non-beautiful human body. If this latter understanding of the puppet's body holds true, then our notion of the "grotesque," as it applies to inanimate *things*, is simultaneously transferred to our perception of our own bodies, or even the actor's body, as a shell without beauty, or, according to Rilke, a duplicitous vessel attached to a half-filled mask. Zich's conceptualization of the puppet dialectic therefore establishes a foundation for a metaphorical discussion of the puppet's relationship to humanity due to its literal, figurative, and symbolic connotations and, in so doing, comes closest to articulating my assertion that the modern actor's inanimate double—the puppet—was also understood by *fin-de-siècle* audiences to represent the pathological body that proliferated in Austrian theater of the same period. Thus, and due to their uncanniness, dolls and puppets could be seen to articulate the grotesque body, in part because of the popularity and prevalence of the hysterical female actress who herself became a theatrical puppet to the pathological aesthetic she needed to adopt stylistically.

In his book *Toward an Aesthetics of the Puppet*, Steve Tillis engages further with Zich's theory of the dichotomous nature of the modern puppet and subsequently constructs a valid argument for the symbolic implications inherent in the puppet aesthetic, or what one might call a "dialectical puppet vision." Building on the assertion that the marionette or puppet embodies a metaphorical dichotomy (or the inverted doppelgänger motif), Tillis contends that the dialectic is actually engaged in a process of double vision, which in turn gives power to the puppet's allegorical manifestations.[36] Although Tillis traces the origins of the double vision of the puppet back to the notion of childhood and doll-play, he nevertheless asserts that,

> the metaphorical relationship of god/person to person/puppet finds far more literary expression than that of child/toy to person/puppet, in that the philosophical ramifications of the former seem far more profound than those of the latter. In the metaphorical sense, people are perceived by other people to have life, while, at the same time, they are imagined to be but objects. The power of the puppet as a metaphor of humanity depends on this inversion, and on the ontological paradox that remains. Ultimately, it is a question of who, or what, creates and controls.[37]

In Tillis' assertion, power and control are at the root of this dual vision of the marionette, and therefore this assessment ultimately bridges the gap between the collective ideas concerning the metaphorical puppet in the writings of Kleist, Bahr, and Rilke. Tillis' belief in the power of the inverted doppelgänger motif additionally allows me to transition to the writings of the hugely influential English dramatist, director, and set designer Edward Gordon Craig, who played a cameo role in Central European theater at the turn of the century. In his most well-known essay "The Actor and the Über-Marionette" (1908), Craig outlines two controversial ideas concerning modern theater, namely that the director is the true artist of the theater, and that actors are irrelevant to a theatrical production, insofar as they are conceived of as mere marionettes on the stage.[38] According to Craig, the actor's doppelgänger—the über-marionette—ought therefore to replace the living actor, given that the puppet can function as the more appropriate artist in a modernist performance. One should not assume, however, that Craig's theorization of the über-marionette suggests that this lifeless object is a more superior double because of its metaphorical or autonomous potential, as we see in the writings of Kleist, Bahr, and Rilke, even though he does assert that the puppet is better equipped to function as an actor than a living person. The distinctive aspect of Craig's notion emerges when he argues that the über-marionette is more ideal than an actor because it is more easily controlled. He asserts further that any actor who might scoff at the puppet, deriding it as a mere plaything, must be reminded that the marionette once had a more generous form than the actor, despite its degeneration throughout the ages. Although he does not explicitly state that he ultimately favors the puppet over the actor due to its lack of autonomy, this belief reverberates throughout Craig's writings on the art of directing, as well as in his subsequent attempts to restructure *fin-de-siècle* modern theater into a largely autocratic enterprise.

Craig's interest in novel approaches to theatrical direction and set design also endeared him to Max Reinhardt and Hofmannsthal, who both collaborated with Craig on a number of productions for the modern stage. In 1904, Craig designed scenes for Hofmannsthal's *Das Gerettete Venedig* (*Venice Preserved*), which opened the following year at Berlin's Lessing Theater.[39] During the 1905 theater season, he similarly prepared designs for Reinhardt's anticipated productions of Shakespeare's *The Tempest* and George Bernard Shaw's *Caesar and Cleopatra*, though these plays were never realized for the Berlin stage since Craig had demanded complete control over the productions, and Reinhardt did not concede to such an arrangement.[40] That same year, Craig produced costumes and set designs for a reprisal of Hofmannsthal's *Elektra* in Berlin, with the Italian actress Eleonora Duse (a close friend of Rilke) poised to star in the title role, though this production, like his previous collaborations with Reinhardt, also did not come to fruition.[41]

Given Craig's proximity to Hofmannsthal's and Reinhardt's modernist productions, which starred theatrical madwomen, it is interesting to supplant Craig's theory of the über-marionette onto such characters as Elektra or Salome, or even onto the figures in paintings by Kokoschka, Schiele, and Koloman Moser. Moreover, if we return briefly to Brooks' contention that Freud attempted to read Dora's body as an articulation of a hysterical sign language, we might say that he essentially treated Dora as though she were a hapless puppet whose body was victimized by her disease. Believing he could translate the language of her hysteria into a scientific formulation of the disorder, Freud assumed control over Dora's symptoms and any consequent interpretation that resulted from this language of signs. Like Craig's autocratic theater, where the director assumes supreme artistic control over every minute aspect of his production, Freud's office might be viewed as a stage where his hysterical über-marionettes were subjugated to his clinical authority. This theorization suggests that the various actresses who performed the role of Elektra or Salome were merely secondary to the more important concept of conveying the aesthetics of the real star of the *fin de siècle*: the *Modekrankheit* of hysteria. In this sense, the identities of the actresses were irrelevant as long as their bodies could accurately communicate a language that could be read as belonging to a pathological disorder. An interesting tautological formula is produced from these various readings of the modern hysterical body: the physician identifies the disease, the photographer documents it, the playwright or poet observes and then articulates it in artistic form, and the actress or puppet performs its morphology/symptomology in the hope that the audience will understand that what it is seeing is the disease, albeit in theatrical form. In parallel to this formula is the understanding that the Viennese modern artist then witnessed the expressive potential of the disease, and painted it.

Aside from the theoretical relationship between the theatrical arts, the puppet, and the pathological body in expressionist painting, which I discuss in greater depth in the final chapter of this book, there are instances when the puppet motif convened in a very clear conflation of the visual and performing arts. One striking example of this is Rilke's essay "Puppets" (1914), which he wrote in response to an exhibition of puppets (or dolls) created by Lotte Pritzel, a Munich-based puppeteer and puppet-maker. Rilke had met Pritzel in the fall of 1913 in Munich and remained in contact with the artist throughout the winter of 1913–14.[42] In the spring of 1914, the artist and the poet met for a second time following the publication of Rilke's essay in the March edition of the expressionist journal *Die Weissen Blätter* (*The White Pages*).[43] Harold Segel has discussed Rilke's thoughts on Pritzel's "dolls" (Segel's preferred translation of the word *Puppen*) in relation to what he identifies as the poet's dual fascination with the symbolic parameters of childhood and his recollection of playing with toys as a small child.[44] This is certainly a relevant examination, as Rilke discusses the puppet/doll in connection to the "world of children" and "puppet-childhood" in the opening pages of his essay.[45]

For the purposes of this study, I am particularly interested in Rilke's specific use of language when describing the symbolic nature of the puppet. One point of interest is the way he turns from his childlike preoccupation with puppets to the adult understanding that a puppet or doll by Pritzel has a *grausige Fremdkörper*, or "ghastly, strange body."[46] What exactly Rilke intended with his use of the adjective *grausige* is somewhat unclear, given that the word can mean "ghastly," "gruesome," or even "macabre," and yet he still conveys an important meaning, suggesting that the puppet body is a bizarre, perhaps even uncanny, imitation of a human figure. This reading of the puppet as it applies to the aesthetics of its *Fremdkörper* is elucidated alongside images of Pritzel's puppets, whose small, elongated, and stringless bodies ostensibly inspired Rilke to write these words (see Figure 5.1). Looking at these dolls, one might assume that their puppet bodies were capable of articulating the concepts of uncanniness, the über-marionette, or pathological otherness even before Rilke offered his analysis of their unsettling iconographies.

Indeed, Rilke's further interpretation of these inanimate but expressive bodies, with their inherent power to control the imagination of the viewer, is apparent in his later discussion of the distinction between puppets and marionettes. Rilke writes:

> It is possible for the poet to be dominated by the marionette, since the marionette is nothing but fantasy. The puppet has none and accordingly is much less a thing, just as the marionette is more a thing. But this being-less-than-a-thing, in its utter incurableness, contains the secret of its superiority.[47]

An initial question that arises from this passage is why Rilke sees such a marked difference between marionettes and puppets, particularly since Pritzel's puppets were not operated as traditional ones would be (by inserting a human hand into the puppet's body), but were wireless/stringless marionettes/dolls controlled and manipulated externally by the hand of the puppeteer. Moreover, Rilke's statement that the puppet lacks fantasy, no doubt a reference to its inescapable objecthood, appears to hold the secret to his belief in its supremacy over the marionette, but not the poet. In being less than a thing, then, the puppet is unable to dominate the poet's mind (or pen) as the marionette does, since the puppet cannot fully embody the fantasy of the marionette. Returning to the fact that the German word *Puppe* can refer to a marionette, a puppet, or a doll, and therefore has a somewhat fluid meaning, it is interesting that Rilke draws such a clear distinction between these similar, though apparently disparate objects. I would argue that the poet's rather enigmatic ideas concerning the nature of the marionette and the puppet are precisely situated within this crisis of language in Viennese modernism, and so much more so since his essay attempts to describe visual metaphors through the written word.

Rilke was not the only turn-of-the-century writer to note that Pritzel's puppets conveyed powerful visual metaphors. Four years prior to Rilke's essay, the Munich-based critic Wilhelm Michel had offered his own analysis of these curious objects in his essay "Puppen von Lotte Pritzel" ("Dolls by Lotte Pritzel," 1910–11), which appeared in *Deutsche Kunst und Dekoration* (*German Art and Decoration*), a journal that circulated widely between 1897 and 1932 in the Scandinavian and German-speaking art worlds.[48] Michel's article is of particular significance to this study since it argues that modern puppets, including Pritzel's *Puppen für die Vitrine*, or cabinet puppets, are objects imbued with a modern aesthetic, a psychological understanding of man, and the concept of the "fallen woman" (this latter point relies on the fact that *die Puppe* uses the feminine article in German).[49] Michel begins his essay by asserting that the puppet has become "a citizen of a new era"—that of the *fin de siècle*:

> Yes, it is true that from so miniscule an occurrence, such as this new affection for puppetness, we find our way to a collective psychology of our epoch. [...] Does not the puppet appear to be the lovable symbolization of a modern aestheticism? Both [the puppet's appearance of living form and its nobleness of inexistence] negate content and life, in favor of form. Both are the final denominators of a satanic sex and nature. Is it an accident then that we find such a strong similarity between Lotte Pritzel's puppets and the physiognomies explored by Aubrey Beardsley?[50]

Prior to this period, Michel suggests that the puppet amounted to nothing more than an inanimate object, a child's plaything, a simple toy, and something to be quickly forgotten. And yet, with the advent of the new epoch, the puppet is welcomed as an inhabitant of the world, capable of articulating a *Gesamtpsychologie*, or a shared consciousness, through its notion of puppethood (*Puppenhaften*). Two years after Michel's essay appeared in the pages of *German Art and Decoration*, the German critic and dramatist Georg Hirschfeld published another article in the same journal on Pritzel's dolls titled "Neue Puppen von Lotte Pritzel–München" ("New Dolls by Lotte Pritzel–Munich," 1912–13). In his essay, Hirschfeld discusses Pritzel's cabinet dolls/puppets in relation to childhood, masks, fairy tales, and the Italian *Commedia dell'arte*, and ultimately concludes that when a human being interacts with these art objects, the dolls appear to "obtain a demonic life of their own."[51] As with the previous examinations of the metaphorical supremacy of the puppet offered by Kleist, Bahr, and Rilke, Michel and Hirschfeld both argue that Pritzel's dolls are symbolic entities, but they differ in the fact that they claim that puppets convey their meaning through a modernist aesthetic and an "inner life," rather than through their complex relationship to the body of a living actor. Suggesting that the puppet was once imbued with notions of a demonic and fallen nature, or the evil sex (*Geschlecht* in German), Michel's and Hirschfeld's reviews, both published in a respected art journal, recall the misogynistic terminology used in Otto Weininger's *Sex and Character* (1903), as well as in other period literature that positioned the femme fatale as an evil seductress throughout the visual and performing arts.

Standing 10 to 26 inches tall, with waxed bodies and silk neo-baroque or rococo costumes and wigs, Pritzel's cabinet puppets were conceived not so much as children's playthings, but as serious works of art.[52] The openly erotic nature of the dolls—an aspect of the "modern aesthetic" that Michel analyzes—is clear to see in a number of photographs reproduced in *German Art and Decoration* alongside Michel's and Hirschfeld's articles. Most telling is the fact that these images illustrate the sexualized manner in which Pritzel arranged her puppets in these photographic compositions, which almost always presented the dolls as though they were on a theatrical stage.[53] One image from 1910 (Figure 5.1) shows a presumably male doll leaning in to capture a kiss from his female lover while noticeably grabbing his groin with his right hand. The female puppet, who appears elated by her lover's attention, seems not to notice his sexually suggestive gesture. Since the gender of these puppets is not entirely known, and of course nonexistent in reality, the photograph also attests to the power of the puppet motif to communicate the modernist interest in androgyny. In this

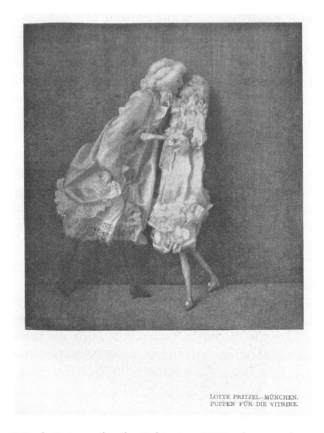

LOTTE PRITZEL–MÜNCHEN.
PUPPEN FÜR DIE VITRINE.

Figure 5.1 Lotte Pritzel, *Puppets for the Cabinet*, c. 1910, photograph reproduced on page
333 in *Deutsche Kunst und Dekoration* (October 1910–March 1911).
Source: Photo: courtesy of the author.

regard, we find a further parallel between Pritzel's genderless puppets, with their elongated limbs, and the androgynous figures that materialize in expressionist artworks (see, for example, Figure 1.2 and Plates 2 and 5). Pritzel's dolls are thus a tangible *fin-de-siècle* example of how the three-dimensional puppet, though inanimate and lifeless, was able to attract the viewer's gaze with a body that was deliberately designed to be sensual and intriguing, perhaps because of its uncanniness.

Richard Teschner and the New Viennese Puppet Theater

Even though Pritzel's dolls were discussed by Rilke—an Austrian—and reviews of her works were published in multiple issues of *German Art and Decoration*—which circulated in the Austrian capital—she herself did not actively exhibit her puppets in *fin-de-siècle* Vienna. Instead, the Bohemian-born Austrian artist, puppeteer, and puppet-maker Richard Teschner emerges as a major figure in modern Viennese marionette theater.[54] Teschner had studied between 1896 and 1899 at the Prager Kunstakademie (Prague Academy of Fine Arts), and in 1900 at the Vienna School of

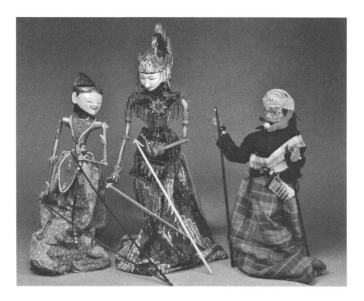

Figure 5.2 Wayang golek, 19th–20th century, fabric and painted wood.
Source: Photo: akg-images / Mark De Fraeye.

Arts and Crafts, before establishing in Prague (in 1906) his first marionette company, which used traditional stringed puppets.[55] He subsequently participated in the 1908 Vienna Kunstschau, and permanently relocated to the Austrian capital a year later, where he worked as a designer and craftsman for the Wiener Werkstätte. In 1911, while traveling in the Netherlands, he was introduced to a number of Javanese rod-puppets that Dutch merchants had brought to Amsterdam from Indonesia. While many of these traditional Indonesian puppets had, by the early twentieth century, been given to museum collections, Teschner was able to purchase a small number of these objects, as well as accumulate literature on Javanese myths and puppetry, from shops in the Dutch capital.[56] Believed to have developed from sixteenth-century Chinese puppet theater, these doll-like figures, known as *wayang golek* in Java and Bali, recall the three-dimensionality of European marionettes, but are uniquely operated by wooden dowels, rather than strings, and often outfitted in traditional Indonesian headdresses and costumes (see Figure 5.2).

Although little is known of the Javanese origins of *wayang* (which, somewhat confusingly, can mean both "shadows" and "puppets"), it is assumed that this form of storytelling grew out of the slightly older Indonesian tradition of *wayang kulit* theater. Unlike *wayang golek*, *wayang kulit* figures take the form of flat rod-puppets made of stretched skin (typically buffalo hide), and are controlled by rods attached to carved buffalo horn handles (see Figure 5.3). According to Indonesian tradition, a *dalang*, or puppeteer, is taught to perform both *wayang kulit* and *wayang golek* by operating the puppets from behind a cotton sheet illuminated by an oil lamp. The purpose of this art form was both to educate and entertain audiences, which, as early as the seventeenth century, included royals and foreign dignitaries at the Javanese court.[57] Although these shadow dramas could be written to honor or dishonor various individuals at court, they were more generally based on Hindu-Javanese tales derived from ancient Indian Sanskrit poems like the *Rāmāyana* and the *Mahābhārata*, or

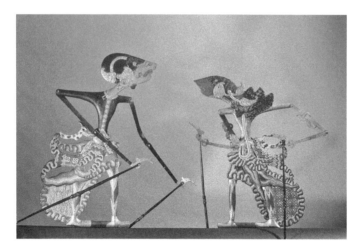

Figure 5.3 Wayang kulit shadow puppets from Java, Indonesia, late 18th–early 19th century, leather, wood and paint. Private Collection.
Source: Photo: Werner Forman / Art Resource, NY.

from Javanese Islamic tales like the relatively modern *Serat Menak Sasak*. Teschner, in turn, became fascinated with the novelty of these non-European creations and their modernist qualities. Otto Koenig, his contemporary, recounts that the puppeteer believed that *wayang* could more adequately communicate the "grand gesture" of their pantomimic movements to the audience than Western marionettes.[58] Accordingly, Teschner is considered to be the first individual to introduce Indonesian puppetry into early twentieth-century Viennese theater culture.[59] This appears to be confirmed by the striking collection of original Javanese *wayang kulit* and *wayang golek* puppets housed in the Austrian Theater Museum, which were bequeathed to the institution by Teschner's estate.[60]

The puppeteer established his second marionette company in Vienna in 1911. Unlike his earlier theater in Prague, which was a public venue that utilized traditional Germanic marionettes for conventional puppet plays, the Viennese company was a private affair, held in Teschner's home, and presented select audiences (including Klimt and Alfred Roller) with the artist's modern, Europeanized versions of *wayang* theater.[61] Known as *Der goldener Schrein* (Golden Shrine, Figure 5.4) and the *Figurenspiegel* (Figure Mirror, Figure 5.5), Teschner's puppet stages showcased *golek*-like puppets controlled by rods (or *Stäbe* in German) that were fitted with additional internal strings that Teschner used to manipulate their joints and limbs more easily. Unlike the stage for the Golden Shrine, which Teschner designed as a miniature proscenium theater, the *Figurenspiegel* was fitted with a muslin sheet hung within a large convex glass lens that protruded from the stage into the viewer's space. Rather than simply operating his puppets from behind a cotton sheet, as in a traditional *wayang* theater, Teschner instead separated his figures from their spectators by operating them from behind (or within) the convex glass apparatus.[62] The invention of the "mirror" stage was important, since it allowed Teschner to experiment with theatrical lighting and cinematic illusions, most notably by illuminating single puppets with spotlights that could then fade in or out to reveal other figures in contrasting perspectives or positions.

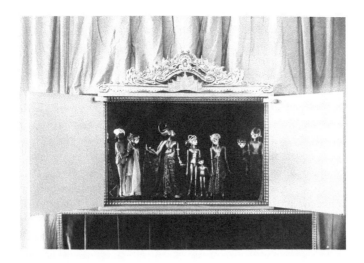

Figure 5.4 Richard Teschner, The Golden Shrine with rod-puppets, c. 1912, photograph. Theatermuseum, Vienna.

Source: Photo: KHM-Museumsverband, Theatermuseum Vienna.

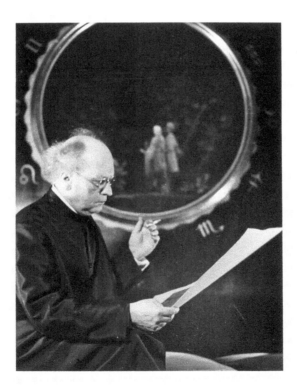

Figure 5.5 Richard Teschner in front of the Figure Mirror, 1941, photograph. Theater-museum, Vienna.

Source: Photo: KHM-Museumsverband, Theatermuseum Vienna.

Once Teschner's marionette company was established in Vienna, he began to produce a series of original puppet plays based on characters or narratives extracted from Javanese *wayang*. These Javanese-Viennese plays included *Nawang Wulan*, *Nabi Isa* (*The Prophet Jesus*), and *Kusomos Opfertod* (*Kusomo's Sacrifice*), all written and performed in 1912. The foreign titles of the three plays readily identify the works as something different from a typical Austrian marionette play that one might watch at a Kasperletheater, or more precisely, at the Wursteltheater in Vienna's Prater amusement park. *Nawang Wulan* focuses on the popular Javanese tale of Joko Tarub who, after falling in love with the moon-princess deity Nawang Wulan, steals her clothes while she is bathing to prevent her from returning to the heavens (see Figure 5.6).[63] Another puppet play, entitled *Nabi Isa*, offered Viennese audiences a further tale of human and divine interaction: in this instance, an Indonesian variation on the story of Jesus Christ (or *Isa*), who was also an important prophet (or *Nabi*) in Islam due to his prediction of Mohammed's coming.[64] In this particular play, Nabi Isa resurrects a devoted man's wife, only to return the woman to death after she flagrantly commits adultery with a prince. The "grand gesture" of the Nabi Isa puppet ultimately conveys to theater goers that divine poetic justice will be exacted on the femme fatale because of her carnal indiscretions. The third of the *wayang*-inspired plays, *Kusomos Opfertod*, has a hybridized title combining Indonesian (Kusomo, the main character of the play) and German (*Opfertod*, meaning "sacrifice" or "sacrificial death"). In the play, Kusomo, a young Tenggerese man, must sacrifice himself to the volcano god Bromo to save his family from death.[65] Interestingly enough, none of Teschner's plays, including the tale of Kusomo, appear to be extracted from the actual repertoire of *wayang* theater, suggesting that the Austrian was borrowing from, but ultimately reinventing, Indonesian myths and puppetry in order to create a quasi-Asian, quasi-European, and wholly unique puppet theater in *fin-de-siècle* Vienna.[66]

In Hans Effenberger's 1913 article titled "Richard Teschners Indisches Theater" ("Richard Teschner's Indian Theater"), which was published in *German Art and Decoration*, scenes from *Nawang Wulan*, *Nabi Isa*, and *Kusomos Opfertod* were visually reproduced for the reader, although Effenberger never actually discusses these

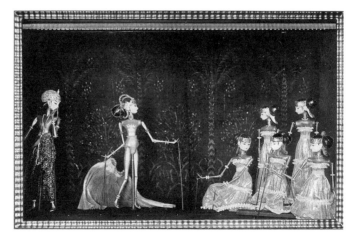

Figure 5.6 Richard Teschner, Scene from *Nawang Wulan*, as performed in the Golden Shrine, 1912, photograph. Theatermuseum, Vienna.
Source: Photo: KHM-Museumsverband, Theatermuseum Vienna.

plays in his essay. Instead, he fills his review with a philosophical critique of Teschner's marionette theater and its relationship to Asian puppetry and the metaphorical automaton. The critic specifically writes: "Our present moment ... seeks to humanize the mechanical ideal of automatons in modern puppet theater. However, rather than offering us the perspective of waxwork figures, Teschner wants to create a new artistic experience."[67] In speaking about the effects of the modern puppet theater on the viewer, Effenberger states further: "We do not sit in front of a puzzling, mysterious mechanism, but rather, we marvel at the infinite grace and deep pathos of [these puppet] gestures, and dream about the immortal fairy tales of humanity."[68] Here, Effenberger's words echo Kleist's sentiments about the gracefulness of the puppet, as well as Wilhelm Worringer's earlier contention in *Abstraction and Empathy* (1908) that "it is from the same rising pathos that exists in all mechanical emulations of organic functions, for example, in marionettes, that expression develops."[69] Tellingly, each of these writers arrives at the conclusion that the marionette theater is more than a staging of automatons, but subsists instead as a deeply expressive presentation of doppelgängers for the human body and the human condition.

However, in 1913, Teschner's puppet plays began to change. No longer based purely on Asian myths or legends, the puppeteer started to write and produce original stories, such as *Prinzessin und Wassermann* (*Princess and Water Elf*, 1913) and *Nachtstück* (*Night Play*, 1913), the latter of which was based on Hoffmann's collection of short stories, similarly titled *Nachtstücke* (*Night Plays*, 1815–17), which included "The Sandman." Photographs of the rod-puppets created for these two plays later appeared in the 1913–14 issue of *German Art and Decoration* alongside an article by the German critic Franz Servaes. Servaes' essay, "Neue Theaterpuppen von Richard Teschner" ("New Theater Puppets by Richard Teschner"), like Effenberger's slightly earlier article in the same journal, discusses Teschner's fascination with the "grotesque stylizations and enigmatic, fairy-tale qualities" of *wayang* rod-puppets and Javanese-Indian puppet theater.[70] One page in particular reproduced a photograph of the prince puppet and multiple views of the princess puppet from *Princess and Water Elf* (Figure 5.7). Even though the play was not thematically based on a Javanese or Indian folktale, the puppets' Orientalist costumes nevertheless suggest that Teschner was still incorporating non-European aesthetics into his post-1912 puppet theater.

In *Princess and Water Elf*, which the *fin-de-siècle* Viennese art critic Arthur Roessler referred to as a "fairy tale play" (or *Märchenspiel*), the cunning water elf hopes to win the heart of the beautiful princess, who is already in love with the prince.[71] In order to seize the princess for himself, the elf hires a magician to imprison the prince, but in the end true love conquers all, and the elf's devious plot is thwarted. Images of the prince and princess puppets printed in the pages of *German Art and Decoration* do not show the puppets' rods, which were ostensibly removed when the photographs were taken. As such, Teschner's rod-puppets here look more like dolls, rather than marionettes or *wayang*-inspired figures—an expedient that inadvertently reinforces the slippery semantics of the various meanings of the word *Puppen*. This notwithstanding, when one views the production photograph of *Nawang Wulan* (Figure 5.6), the thin rods are clearly visible, as they would have been to Viennese audiences attending live performances of Teschner's plays.

In turning to images of the princess puppet, I am chiefly intrigued by Teschner's decision not only to photograph the female puppet without clothing, but to then disseminate these "nude" images throughout the art world. This choice is particularly striking since the prince and the other humanlike puppets were not depicted without

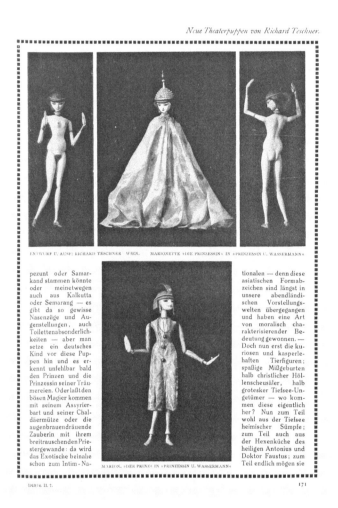

Figure 5.7 Richard Teschner, Princess and prince rod-puppets from *Princess and Water Elf*, 1913, photograph reproduced on page 171 in *Deutsche Kunst und Dekoration* (October 1913–March 1914).

Source: Photo: courtesy of the author.

garments in the pages of the journal. What is more, the photographs of the princess reveal that the puppeteer was striving for anatomical "accuracy," since the figure contains breasts with painted nipples, defined buttocks, and painted pubic hair. A production photograph of *Princess and Water Elf*, which was not reproduced in *German Art and Decoration*, nevertheless reveals that the male magician appeared naked during one scene in the play (Figure 5.8), yet the body of this puppet lacks conspicuous male genitalia or even the semblance of pubic hair. Perhaps Teschner created the princess as a corporeally "complete" puppet in case the puppet needed to appear without clothing in the play, like Nawang's character in *Nawang Wulan*, whose garments are stolen by Joko (see Figure 5.6). Alternatively, Teschner may have planned to reuse the naked female puppet in a different, or even later, play. Regardless of Teschner's intentions, it is clear that this particular puppet was fashioned as a doppelgänger for a sexualized woman. First, "she" possesses a fully rendered body beneath her dress, rather than the more generalized humanlike form used for the male magician. Second, her anatomy and body hair imply that she—a lifeless thing—has gone through puberty, albeit in the hands of the puppet master. These signs of a sexually mature human supplanted onto the inanimate body of the puppet hint, moreover, at the eroticism of Pritzel's dolls (Figure 5.1), as well as the idea that these uncanny objects can no longer be regarded as innocent children's toys, least of all on Teschner's modern stages.

Teschner was understandably secretive about the fabrication and execution of his new Viennese marionette theater—particularly about the Figure Mirror—suggesting further that he was intent on maintaining the uniqueness of his practice in the German-speaking theater world.[72] Accompanied only by incidental music that enhanced the *Gesamtkunstwerk* effect of the performance, Teschner's productions all relied heavily on the puppets' pantomime to convey meaning through gesture and successfully reveal the narrative of the plot—from the opening scene to the closing curtain—to each of his spectators. In this respect, the sign language of the puppet's body (in both the non-verbal/linguistic and semiotic understanding of this mode of communication) was the primary focus in each play since the viewer principally focused his or her attention on the movements of the puppets, instead of listening to a scripted dialogue. The presence of a dialogue would have arguably taken precedence in the hegemony of language had it been used in these plays, and its absence thus cleverly allowed Teschner to inundate his audiences with the polyvalent signs invoked by the language of gesture, rather than words.

Teschner's hybridized puppet theater, moreover, cannot be interpreted as divorcing the polyvalence of its signs from either of its cultural contexts. First, his European-Javanese puppets are not Indonesian. Second, his Viennese marionette company cannot suppress its role in Austro-Hungarian culture as historically bound to its transcendental signified. This realization on the part of the (Viennese) viewer is what would have made Teschner's puppets so strongly metaphorical. As previously discussed, Bahr writes that the marionette theater, rather than a traditional theater like the Vienna Burgtheater, exists as an appropriate didactic tool for artists and actors wishing

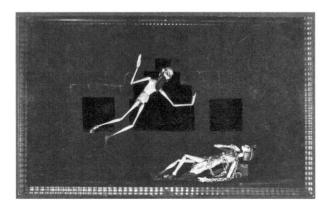

Figure 5.8 Richard Teschner, Scene from *Princess and Water Elf*, with the naked magician levitating above the chained prince, 1913, photograph. Theatermuseum, Vienna.
Source: Photo: KHM-Museumsverband, Theatermuseum Vienna.

to learn the art of dramatic storytelling through theatrical gestures and expressive movements.[73] One wonders if Bahr was in fact thinking of Teschner's Viennese marionette theater, given that the critic does not identify a specific company in his essay. Although Bahr's celebration of the Austrian marionette theater largely revolved around his praise for the metaphorical and emotive nature of inanimate *Puppen*, it is appropriate to highlight how his "Marionettes" essay also recalls the vision dialectic that is so prevalent in Kokoschka's writings. As noted in Chapter 1, Bahr advocated for the primacy of inner vision over corporeal sight in his book *Expressionism* (1916), asserting that the expressionists, in spite of their detractors' criticisms, only painted what they saw.[74] However, by acknowledging that a conundrum arises when these related yet disparate painters and their advocates attempted to define the essence of vision, Bahr ultimately sets the stage for a plethora of divergent meanings that were later attached to this concept of "seeing" and its relationship to modernist painting. The totality of Bahr's writings thus reveals the dialectical nature of expressionistic vision, particularly when he suggests in "Marionettes" that the expressionists should use their optical vision to study the physicality and expressiveness of puppet bodies, only to state later in *Expressionism* that these same artists must call upon their inner vision when generating expressive forms in a modern work of art, be that a painting or a dramatic performance.

   When read alongside one another, Bahr's texts offer a reformulation of Kokoschka's conception of the semblance of things, insofar as the artist (in Bahr's texts) must observe puppet gestures with his corporeal eye in order to create art that is then molded by the inner visions generated by these visual stimuli. Perhaps the discrepancy in Bahr's argument can simply be explained as a changing viewpoint regarding the role of opticality in relation to expressive movement in the performing and visual arts, though I think it more accurately elucidates the tenuous nature of turn-of-the-century attempts to place expressionistic vision into a single, definitive classification. As a result, we are again reminded that Kokoschka's dialectic may be the most competent formulation of expressionistic vision. If historians of Viennese expressionism had been charged only with decoding the meanings ascribed to abstract forms, rather than representations of the human body, it would be easy to conclude that Austrian painters were, for the most part, rejecting corporeal sight in favor of inner vision. But since this is not the case, and we are indeed confronted with images of human bodies, it is difficult to state conclusively that these artists were anti-optical in their approach to modernist painting, particularly when critics (Bahr included) were reinforcing the benefits of optically observing theatrical bodies, including those belonging to Teschner's puppets.

Hofmannsthal, Gütersloh, and the Language of Signs

Hofmannsthal's writings offer some additional indications as to how the uncanny body of the *Puppe*, be that a doll, puppet or marionette, participated in the crisis of language in Viennese modernism and thus became a powerful visual metaphor for *fin-de-siècle* artists. In "The Letter of Lord Chandos" (1902), Hofmannsthal writes:

> My situation, in short, is this: I have utterly lost my ability to think or speak coherently about anything at all. [...] To me, then, it is as though my body is made

up of nothing but ciphers that give me the key to everything; [...] I could present in sensible words as little as I could say anything precise about the inner movements of my intestines or a congestion of my blood.[75]

Hofmannsthal—who Rilke considered the most "eminent" modern Austrian poet by 1908—paradoxically asserts (using linguistics nonetheless) that his words, his thoughts, and his mouth's ability to formulate speech can no longer properly or coherently articulate meaning.[76] However, his contention belies its intended effect. His words instead convey a precise meaning through the notion that acknowledging the dissolution of meaning (between signs and their signifieds) might elucidate a deeper, more profound understanding of how ideas are communicated by way of the body. In Hofmannsthal's analysis, then, the human body becomes a complex system of signs or ciphers, which, when decoded, reveal their mysteries and meanings about the world he inhabits. When analyzed alongside his earlier contention that words cannot sensibly convey meaning, it appears clear that Hofmannsthal suggests that the interpretation of our gestures, our movements, or our bodily signs is an alternative instrument that we might utilize to communicate our thoughts effectively, and reciprocally understand the codes that construct societal meanings. It is as though the writer is also arguing that the hand can be conceptualized as a cipher for the artist's true meanings: that is, as an external and physical instrument used to decode inner visions and emotions. His nonverbal body must thus communicate what the mind and tongue can no longer linguistically utter.

Hofmannsthal, whose very livelihood depended on the power of the written word to communicate meaning to his readers or theatrical audiences, had explored this paradoxical love–hate relationship with language seven years prior to writing the Chandos letter. Penned in 1895, the following passage from Hofmannsthal's early musings on the problem of linguistics demonstrates his belief that this crisis was already deeply imbedded in the cultural fabric of Vienna. As in "The Letter of Lord Chandos," Hofmannsthal questions the primacy of verbal or written language in the communicative process. He writes:

> People are indeed tired of hearing speech. They are deeply revolted by words: for words have placed themselves before things. [...] And thus there awakens a desperate love of all those arts which are exercised in silence: music, dancing and all the arts of acrobats and jugglers.[77]

Hofmannsthal praises dancing as one of the "silent" languages capable of delighting modern audiences. This love of the theatrical art of dance is made clear in "Die unvergleichliche Tanzerin" ("The Incomparable Dancer," 1906), an essay that celebrates avant-garde performances by the American dancer Ruth St. Denis.[78] In a later article entitled "Über die Pantomime" ("On the Pantomime," 1911), which was (self-indulgently) written as a review of the pantomime *Das fremde Mädchen* (*The Strange Girl*) that he had personally composed for the Viennese modern dancer Grete Wiesenthal, Hofmannsthal celebrates the ability of gestures to communicate an unspeakable, or unutterable, language to the viewer.[79] In all three of these writings—that is, his essays from 1895, 1906, and 1911—Hofmannsthal exalts the language of the body over the language of words, arguing that things (and here we can infer that Hofmannsthal is also implying bodies) should be placed before words. This hegemonic inversion further implies that the ear has become tired of hearing words, whereas the eye has only just begun to see the language of modernism—that is, the language of the modern body and its codified gestures and meanings. If Hofmannsthal meant for the listener/viewer to *observe* language, rather than to read or hear it, then it is clear that the body was being conceived of as a text capable of being translated. In other words, when the body moves, it also speaks.

In his theoretical response to the crisis of traditional language, Hofmannsthal conceptualizes a language of abstraction that can be mapped onto the body, and one that I would argue can be translated onto both human and puppet bodies. If Hofmannsthal had only cited music, rather than music and dance, as the only silent language, it would be easy to conceive of this complicated semiotic system as an abstracted system that creates meaning in the mind beyond words. The body in motion, by contrast, is akin to music, insofar as the body does not speak *through* words, yet the language of the dancer's or actor's body is always contingent upon its corporeal shell. As such, the language of the body can never be divisible from its host. To a certain degree, the German philosopher Walter Benjamin later reinforced this reading in the essay "What is Epic Theatre?" (1939), in which he suggests that a pause between gestures is paramount to a successful theatrical performance, since this silence allows the preceding and subsequent body gestures to become "quotable" by the audience.[80] It is precisely this "quotability" that I find most advantageous in Hofmannsthal's theory of an observable (or visually quotable) body language, given its applicability to corporeal gestures appearing in paintings by expressionist artists, especially Kokoschka and Schiele, and in the dolls or marionettes created by Pritzel and Teschner.

In 1911, the artist and writer Albert Paris von Gütersloh, who had been a member of the New Art Group with Schiele, wrote a monograph entitled *Egon Schiele* that is still considered a landmark, turn-of-the-century study on the role of gestures in modern painting. Seven years later, Schiele tellingly painted Gütersloh's own gestural language in *Portrait of Albert Paris von Gütersloh* (1918, Plate 7). Printed as a pamphlet-like publication containing an essay and multiple reproductions of Schiele's paintings from the previous year, Gütersloh's text is arguably the first to have discussed Schiele as an autonomous artist, now separated from Klimt, the Academy, and the short-lived Neukunstgruppe. Gütersloh's essay in *Egon Schiele* sets out two avant-gardist aims: to paint Schiele as an artistic "prophet," capable of leading *fin-de-siècle* Vienna into the future with his modernist vision; and to establish Gütersloh as a critic conversant with this modernist aesthetic. The critic observes that some viewers may be frightened by the painter's jarring canvases and peculiar psyche, but he reasons that this is only because they do not realize that they have been waiting for a visionary like Schiele to emerge from society.[81] The writer explains that the public's fear of Schiele's aesthetic—in other words, its discomfort with his grotesque bodies—can be linked to the painter's "knowledge of pathological nomenclature."[82] Given the primacy of Gütersloh's text within the extant literature on Schiele's unique aesthetic, it is all the more curious that previous scholars have neglected the work, particularly when one considers that the critic definitely ties the iconography of Schiele's figures to representations of the pathological body.

Gütersloh's ideas concerning the cryptic language of Schiele's painted bodies do not terminate here though, as the writer was intent on explaining how these corporeal gestures might function in the artist's resultant canvases. Gütersloh argues that, "alongside one sense of the morbidity, depravity and obscenity of a figure, a line or a gesture, lies another deeper meaning like a cipher or a system of symbols."[83] Hofmannsthal's theorization of the modern body as a system of ciphers once more comes to mind at this point, and I would be hard-pressed to imagine that Gütersloh was not in fact thinking of Hofmannsthal when he conceived of Schiele's bodies as embodying a complex system of signs. Gütersloh reiterates the notion that the body can speak a nonverbal language that only the painter, as a sort of visual poet, is capable of writing. He states:

> The loudest ecstatics seem to sense that paintings yearn only for gestures. And if we must speak [of paintings], our words are only the staggered and haphazard tonal gestures of the body, which man verbally accumulates in the ignorance of his ways. A painting, then, develops when the initial agitated pantomime of ideas begins to solidify in the painting's intermediate spaces and in the places of its action.[84]

When Gütersloh uses the word "ecstatics" in the essay, he is referring to individuals who speak through their actions, rather than their words. In this regard, Gütersloh again seems to channel Hofmannsthal when he argues that words, or "tonal gestures," are subservient to the body and thus only legible through the body's specified language of movements. Incredibly, Gütersloh hypothesized (as early as 1911) that expressionist painting might be contingent on corporeal movements; not just ordinary, meaningless gestures, but those that develop from an "agitated pantomime," or a nonverbal performance capable of conveying meaning through a language of theatrical, pathological signs.

If one directs this analysis to Schiele's *Portrait of Albert Paris von Gütersloh*, one finds that the artist has taken Gütersloh's prescription for gesture in modernist painting and applied it directly to the body of the critic. Rather than permitting Gütersloh's words to speak through his pen, as controlled by his hands, Schiele instead makes his hands speak through their puppet-like gestures in a silent painting. It is clear that Schiele had a profound respect for Gütersloh, given that the two men were close friends, though I cannot help but speculate that the painting represents the artist's attempt to resolve the crisis of language in Viennese modernism by definitively asserting that the painter—and not the writer, poet, actor or playwright—was ultimately the only artist capable of fully developing this new language of the body. In this sense, Schiele's portrait of the critic symbolically concludes that the painter was more capable than even Gütersloh of conveying the poetry of the writer's own hands, particularly when one considers that Gütersloh was unavoidably dependent on words to execute *his* art form. Schiele's canvas thus affirms that if one wanted to be regarded as a modernist poet in turn-of-the-century Vienna, one would be well advised to become an avant-garde painter. It is also the reason why, I believe, one can identify a kinship between the unique iconographies of modern puppets—with their language of expressive, though inaudible words—and the bizarre corporeal gestures that appear in Wiener Moderne paintings, including Schiele's portrait of Gütersloh.

Conclusion

It is important to reiterate that the strange, enigmatic gestures that became so prominent in Viennese expressionist paintings can literally and figuratively be seen to speak a language of modernity, as filtered through the modern or pathological body. Like a specialized sign language, this modern body was perhaps only legible (or for that matter, relevant) to the artists, playwrights, actors, and writers who utilized gestures to develop a language of the new era that was no longer contingent on words to communicate meaning to their audiences. In this respect, writers and puppeteers working alongside the expressionists in Vienna were capable of uniting a linguistic avant-gardism with a pictorial or visual modernism. This aesthetic idiom of the metaphorical puppet, doll, or marionette has been scrutinized by scholars in later artistic movements like German Dada and surrealism, yet less attention has been paid to its relation to Viennese expressionist painting—a gap that I address in the final chapter of this book.[85]

Thus far, I have argued that the theatrically hysterical body articulated a *Modekrankheit* to *fin-de-siècle* audiences in large part because of the crisis of language that became a key aspect of Viennese visual culture. My theorization of the dialectics of expressionistic vision also reinforces the importance of optical vision to expressionist artists working in various media at the turn of the century, particularly when one considers that the representation of the modern body in a painting was believed to articulate a nonverbal language that was reliant on a recognition of gestures simultaneously on display in the performing arts. Because this understanding of corporeal gesture allowed Viennese artists, playwrights, and writers to continue to explore the expressive qualities of the human form, rather than turning toward abstraction, this vision dialectic was paramount to their somewhat paradoxical activities, ultimately allowing *fin-de-siècle* viewers to witness the vogue for the modern, pathological body on the canvas and the stage, including the puppet stage.

To illustrate this point, I want to return briefly to Kokoschka's *Hans Tietze and Erica Tietze-Conrat* (Plate 1) and Schiele's *Portrait of Albert Paris von Gütersloh* (Plate 7). Each of these paintings, which were created nearly a decade apart, incorporates expressive hand gestures performed by an art critic or art historian. Both works depict their subjects in contemporary clothing, and both place the human body against an abstracted background of flattened colors. Even in terms of artistic conventions, such as the deceptively subtle impasto application of paint typical of much expressionist brushwork, the paintings are strikingly similar for works created by artists with such different styles. In Kokoschka's painting, the importance of vision is made clear by the complicated relationship between the two sitters who fail to make eye contact with one another or the viewer. This disruption of corporeal sight in the subject-to-subject relationship, as well as the subject-to-viewer or viewer-to-subject relationship was, I think, a deliberate tactic on the part of the painter to compel his viewers to find meaning in the sitters' curious hand gestures, given that these corporealities become the focal point of the canvas. In my opinion, one of the more fascinating aspects of Kokoschka's work is the idea that his subjects are aware of what their gestures do or do not signify, even though the viewer is frustratingly left to decipher their meaning, assuming there is any meaning at all. The fact that the gestures taunt us, drawing us into the painting by suggesting that they are the primary form of communicative language deployed in the work, creates an enigma that makes them all the more alluring. The end effect is that Hans and Erica Tietze's hands speak a language that we desperately want to understand, but cannot quite decipher.

The same can be said for Schiele's portrait of Gütersloh, which appears to mimic the Tietzes' mysterious sign language, as if attempting to communicate something equally profound to the viewer, whose gaze he returns intensely. The fact that both Schiele's and Kokoschka's paintings invoke the body language of individuals whose livelihoods revolved around the interpretation and criticism of art is all the more telling since the public, which might struggle to read and understand such gestures, would normally have turned to these art aficionados for erudite explanations. Despite the fact that Schiele was a personal friend of Gütersloh, and in spite of the fact that Kokoschka shared a close relationship with the Tietzes, both paintings insist that the modern artist, rather than the art critic, ultimately dictates who controls meaning in a Viennese modern painting, deciding to what extent this meaning was or was not decipherable by anyone other than themselves. The bodies and gestures in Kokoschka's and Schiele's canvases can thus be seen as metaphorical possessions of the artist, rather than of the individuals they represent. This notion that the body had become a manipulated, puppet-like object in the hands of Viennese expressionists suggests moreover that the modern artist functioned as an omnipotent *Puppenspieler*, or puppet master, controlling a semiotic system built around the complexities of enigmatic body gestures. Accordingly, the final chapter turns to specific case studies of expressionist paintings and drawings by Kokoschka and Schiele that incorporate the language of pathological puppets, and similarly examines plays by Kokoschka and Arthur Schnitzler, who likewise explored the *Puppenspieler* motif in their theatrical works.

Notes

1 Hugo von Hofmannsthal, *The Lord Chandos Letter*, trans. Russell Stockman (Marlboro: The Marlboro Press, 1986), 19, 27.

2 Hermann Bahr, "Marionetten," in *Das Hermann-Bahr-Buch* (Berlin: S. Fischer, 1913), 214. The original German reads: "Wir haben jetzt ein Theater, das Schauspieler besuchen sollten: sie können da, ja alle Künstler können da lernen. Das ist das Theater der Marionetten."

3 Various discussions with Kimberly Smith and Laura Muir helped to refine the arguments I have made in this chapter on the nature and extent of the language crisis in Viennese literature. In many ways, this chapter is also an extension and re-evaluation of the ideas outlined in Michael Huter, "Body as Metaphor: Aspects of the Critique and Crisis of Language at the Turn of the Century with Reference to Egon Schiele," in *Egon Schiele: Art, Sexuality, and Viennese Modernism*, ed. Patrick Werkner (Palo Alto: The Society for the Promotion of Science and Scholarship, 1994), 119–29. With regards to Hofmannsthal, Jill Scott has argued that this language crisis can be situated alongside dramatic action in *Elektra*, as well as in modern dance and musical forms. See Jill Scott, *Electra after Freud: Myth and Culture* (Ithaca: Cornell University Press, 2005), 85.

4 Hermann Bahr, *Expressionismus* (1916; Munich: Delphin-Verlag, 1919), 50–51; and Hofmannsthal, *The Lord Chandos Letter*, 19.

5 Andreas Huyssen, "The Disturbance of Vision in Vienna Modernism," *Modernism/Modernity* 5, no. 3 (1998): 35.

6 Huyssen, "The Disturbance of Vision in Vienna Modernism," 34.

7 Gemma Blackshaw, "The Pathological Body: Modernist Strategising in Egon Schiele's Self-Portraiture," *Oxford Art Journal* 30, no. 3 (2007): 377–401.

8 Itzhak Goldberg, "Talking Hands," in *Vienna 1900: Klimt, Schiele, Moser, Kokoschka*, ed. Marie-Amélie zu Salm-Salm (London: Ashgate, 2005), 75–76.

9 Goldberg, "Talking Hands," 76.

10 Huter, "Body as Metaphor," 119–29.

11 See, for example, Arthur Symons, "Aubrey Beardsley," *Ver Sacrum: Organ der Vereinigung bildender Kuenstler Österreichs*, trans. Anna Muthesius 6, no. 6, trans. Anna Muthesius (March 15, 1903): 117–38; Armin Friedmann, "Feuilleton: Bildende Kunst. Salon Miethke: Beardsley," *Wiener Abendpost: Beilage zur Wiener Zeitung*, no. 1, January 2, 1905, 1;

Hugo Haberfeld, *Aubrey Beardsley: Galerie Miethke Ausstellung von Werken alter und moderner Kunst* (Vienna: Galerie Miethke, 1905), 2; and Rainer Maria Rilke, *Auguste Rodin*, vol. 10, *Die Kunst* (Berlin: Bard, 1903).

12 Huyssen, "The Disturbance of Vision in Vienna Modernism," 35–36. For Freud's essay, see Sigmund Freud, "The Uncanny," in *The Standard Edition of the Complete Psychological Works of Sigmund Freud*, trans. and ed. James Strachey, vol. 17 (London: The Hogarth Press and the Institute for Psycho-Analysis, 1953–74), 219–56. For Hoffmann's story, see E. T. A. Hoffmann, *The Best Tales of Hoffmann*, ed. E. F. Bleiler (New York: Dover Publications, Inc., 1967), 183–214. Sue Taylor offers a good summation of critical responses on the relationship between Freud's and Hoffmann's texts in Sue Taylor, *Hans Bellmer: The Anatomy of Anxiety* (Cambridge, MA: The MIT Press, 2002), 66–69.

13 Freud, "The Uncanny," 231–33.

14 Peter Brooks, *Body Work: Objects of Desire in Modern Narrative* (Cambridge, MA: Harvard University Press, 1993), 234–44.

15 Jentsch's essay on the uncanny was published serially across two issues in the journal *Psychiatrisch-Neurologische Wochenschrift*. See Ernst Jentsch, "Zur Psychologie des Unheimlichen," *Psychiatrisch-Neurologische Wochenschrift* 8, no. 22 (August 25, 1906): 195–98; and no. 23 (September 1, 1906): 203–05. For an English translation, see Ernst Jentsch, "On the Psychology of the Uncanny (1906)," *Angelaki: A New Journal in Philosophy, Literature, and the Social Sciences* 2, no. 1, trans. Roy Sellars (1996): 7–16.

16 Jentsch, "On the Psychology of the Uncanny," 12.

17 Jentsch, "On the Psychology of the Uncanny," 13.

18 Jentsch, "On the Psychology of the Uncanny," 12.

19 Heinrich von Kleist, *Über das Marionettentheater: Aufsätze und Anekdoten*, Second edn (Frankfurt am Main: Insel, 1982). Kleist's work published serially across several issues of the *Berlin Evening Paper*, rather than as a single essay. See von Kleist, "Über das Marionettentheater," *Berliner Abendblätter*, nos. 63–66, December 12–15, 1810, 247–61. For a good English translation of the essay, see Heinrich von Kleist, "On the Marionette Theatre," *The Drama Review* 16, no. 3, The "Puppet" Issue, trans. Thomas G. Neumiller (September 1972): 22–26.

20 Rilke's interest in Kleist's works has been examined by a number of scholars, all of whom note the influence of Kleist's romanticism on Rilke's modernism. A specific indicator of this relationship is Rilke's 1898 poem *An Heinrich von Kleist's wintereinsamem Waldgrab in Wannsee*, in which the young poet draws a direct parallel between Kleist's life and his own. This poem, along with the parallel between Rilke's *Duino Elegies* and Kleist's "Über das Marionettentheater" is further analyzed by Kurt Bergel in "Rilke's Fourth Duino Elegy and Kleist's Essay Über das Marionettentheater," *Modern Language Notes* 60, no. 2 (February 1945): 73–78.

21 Kleist, *Über das Marionettentheater*, 338. The original German reads: "Ich sagte ihm, daß ich erstaunt gewesen wäre, ihn schon mehrere Male in einem Marionettentheater zu finden, das auf dem Markte zusammengezimmert worden war, und den Pöbel, durch kleine dramatische Burlesken, mit Gesang und Tanz durchwebt, belustigte. Er versicherte mir, daß ihm die Pantomimik dieser Puppen viel Vergnügen machte, und ließ nicht undeutlich merken, daß ein Tänzer, der sich ausbilden wolle, mancherlei von ihnen lernen könne." For the English translation, see Kleist, "On the Marionette Theatre," 22.

22 Kleist, "On the Marionette Theatre," 24.

23 Kleist, "On the Marionette Theatre," 26.

24 Paul de Man, *The Rhetoric of Romanticism* (New York: Columbia University Press, 1984), 266.

25   See Kleist, *Über das Marionettentheater*, 341–42.

26 Bahr, "Marionetten," 214.

27 The concept of the *Übermensch*, which is arguably one of the most significant motifs/principles in Nietzsche's thoughts about mankind, is briefly discussed in the prologue to *Thus Spoke Zarathustra*. For a good English translation of this work, see Friedrich Nietzsche, *Thus Spoke Zarathustra: A Book for Everyone and No One*, trans. R. J. Hollingdale (New York: Penguin, 1969).

28 See Wolfram Groddeck, "Nachwort," in *Duineser Elegien, Die Sonette an Orpheus* (Stuttgart: Philipp Reclam, 1997), 140–41.

29 There appears to be some discrepancy in the dates attributed to the completion of the *Fourth Elegy*, though all scholars agree it was finished in Munich. Groddeck suggests it was completed in 1914, just one year after Rilke returned from Paris, in Groddeck, "Nachwort," 141. Harold Segel, who also examines Rilke's Fourth Elegy and its connection to the puppet motif, suggests that it was written on 22 and 23 November 1915, in Harold B. Segel, *Pinocchio's Progeny: Puppets, Marionettes, Automatons, and Robots in Modernist and Avant-Garde Drama* (Baltimore: Johns Hopkins University Press, 1995), 43. For Segel's entire analysis of the *Fourth Elegy*, see pages 43–49.

30 Rainer Maria Rilke, *The Duino Elegies*, trans. John Waterfield (Lewiston: Edwin Mellen Press, 1999), 49, 51. Of the many translations of Rilke's elegies currently in print, Waterfield's is by the far the most faithful to Rilke's original intent and structure. The original German reads: "Wer saß nicht bang vor seines Herzens Vorhang? Der schlug sich auf: die Szenerie war Abschied. Leicht zu verstehen. Der bekannte Garten, und schwankte leise: dann erst kam der Tänzer. Nicht der. Genug. Und wenn er auch so leicht tut, er ist verkleidet, und er wird ein Bürger und geht durch seine Küche in die Wohnung. Ich will nicht diese halbgefüllten Masken, lieber die Puppe. Die ist voll. Ich will den Balg aushalten und den Draht und ihr Gesicht aus Aussehn. Hier. Ich bin davor," in Rainer Maria Rilke, *Duineser Elegien, Die Sonette an Orpheus* (Stuttgart: Philipp Reclam, 1997), 19–20.

31 For Rilke's mention of the *Puppenbühne*, see Rilke, *Duineser Elegien*, 20.

32 Man, *The Rhetoric of Romanticism*, 266.

33 Otkar Zich, from his book *The Aesthetics of Dramatic Art*, quoted and translated in Peter Bogatyrëv, "A Contribution to the Study of Theatrical Signs," trans. John Burbank, Olga Hasty, Manfred Jacobson, Bruce Kochis, and Wendy Steiner, in *The Prague School: Selected Writings, 1929–1946*, ed. Peter Steiner (Austin: University of Texas Press, 1982), 58.

34 Scott Cutler Shershow, *Puppets and "Popular" Culture* (Ithaca: Cornell University Press, 1995), 214–18.

35 Otkar Zich, quoted in Bogatyrëv, "A Contribution to the Study of Theatrical Signs," 58.

36 Steve Tillis, *Toward an Aesthetics of the Puppet: Puppetry as a Theatrical Art* (Westport: Greenwood Press, 1992), 159.

37 Tillis, *Toward an Aesthetics of the Puppet*, 160.

38 Edward Gordon Craig, "The Actor and the Über-Marionette," *The Mask: A Monthly Journal of the Art of the Theatre* 1, no. 2 (April 1908): 3–8.

39 Christopher Innes, *Edward Gordon Craig: A Vision of the Theatre*, Second edn (Amsterdam: Hardwood Academic Publishers, 1998), 311.

40 Innes, *Edward Gordon Craig*, 311.

41 Innes, *Edward Gordon Craig*, 311.

42 Segel, *Pinocchio's Progeny*, 47.

43 Segel, *Pinocchio's Progeny*, 47.

44 Segel, *Pinocchio's Progeny*, 47–48.

45 Rainer Maria Rilke, *Puppen* (Munich: Hyperionverlag, 1921), 5. The original German reads: "die Welt der Kinder" and "Puppen-Kindheiten." Although Rilke's essay first appeared in the March 1914 edition of *Die Weissen Blätter*, I am working from the reprint edition of the essay in Rilke's book *Puppen*, which contains illustrations by Pritzel. *Die Weissen Blätter* was a literary review published between 1913 and 1920, and was principally devoted to reproducing German modernist/expressionist texts. The journal's publishers and contributing writers generally rejected the ideals of the liberal and moderately conservative bourgeoisie, and instead adopted an anti-bourgeois pacifist credo.

46 Rilke, *Puppen*, 8.

47 Rilke, *Puppen*, 11. The original German reads: "Es könnte ein Dichter unter die herrschaft einer Marionette geraten, denn die Marionette hat nichts als Phantasie. Die Puppe hat keine und ist genau um so viel weniger als ein Ding, als die Marionette mehr ist. Aber dieses Wenigersein-als-ein-Ding in seiner ganzen Unheilbarkeit, enthält das Geheimnis ihres Übergewichts."

48 Founded in 1897, *Deutsche Kunst und Dekoration* was a Germanic art journal devoted to Jugendstil, art nouveau, and the decorative arts.

49 Wilhelm Michel, "Puppen von Lotte Pritzel," *Deutsche Kunst und Dekoration* 27 (October 1910–March 1911): 329–38. For the sake of brevity, and since Michel's article has never before been translated into English, I am only reproducing passages from his essay that reiterate my contention that the appearance of the metaphorical puppet was a significant and meaningful aesthetic for modern writers, playwrights, and artists working in *fin-de-siècle* Central Europe. In addition, Paul Westheim provides a postscript to Michel's essay on page 338 of the journal.

50 Michel, "Puppen von Lotte Pritzel," 329. The original German reads: "Die Puppe ist eine Bürgerin der neuen Zeit. [...] Ja, es ist wirklich wahr, daß von so einer winzigen Erscheinung wie es die neue Liebe zum Puppenhaften ist, Wege führen zur Gesamtpsychologie unserer Epoche. [...] Sieht sich die Puppe nicht ganz wie eine liebenswürdige Symbolisierung des modernen Ästhetizismus an? Beide verneinen den Inhalt, das Leben, zugunsten der Form. Beide sind letzten Grundes von satanischem Geschlecht und Wesen. Ist es ein Zufall, daß hier bei Lotte Pritzels Puppen immer dieselbe, an Beardsley erinnernde Physiognomie widerkehrt?" The word "beide" (or "both") in this passage refers to concepts expressed in the preceding sentence in Michel's essay, which I am not reproducing in this text.

51 Georg Hirschfeld, "Neue Puppen von Lotte Pritzel–München," *Deutsche Kunst und Dekoration* 31 (October 1912–March 1913): 254–60. Hirschfeld writes: "Hält man Lotte Pritzels Puppen einzeln in der Hand, so sind sie ein Spielzeug, mit dem man machen kann, was man will. Läßt man sie frei aufeinander wirken, so gewinnen sie dämonisches Eigenleben, und ihre Bewegungen geben mehr als starre Bildwerke."

52 Harold Segel states that Pritzel's dolls were life-size, in Segel, *Pinocchio's Progeny*, 47.

53 Michel, "Puppen von Lotte Pritzel," 330.

54 For literature on Teschner, see "Richard Teschner's Figure Theatre," *Theatre Arts Monthly* 23, no. 7 (1928): 490–95; Arthur Roessler, *Richard Teschner* (Vienna: Gerlach und Wiedling, 1947); Franz Hadamowsky, ed., *Richard Teschner und sein Figurenspiegel* (Vienna: Eduard Wancura, 1956); Jarmila Weißenböck, *Der Figurenspiegel Richard Teschner* (Vienna: Böhlau, 1991); Hannah Kohn, "Richard Teschners Figurenspiegel als Spiegel des Zeitgeistes einer Epoche," M.Phil. thesis, University of Vienna, 2012; and *Die Bühnen des Richard Teschner* (Vienna: Österreichisches Theater Museum, 2013).

55 Roessler, *Richard Teschner*, 20.

56 Matthew Isaac Cohen, "Contemporary Wayang in Global Contexts," *Asian Theatre Journal* 24, no. 2 (Fall 2007): 345.

57 For the role of *wayang* theater at the Javanese court, and its subsequent appeal to European guests who were invited to view these performances as early as the seventeenth century, see Ann Kumar, *Java and Modern Europe: Ambiguous Encounters* (Richmond: Curzon Press, 1997), 28.

58 Otto Koenig, quoted in "Richard Teschner's Figure Theatre," 492n.

59 Indonesian puppet plays were performed throughout Europe at the *fin de siècle*, though it is not known if Teschner actually attended a play during his stay in Holland, or if he only encountered these puppets in Amsterdam museums. For readings on the historical and contemporary aspects of Javanese puppet theater, see Richard Schechner, "Wayang Kulit in the Colonial Margin," *TDR* 34, no. 2 (Summer 1990): 25–61; and Jan Mrázek, "Javanese Wayang Kulit in the Times of Comedy: Clown Scenes, Innovation, and the Performance's Being in the Present World: Part One," *Indonesia* 68 (October 1999): 38–128.

60 Provenance records at the Austrian Theater Museum substantiate that these puppets had once belonged to Teschner.

61 Cohen argues that Teschner's Viennese theater was held in his home to intentionally limit his audiences. See Cohen, "Contemporary Wayang in Global Contexts," 348. Regarding Klimt's and Roller's attendance, see Klaus Behrendt, "Austria: Puppet Theatre," in *The World Encyclopedia of Contemporary Theatre*, eds. Don Rubin, Péter Nagy and Philippe Rouyer, vol. 1: Europe (London and New York: Routledge, 1994), 72.

62 Cohen discusses the make-up of the stage in Cohen, "Contemporary Wayang in Global Contexts," 351.

63 Kumar, *Java and Modern Europe*, 133; and Cohen, "Contemporary Wayang in Global Contexts," 347.

64 Paul Carus, "Indonesian Legend of Nabi Isa," *The Open Court* 22 (1908): 499–502; and Cohen, "Contemporary Wayang in Global Contexts," 346.

65 Cohen, "Contemporary Wayang in Global Contexts," 346.

66 Cohen has analyzed the *wayang* repertoire, concluding that Teschner's plays do not appear in the historical or contemporary literature. See Cohen, "Contemporary Wayang in Global Contexts," 347.

67 Hans Effenberger, "Richard Teschners Indisches Theater," *Deutsche Kunst und Dekoration* 32 (April–September 1913): 218. Effenberger writes: "Unsre Zeit, die sich über das ewige Homunkulus-Problem mit dem Automaten hinweghilft, sucht im modernen Puppentheater das Ideal des Automatischen zu vermenschlichen. Teschner will, im Gegensatz zu diesem Panoptikum-Standpunkt, ein neues künstlerisches Erlebnis gestalten."

68 Effenberger, "Richard Teschners Indisches Theater," 222. The original German reads: "Wir sitzen nicht vor den Rätseln eines geheimnisvollen Mechanismus, sondern staunen über die unendliche Anmut und das tiefe Pathos der Geberden und träumen die unsterblichen Märchen der Menschheit."

69 Wilhelm Worringer, *Abstraktion und Einfühlung: Ein Beitrag zur Stilpsychologie*, Third edn (1908; Munich: R. Piper & Co., 1911), 117.

70 Franz Servaes, "Neue Theaterpuppen von Richard Teschner," *Deutsche Kunst und Dekoration* 33 (October 1912–March 1913): 169. The original German reads: "Bis bendlich die javanisch-indische Puppenwelt mit ihrer grotesken Stilisierung und rätselvollen Märchenseele und mit ihren durch Stäbchen von untenher dirigierten Bewegungen den Künstler entzückten, und ihn sozusagen die Knöpfe von den Augen springen ließ und seine eigene reiche Einbildungskraft entfesselte."

71 Roessler, *Richard Teschner*, 35.

72 Cohen, "Contemporary Wayang in Global Contexts," 348.

73 Bahr, "Marionetten," 214. The original German reads: "Wir haben jetzt ein Theater, das Schauspieler besuchen sollten: sie können da, ja alle Künstler können da lernen. Das ist das Theater der Marionetten."

74 Bahr, *Expressionismus*, 50–51.

75 Hofmannsthal, *The Lord Chandos Letter*, 19, 27.

76 Rilke referred to Hofmannsthal in this manner in a number of letters written to Auguste Rodin in 1907 and 1908. See Rainer Maria Rilke, *Briefe an Auguste Rodin* (Leipzig: Insel-Verlag, 1928), 36, 44.

77 Hugo von Hofmannsthal, *Prosa*, vol. 1 (Frankfurt: S. Fischer, 1956), 228. An English translation of this poem is provided by David Levin in Anton Kaes, "The Debate about Cinema: Charting a Controversy (1909–1929)," *New German Critique* no. 40, Special Issue on Weimar Film Theory (Winter 1987): 25. Kaes' article also examines Hofmannsthal's response to the problem of language in Viennese modernism, particularly on page 25.

78 Hugo von Hofmannsthal, "Die unvergleichliche Tänzerin," in *Reden und Aufsätze I: 1891–1913*, vol. 8, *Gesammelte Werke*, ed. Bernd Schöler (Frankfurt: Bernd Schöler, 1979), 496–501. A good English translation can be found in David Berger, "Her Extraordinary Immediacy," *Dance Magazine* XLII (September 1968): 36–38.

79 Hugo von Hofmannsthal, "Über die Pantomime," *Süddeutsche Monatshefte* 9, no. 1 (October 1911): 100–3.

80 For Benjamin's discussion of gesture as a form of theatrical language, see Walter Benjamin, "What is Epic Theatre?" in *Illuminations*, ed. Hannah Arendt (New York: Schocken Books, 1977), 147–54, here 51.

81 Albert Paris von Gütersloh, *Egon Schiele* (Vienna: Brüder Rosenbaum, 1911) 2. Gütersloh writes, "Ich gebe ihnen die Bilder von Egon Schiele. Ich gehe, meinem neuen Wege gemäß, die Psyche dieses Malers entlang, und siehe, er kommt mir schon entgegen. Das erschreckt so viele. Sie wußten nicht, daß sie erwartet wurden."

82 Gütersloh, *Egon Schiele*, 4. In German, this passage reads: "seine Kenntnis der pathologischen Nomenklatur."

83 Gütersloh, *Egon Schiele*, 4. The original German reads: "Denn auch das Morbide, Lasterhafte, Zotige einer Figur, einer Linie, einer Geste hat neben dem Auch-Sinn noch einen Hintersinn ist Chiffre und Stenogramm."

84 Gütersloh, *Egon Schiele*, 1. The original German reads: "Leute, die Gruppen stellen nach berühmten Bildern, sind seiner Urwirkung näher, als die lauten Ekstatiker, weil sie zu ahnen scheinen, daß Bilder nur Gebärden verlangen. Und wenn wir doch sprechen, sind unsere Worte nur die versetzten und zufällig tönenden Gebärden des Körpers, die man in Unkenntniß ihres Willens in der Mundhöhle zusammengedrängt hat. Irgend ein Bild entsteht, wenn die anfänglich erregte Pantomime der Einfälle beginnt in ihrem Lichte und auf dem Orte ihrer Aktion zu erstarren."

85 See sources listed in Chapter 6, note 2.

6 Pathological Puppets
The Body and the Marionette in Viennese Expressionism

> When I offered him the choice of any Javanese shadow puppet to make him happy, he chose the grotesque figure of a diabolical demon with an adventurous profile.[1]
> —Arthur Roessler, referring to Egon Schiele, 1922

As explored in the previous chapter, the modern marionette theater provided yet another opening through which expressive gestures entered Viennese visual culture. This conclusion challenges earlier findings that the photographs of hysterical patients published by Jean Martin-Charcot were the primary (or only) means by which the abnormal, grotesque, or pathological body was made available to artists associated with Viennese Secessionism and expressionism. Charcot did, of course, initiate the dialogue on the theatrics of human pathology, but he was not the only participant. I argue instead that taxonomies of the expressive, hysterical body followed a circuitous route before finding their place in Viennese expressionist painting. This body was first conceived in the Parisian clinic, then the Parisian stage, before moving to the German stage, and eventually to Viennese opera, theater, and cabaret performances. There, hystero-theatrical gestures were dramatized by living actors in the guise of hysterical madwomen or, in the case of Hugo von Hofmannsthal's *Oedipus Rex* (1906), a mad man. Expressive movements were simultaneously explored through the inanimate and uncanny puppet, which served as a metaphor for human nature interpreted in the modern marionette theater, especially as envisioned by Richard Teschner in the Austrian capital.

In terms of art historical discourse, the metaphorical *Puppe* played an important role in constructing narratives of modern art in post-expressionist styles, especially German Dada and surrealism. To focus narrowly on the significance of these metaphorical bodies in Hannah Höch's Dada dolls, Oskar Schlemmer's mechanized dancers in the Triadic Ballet, Hans Bellmer's photographs of his fabricated *Puppen*, or Max Ernst's painted automatons and their respective relationship to Freud's writings, is nevertheless to overlook the centrality of the *Puppe* motif in earlier articulations of modernist theater and painting.[2] The debt owed by Bellmer to Oskar Kokoschka's (sex) doll, appropriately called "Der Fetisch" (The Fetish, 1919), and Schlemmer's and Tristan Tzara's interest in Kokoschka's puppet-inspired plays, cannot be neglected.[3] In fact, it is clear that the expressionists adopted the doll, the puppet, and the marionette before the Dadaists and the surrealists began using them as appropriate metaphors for the human body, diseased or otherwise.[4]

The present chapter presents a more nuanced interpretation of the semiotics of gestures enacted by both living and inanimate bodies as a means to confront further representations of the modern body and its relation to the crisis of vision and language that unfolded in turn-of-the-century Vienna. More specifically, this examination explores theatrical productions created by Kokoschka and Arthur Schnitzler that included actors in the guise of pathological puppets or metaphorical marionettes. Kokoschka and Egon Schiele likewise serve as key figures in the realm of the visual arts, given that a number of their images incorporate representations of actual dolls, or of human bodies fashioned into depictions of the pathological puppet. What is more, Kokoschka's artistic activities at the famed Cabaret Fledermaus often blurred the boundary between avant-garde art and theater, since a number of his early expressionist plays highlighted the puppet-like or hystero-theatrical gestures "enacted" by subjects in his paintings. However, before delving into Kokoschka's complex and multifarious works, or Schiele's analogous exploration of diseased puppets in painted form, it is worth surveying the psychologically charged puppet plays and pantomimes written by one of Kokoschka's contemporaries, Arthur Schnitzler, who set the stage for expressionist explorations of humans as marionettes in *fin-de-siècle* Viennese theater.

Playing God: Schnitzler and the Puppet Master Motif

Schnitzler is best remembered today as a prominent turn-of-the-century Austrian novelist and playwright, due in large part to the success of his early play *Reigen* (*Roundelay*, or *Hands Round*, 1897) and the novella he wrote in his mature years, *Traumnovelle* (*Dream Story*, 1926). Given his acumen for dramatic literature, it is perhaps surprising that Schnitzler's early professional life was not founded in the world of books or theater. Instead, he received a prestigious medical degree from the University of Vienna in 1885 and worked as a physician and psychiatrist at Vienna's General Hospital in the last years of the nineteenth century. In this sense, Schnitzler's early career draws a distinct parallel to Freud's, even though the two men had not even met by 1922.

The similarities between Schnitzler and Freud have been well documented in the academic literature: both had been assistants to the Austrian neurologist Theodor Meynert at the University of Vienna, both were from prominent Austro-German Jewish families, and both had studied hypnosis and dream analysis by the turn of the century.[5] Schnitzler had reviewed Freud's translation of Charcot's texts, and scholars have also argued that Freudian theories greatly contributed to the development of Schnitzler's unique prose style and psychologically charged characters.[6] In a now-famous letter from 14 May 1922, Freud addressed Schnitzler as his elusive "doppelgänger," stating: "Your determinism, like your skepticism, your affection for the truths of the unconscious, for the instinctual nature of man, your dismantling of culturally conventional certainties, [and] the adherence of your thoughts on the polarity of life and death: all of this touched me with an uncanny familiarity."[7] Urszula Kawalec has argued that Freud's translation of Charcot's twenty-third and twenty-fourth lectures in *Leçons sur les maladies du système nerveux* (*New Lectures on the Diseases of the Nervous System, Concerning Hysteria*, 1886) had a profound effect on Schnitzler's understanding of hypnosis, since Charcot believed hypnosis was primarily effective on hysterical patients.[8] Unlike Freud, however, Schnitzler never published his thoughts on hypnotism as a formal treatise. Instead, he embraced hysterical gesticulations as an expressive body language and explored the theatricality of hypnotized bodies in his various plays, pantomimes, and stories. It is all the more telling that all of Schnitzler's publications on modern psychopathology were written as theatrical or literary works, and not as medical or scientific studies.[9]

Schnitzler's fascination with hypnosis thus stemmed from his dual interest in psychology and theater or, perhaps, the drama of modern psychology. He consequently incorporated demonstrations of hypnotism into two of his earliest plays: the one-act drama entitled *Anatol* (1888–92, performed in 1889, published in 1893), in which the titular character hypnotizes his female lover in order to learn of her supposed infidelity, and the contemporaneous one-act play titled *Paracelsus* (1898), which Schnitzler wrote as a tragic pantomime incorporating the convulsive gestures of a hypnotized actress who becomes mesmerized by Paracelsus, the sixteenth-century Swiss-German Renaissance physician and occultist.[10] These early "hypnotic" plays also make clear that Schnitzler, like Hofmannsthal, helped to introduce Viennese theater culture—via dramatic texts, rather than medical publications—to the aestheticized movements of hysteria. This interest in theatrical hypnosis as a means of mimicking pathological maladies also found its way into other dramatic works by Kokoschka, Hofmannsthal, and Richard Beer-Hofmann, all of whom explored this aspect of the modern body in pantomimes staged at the Fledermaus in the early years of the twentieth century.[11]

The prevalence of hysterical and hypnotic gestures in Schnitzler's "pathological" pantomimes was also a feature of his numerous puppet plays. Foremost among these particular works is the *Marionetten* (*Marionettes*) trilogy of 1906, which reveals the dramatist's recurring interest in the symbolic theme of the *Puppenspieler*, or puppet master. Although Schnitzler conceived of *Marionettes* as a single work comprised of three separate acts, the trilogy was in fact organized around three earlier one-act plays: *Der Puppenspieler: Studie in einem Aufzug* (*The Puppet Master: Study in One Act*, 1903), *Der tapfere Cassian: Puppenspiel in einem Akt* (*The Gallant Cassian: Puppet Play in One Act*, 1904), and *Zum großen Wurstel: Burleske in einem Akt* (*The Great Prater Puppet Theater: Burlesque in One Act*, 1905). Prior to being consolidated into a single cycle, each of these plays was published independently in Viennese newspapers and journals, and also appeared on the theatrical stage between 1903 and 1906 in Berlin and Vienna.[12] The works were not, however, the first of Schnitzler's plays to explore the *Puppenspieler* motif, as he had also incorporated this theme into *Paracelsus*, whose eponymous character uses mesmerism to manipulate others as though they were his puppets.[13] The role of Schnitzler's manipulative puppet master was subsequently developed through other characters, including "Georg Merklin" in *The Puppet Master*, "Martin" in *The Gallant Cassian*, "The Unknown" in *The Great Prater Puppet Theater*, and "Pierrot" in Schnitzler's later pantomime entitled *Die Verwandlungen des Pierrot* (*The Metamorphoses of Pierrot*, 1908).[14] It is also important to note that many of Schnitzler's puppet-inspired plays predate Teschner's marionette company, and may therefore subsist as the earliest manifestation of modern puppet theater in *fin-de-siècle* Vienna.

In the *Marionettes* trilogy, each act integrated the artistic device of metatheatricality, or the motif of a play-within-a-play, which deliberately added a level of confusion for the actual *fin-de-siècle* audiences who saw these plays performed. Schnitzler often blurred the boundary between what was "real" and what was illusory, a distinction that is always somewhat paradoxical in theater. Harold Segel has argued that the "illusion-versus-reality dichotomy" in Schnitzler's work is at the very heart of *fin-de-siècle*, neo-romantic agendas, though it is equally important to recognize that it was not necessarily intended to juxtapose the semblance of reality against the theatricality of illusion; instead, it highlights Schnitzler's attempt to distort the audience's notions of reality and illusion in *any* dramatic production, particularly when meta-theatricality was used to showcase a puppet play within the larger play.[15] The simple fact that the trilogy occasionally incorporated human actors in the guise of marionettes suggests that the living actor had, quite ironically, become the puppet's doppelgänger, rather than the reverse.

This was certainly the case with the third act of the cycle (or third play), *The Great Prater Puppet Theater*, in which real actors played the part of marionettes suspended from visible strings controlled by "The Unknown," a character that assumes the role of the puppet master, but is symbolically understood to be Fate or Death.[16] At the conclusion of the play, The Unknown appears on stage and cuts the strings of the actors-as-puppets, thereby causing the "marionettes" to fall into a massive heap at the feet of the play's "false" audience—that is, at the feet of actors playing the part of audience members watching the "puppet" drama). More importantly, the actors who were playing the part of the audience were meant to parody real-life Viennese audiences and their conservative bourgeois attitudes toward Schnitzler's sexually provocative and psychologically driven plays.[17] What is particularly fascinating about the use of actors in the guise of marionettes in *The Great Prater Puppet Theater* is the realization that puppets or marionettes no longer serve as metaphorical body doubles for humans controlled by external forces. Instead, Schnitzler required human actors to mimic the lifelessness of inanimate objects in order to raise existential questions about humanity's presumed autonomy in the world. The actors therefore had to communicate that they, as symbolic representatives of mankind, had, in fact, become manipulated puppets.

In Schnitzler's second puppet play, *The Gallant Cassian*, one finds an important link between cabaret, marionette theater, and burlesque entertainment, as well as the popular *fin-de-siècle* trope of the femme fatale.[18] In nineteenth and early twentieth-century Vienna, burlesque (like some cabaret and marionette performances) was a form of theatrical entertainment that utilized humor, satire, and even grotesque exaggerations to amuse audiences—all features that intrigued Schnitzler. Unlike the other two puppet plays in his trilogy, *The Gallant Cassian* was specifically written as a marionette performance, or *Puppenspiel*, though it could feasibly have been performed by living actors in the guise of puppets, as in *The Great Prater Puppet Theater*.[19] As the drama unfolds, we learn that Martin, the would-be puppet master, manipulates his girlfriend Sophie into believing he loves her, when in reality he is only using her as a temporary romantic distraction. The audience soon discovers that Martin is instead madly obsessed with a ballet/burlesque dancer named Eleonora Lambriani. As an avid gambler and a generally duplicitous character, Martin decides to secretly abandon Sophie in order to travel to Homburg to win a small fortune and then tempt the sensuous dancer away from her current lover, the Duke of Altenburg. As his infatuation matures, Martin becomes fixated on winning the beguiling ballerina for himself, and consequently vows (in a private conversation with his cousin, Cassian) to offer Eleonora his money, his heart, and his life. Martin even declares at one point to "love her like a madman," even though the two have never once spoken to one another.[20] The root of his mad obsession, he explains, resides in the fact that the beautiful Eleonora danced, and in so doing, altered his mind and his heart.

Consistent with Schnitzler's use of foreshadowing and irony as effective theatrical devices within his puppet plays, the audience begins to sense that things might not fare so well for the manipulative puppet master. Toward the beginning of the play Sophie confronts Martin about his supposed interest in the exquisite ballerina, which Martin denies. Sophie, however, is not reassured by his cool answer and proclaims:

> How I see her there before me! Like quivering snakes in snow, her black locks curled over her shoulders. Everyone who saw her was mad with delight. And the crown prince threw red roses to her down on stage. Oh, I recall it still![21]

Martin again declares that he does not remember the dancer or her name, provoking Sophie to advise him not to be enticed by false women or seductive dancers who wander the world without a home.[22] When Sophie leaves to prepare supper for Martin and their guest, Cassian, the latter confronts Martin about his love-struck feelings for the young Eleonora. Throughout Cassian's conversation with Martin, the seductive dancer is revealed to be a dangerous femme fatale, and Martin to be a dim-witted fool, as the following excerpt shows:

CASSIAN: What's wrong with you?
MARTIN: I get giddy whenever I speak her name.
CASSIAN: Eleonora Lambriani?—The mistress of the Duke of Altenburg?
MARTIN: Was [his mistress]!
CASSIAN: She who danced at night in the garden of the Palace of Fontainebleau before the King of France and his officers without a veil—?
MARTIN: [Speaking about the king] An idiot, who understands nothing! She was intoxicated by her own beauty.
CASSIAN: She who threw the Count of Leigang out the window, into the courtyard, so that the dogs rushed upon him and tore off an ear—?
MARTIN: It was only one story high, and he still has the other one—
CASSIAN: She who once swore that for ninety-nine nights she would make a new lover happy every night, none of whom was allowed to be less than a prince—who kept her oath, and on the hundredth night took a Savoy boy with his street organ to her bedchamber?
MARTIN: Yes, it's her, it's her! The woeful, the most glorious, the most beautiful! And I want her—I must have her! And then die![23]

Throughout this amusing *tête-à-tête* regarding Eleonora's virtues and vices, the audience learns that the sensuous performer has not only lured Martin toward literal and figurative madness, but has equally caused him to accept death as a worthy price for the opportunity to win her love, or at least her loins. When Cassian cautions Martin against Eleonora's ruinous attributes and past indiscretions, particularly with the unfortunate Count of Leigang, Schnitzler cleverly alludes to the conclusion of the play, when both Sophie and Cassian jump from a window as a result of scorned love. This particular plot twist develops when Martin, the great gambler, bets and loses Sophie—who has now fallen in love with Cassian—in a game of dice. Martin soon becomes distraught and challenges Cassian to a duel, which he loses. Cassian, running Martin through with his sword, then mockingly enquires about Eleonora's whereabouts while Martin lies bleeding on the floor, suggesting that he, Cassian, will take his cousin's place in Homburg and ultimately win the alluring dancer for himself. Overcome by the news that her new love interest will also leave her for Eleonora, Sophie throws herself from the window, only to be caught by the gallant Cassian, who leaps out to rescue her. In end effect, Martin is unsuccessful in controlling Cassian and Sophie as his puppets and, as alluded to earlier in the play, ultimately pays with his life for having loved and lusted after the dancing femme fatale. In the ironic climax of the play, Martin, the would-be puppet master, is instead revealed to be the one who is manipulated, having become the puppet of Sophie, Cassian, Eleonora, and poetic justice.

Although there are no known photographs of performances of the play at the Fledermaus, or of its premiere on 22 November 1904 at the Kleines Theater in Berlin, it is easy to surmise that the gestures enacted by Schnitzler's marionettes were instrumental in conveying the *Puppenspieler* motif with clarity, as well as communicating Martin's madness for Eleonora, which was no doubt exaggerated by the mechanically awkward movements of the marionette's limbs. It is unlikely, however, that Schnitzler's inanimate objects replicated the hystero-theatrical gestures enacted by actresses like Anna Bahr-Mildenburg or Maud Allan in *fin-de-siècle* Vienna with any precision. This notwithstanding, characters in *The Gallant Cassian* highlight the fact that modern psychology—as revealed through the recurrent puppet master theme and in Martin's attempts to manipulate his fellow puppets, as well as in the theatrical femme fatale represented by the enigmatic Eleonora Lambriani—had a direct impact on other forms of avant-garde theater, including plays and pantomimes focused on the metaphorical *Puppe*. In this instance, Schnitzler's "high" theatrical works were referencing, incorporating, and even mimicking "low" puppet plays. It was through this reversal of artistic and cultural hegemony that Viennese audiences no doubt understood Schnitzler's *Marionettes* trilogy to be particularly modern.

Tellingly, Schnitzler's interest in the marionette theater, which had previously been relegated to the apparently less important world of children's entertainment, developed at a time when the Vienna Secession and Jung Wien were collectively embracing childhood and youthfulness as periods of artistic inspiration. As previously analyzed, the Secession emphatically adopted the mantra of rebellious adolescence, embracing the theme of childlike creativity in its 1902 exhibition *The Child as Artist*. Schnitzler's *Marionettes* trilogy reveals, however, that his interest in puppet gestures was not simply focused on the marionette as a plaything for children, but rather, that the puppet—acting as a doppelgänger for the human actor—could possess and convey adult sexual desire, as with Martin in *The Gallant Cassian*. The stylized and manipulated movements of Schnitzler's psychological marionettes (whether in the form of human actors or actual puppets) can therefore be seen to parallel—though not recreate verbatim—the expressive gestures enacted by human actors in Vienna, including Bahr-Mildenburg and Allan, who employed these pathological movements as instruments with which to disseminate a semiotic language of the modern body.

Kokoschka's Uncanny Puppets and Dolls

Like Schnitzler, Kokoschka investigated the potential for inanimate bodies to convey a sense of modernity in puppet plays and burlesques staged at the Fledermaus, with the difference that his artistic goal was to blur the line between avant-gardist drama and visual art. Following his studies at the Vienna School of Arts and Crafts—where

Teschner and Gustav Klimt had also studied—Kokoschka gravitated toward the Wiener Werkstätte, where he worked as a student artist between 1907 and 1909. Through his involvement with the Werkstätte, he participated in a number of collaborative projects, including the creation of the Fledermaus as a modern Viennese example of the *Gesamtkunstwerk*. Kokoschka worked as an artist, designer, and playwright at the cabaret, thus revealing his desire to synthesize the visual and performing arts into a single *oeuvre*. His latently erotic, illustrated poem *The Dreaming Youths* (1907–08, see Figure 1.2)—the lithographs for which were produced by the Werkstätte and first exhibited at the 1908 Kunstschau—had actually debuted half a year earlier in 1907 in the form of a dramatic reading (without images) given at the newly opened Fledermaus.[24] Three additional theatrical works quickly followed: a shadow puppet play called *Das getupfte Ei* (*The Speckled Egg*, first performed at the *Fledermaus* in October 1907, and again in March 1909); *Sphinx und Strohmann: Komödie für Automaten* (*Sphinx and Scarecrow: A Comedy for Automatons*, conceived in 1907, and performed at the Fledermaus in 1909); and his most famous one-act expressionist play: *Mörder, Hoffnung der Frauen* (*Murderer, Hope of Women*, first performed at the Kunstschau in 1909). While *Murderer, Hope of Women* was written as a spectacle of theatrical gesture and movement, and was therefore less concerned with spoken word content, the first two plays were designed as more traditional theatrical pieces, rather than expressive poetry for the stage. More interestingly still, both *The Speckled Egg* and *Sphinx and Scarecrow* revolved explicitly around the theme of the manipulated marionette.

Sphinx and Scarecrow was historically performed as an unrestricted, quasi-improvisational theatrical piece by students at the School of Arts and Crafts in 1907, and was later produced as two, more-refined, full-scale productions held at the Fledermaus in 1909.[25] Two years later, visual illustrations for the play reached a wider Germanic audience when Kokoschka published an etching, appropriately titled *Sphinx und Strohmann*, on the front cover of the 11 March 1911 issue of the Berlin-based modern art magazine *Der Sturm* (*The Storm*), to which he regularly contributed throughout the *fin de siècle*.[26] Like Schnitzler's *The Great Prater Puppet Theater*, Kokoschka's *Sphinx and Scarecrow* was imbued with the theatrics and metaphorical connotations of a play performed by actors in the guise of marionettes. Its subtitle, *A Comedy for Automatons*, makes this point clear, even though living actors, not puppets, consistently performed the role of the automatons during the play's early incarnations at the art school and the cabaret.[27] Rather than presenting a meta-theatrical motif, or suggesting that Fate was responsible for manipulating the strings of the puppet-like actors, Kokoschka instead focused on the idea that the body (whether puppet, human, or a hybrid of both) is controlled by one's libidinal desires, which in turn are manipulated by other humans.

In the play, the male protagonist, Firdusi, is a victim to his carnal nature, and is thus manipulated by his alluring and adulteress wife, Lilly, the "sphinx" in the work's title.[28] Firdusi, who wears a large, straw-filled, scarecrow-like head throughout the play, is revealed as a witless man who is all too easily controlled by the wiles of his seductive and unfaithful wife. The power of the femme fatale over her simple-minded husband is portrayed comically when Firdusi, believing Lilly to be another woman altogether, unknowingly marries his wife for a second time. Kokoschka's refashioning of the popular symbolist motif of the seductive and destructive sphinx suggests that the Viennese artist regarded this particular incarnation of the femme fatale—now acting as a puppet master—as fertile territory for expressionist drama. By attempting to recapture the dialectics of this metaphorical construct, however, Kokoschka essentially reinforced the idea that the fatal woman manipulates men, and in turn is controlled by her carnal, murderous desires. Accordingly, Kokoschka's play proposes that a sphinx does not have to materialize as a mythological, hybrid creature but can more cunningly survive as a mortal woman: the femme fatale in plain sight, but in the guise of a man's wife, rather than an ancient monster.

It is equally plausible that the male and female characters in *Sphinx and Scarecrow* were meant to represent adult versions of the stringless, adolescent "marionettes" that appear in *The Awakening*, a lithograph from *The Dreaming Youths* (Figure 1.2). In this fantastical, dreamlike image, Kokoschka places four pubescent youths—three who are presumably maidens, and one androgynous figure at the left of the composition—in a skewed landscape replete with bizarre plant formations that recall the golden, Orientalist foliage in Klimt's *Judith I* (1901, Plate 6). In terms of style, the image seems to reference European folk art or Japanese woodblock prints, both of which were used as artistic sources at the turn of the century by Europeans seeking to capture a purity believed to be inherent in the expressiveness of "primitive," outsider, or non-European art. So-called "primitive" aesthetics also aligned with expressionism's interest in youth as a symbolic period in which innocence dictated a deeper sense of reality free from the strict and often hypocritical mores that governed bourgeois Viennese society.[29] Metaphorically, *The Awakening* thus suggests that adolescence is a bridge between incorruptibility and innocence lost, between man's "primitive" nature and society's "civilized" constraints. In this way, Kokoschka's exploration of burgeoning adolescence in the original dramatic reading of *The Dreaming Youths*, as well as the later printed suite, is comparable to modernist plays by Schnitzler and Frank Wedekind (think of Wedekind's *Spring Awakening*), which challenged social mores in order to confront *fin-de-siècle* audiences with culturally taboo topics.[30] This understanding of *The Dreaming Youths* as an "inappropriate" exploration of adolescent sexuality was tellingly addressed in the contemporary critical press in Vienna, which, like the negative reviews that later surrounded Kokoschka's Hagenbund paintings, largely disliked the print cycle.[31]

By viewing *The Awakening* as a synecdoche for Kokoschka's larger print series, I want to assert that the deliberately androgynous figures in the image can be read as further examples of *fin-de-siècle* marionettes, albeit ones given a flattened and graphic form, and whose libidinal bodies Kokoschka purposefully manipulates in his role as the omnipotent puppet master. Like Firdusi and Lilly in *Sphinx and Scarecrow*, the figures in *The Awakening* cannot be understood as autonomous characters in control of their own fates or bodies, but must be viewed as two-dimensional puppets or dolls controlled by the artist's visual language. Kokoschka referenced this motif temporally during contemporary performances of *Sphinx and Scarecrow*, where the choreography performed by the acting troupe was symbolically, if not literally, read as the mechanized movements of automatons. In this sense, a further parallel can be drawn between Schnitzler's emphasis on the sexualized puppet, particularly in *The Gallant Cassian*, and Kokoschka's analogous exploration of eroticized puppet bodies. In *The Awakening*, this metaphor is revealed visually through androgynous physiques that confuse the viewer's understanding of what kind of body he or she is looking at. If read through the language of semiotics, this disjuncture between the signified (the idea or notion of what a gendered body should look like) and the sign (the artist's construction of pubescent bodies in printed form) becomes somewhat arbitrary, since the signifier (the body) theoretically has no fixed meaning, particularly in a work of art that does not contain actual bodies anyway.

It is precisely the lack of any fixed meaning that was undoubtedly upsetting to Kokoschka's contemporary audiences. One must therefore question whether *The Awakening* contains pre-pubescent childlike bodies, or instead shows post-pubescent adult bodies. The title of the work suggests that the figures are children rather than adults, but the lack of a strong understanding of age and gender ultimately leaves this question unanswered. It is clear, however, that Kokoschka mapped aspects of the uncanny puppet body onto the human bodies in the print, as witnessed in the static and awkward positioning of the figures' limbs—particularly their raised, bent, or outstretched arms—which look as though they are being controlled by invisible strings or rods. These gestures, though not expressly hysterical, bring a contrived and theatrical element to the work, and visually imply that the bodies are affixed to appendages that can easily be manipulated by the hands of the artist. As such, it is not so much that Kokoschka's puppets materialize as pathological agents, but that he, as the ultimate puppet master and creator of the image, is exposed as the "abnormal" artist who has sexualized what ought to have remained asexual: that is, the body of pubescent youths.

As discussed in the previous chapter, a crisis of language struck Vienna in the early twentieth century, leaving it in a predicament that shaped the relationship between written and spoken words, visual or gestural languages, and the artistic body. Given that Kokoschka's *The Dreaming Youths* was printed as an illustrated story, rather than as an autonomous print cycle, or left as an image-less dramatic reading (as in its earliest incarnation), it is clear that this particular work was caught in the historical interplay between words and images. To reinforce this point, the expressive quality of the work's printed text is dictated by the poem's omniscient narrator, a character often interpreted as the symbolic incarnation of Kokoschka as an adolescent boy. At one moment in the story, the narrator addresses a girl named Li, stating: "I want to visualize the childlike tremors of your shoulders and see how your mouth seeks to speak for me without words."[32] Given the emphasis on "visualizing" and "seeing" in the boy's statement, each clause in the sentence ties his words to the temporal world, suggesting that if a metaphorical realm does exist within the work, it is in addition to the corporeal experience to which these youths bear witness. What the boy visualizes or hopes to see is the female body undergoing a change from youthful androgyny to sexual maturity. Given the boy's desire for the girl to grow into a sexual being, presumably for his own erotic benefit, it is intriguing to wonder if Kokoschka intended the girl Li to emerge in *The Dreaming Youths* as a child version of the sexualized Lilly in *Sphinx and Scarecrow*. Kokoschka initially conceived the two works together in 1907, and the names of the two main female characters are certainly connected ("Li" and "Lilly"), so perhaps he envisioned *The Dreaming Youths* to serve as a prequel to *Sphinx and Scarecrow*, and the girl Li to represent the innocent incarnation of the femme fatale in the play.

With this in mind, Kokoschka's text can also be seen to imply that the biological or sexual development of Li/Lilly's pubescent female body in *The Dreaming Youths* can be witnessed directly through the tremors of her shoulders. In the boy's statement, the first half of the sentence establishes the erotic overtones of the work, which merge into a more complete understanding of the work as a series of images and texts that visually and linguistically represent the intangible notion of burgeoning sensual love. The second half of the boy's statement, on the other hand, establishes the symbolic and poetic realm in which the characters reside: a place where young males and females are able to communicate with one another without words. This seems to suggest that the body and its gestures have replaced the mouth and the mind as the primary agents of communication, and that the girl's aural expressions are ultimately unnecessary, since her body can be controlled (as one would manipulate a doll or puppet) to communicate her libidinal desires to the boy. Her ability to speak without words suggests that an unseen ventriloquist is controlling her mouth and actions, and allows us to return to Hofmannsthal's belief that the language of the modern body was more expressive and more powerful than spoken words. In *The Dreaming Youths*, this device ultimately reveals Kokoschka's dual role within his illustrated story: he is both narrator (the youthful boy) and puppet master (the creator of meaning through words and images).

The centrality of the puppet motif in Kokoschka's early dramatic works was further expressed in his shadow puppet show *The Speckled Egg* (1907), and in a later piece entitled *Der Weisse Tiertöter* (*The White Animal Slayer*, 1909), both of which provided literal and figurative examinations of the inanimate body in motion. In his book *Pinocchio's Progeny* (1995), Harold Segel suggests that *The Speckled Egg* was based on Indian folklore, and thus reveals Kokoschka's interest in Oriental miniatures, whereas Robert Whalen argues, somewhat differently, that the play was created in response to Balinese shadow theater.[33] First unveiled at the Fledermaus a week after the cabaret opened its doors, *The Speckled Egg* presented audiences with the first known public performance of an Asian-inspired, shadow puppet play in the Austrian capital, a novelty that must have added to the appeal of Kokoschka's piece. The puppets, however, were not precisely modeled on Asian shadow figures, since Kokoschka created the flat figures from painted paper glued to slim copper sheets. Like traditional European marionettes, his thin shadow puppets were constructed with movable joints that could be controlled by the puppet master via a spring mechanism. Kokoschka then placed the figures inside a lighted box containing a large mirror, and when the silhouettes of the puppets were projected to the audience, the overall effect was similar to that of an Indian or Indonesian shadow show. *The White Animal Slayer*, which followed two years later and was performed alongside a reading of *The Dreaming Youths* at the Fledermaus in March 1909, was, by contrast, created as a more conventional puppet play, in which flat painted figures cut from paper were moved by hand within a small box resembling a proscenium stage, not unlike Teschner's Golden Shrine.[34] Although Teschner was working in Prague during the premiere of *The Speckled Egg*, it is conceivable that he saw Kokoschka's *The White Animal Slayer* and incorporated aspects of Kokoschka's various puppet stages into his own by 1911.

Furthermore, Kokoschka's introduction of Asian puppet theater into Viennese visual culture, which occurred before the establishment of Teschner's second marionette company, was very much in keeping with similar practices popularized in clubs and cabarets throughout turn-of-the century Europe.[35] Segel has explored the intricate relationship that developed between European puppet theater, avant-garde cabarets, and modernist literature produced during the late nineteenth and early twentieth centuries, arguing that the first two were "an area of creativity" for the latter.[36] When combined with additional investigations offered by Peter Jelavich and Scott Shershow, Segel's research paints a clearer picture of the importance given to puppets and marionettes in *fin-de-siècle* visual culture. According to Jelavich, the first modern European puppet plays—performed, incidentally, as burlesques—were staged at Le Chat Noir (The Black Cat) in Paris in 1885.[37] Recognizing that his wealthy bourgeois clientele were readily attracted to these flamboyant burlesques and shadow shows, Rodolphe Salis, with the help of Henri Rivière, transformed his club's small and peripheral *cabaret artistique* into a thriving, profitable, and fashionable *théâtre d'ombres* (shadow theater) by the mid-1880s.[38] Despite the puppet theater's association with Le Mirliton (The Reed Pipe: a more vulgar Parisian cabaret of the period), both of these clubs remained "artistically respectable" venues for more than a decade.[39]

Having thrived in the nightclubs of Paris—the litmus test for most profitable avant-gardist activities in the late nineteenth century—these modern, often crude puppet dramas eventually made their way to cabarets in Berlin, Munich, and Vienna.[40] Günter Böhmer notes that shadow puppetry had a significant influence on the Austro-German romantic movement, and subsequently found fertile ground in Germanic cabarets, even becoming a significant part of the theatrical repertoire of Munich's Schwabinger Schattenspiele (Schwabing Shadow Theater) by 1906.[41] Segel argues, however, that the raw energy, morbid poetry, shadow shows, and pantomimes that attracted the bourgeoisie in Paris, Barcelona, and Munich to these avant-garde clubs "found little resonance in the aristocratic elegance and bourgeois liberalism of turn-of-the-century Vienna."[42] It appears then, that anti-bourgeois puppetry, which in truth was embraced by a number of young expressionists in Vienna, including Kokoschka and Schiele, emerged not as crude burlesques, but as "serious" expressionist plays by Kokoschka, Schnitzler, and Teschner, who either explored the *Puppenspieler* motif in actual puppet plays, or in theatrical productions that employed living actors playing marionettes.

Kokoschka was not only interested in the puppet theme in the realm of theater. He also explored the symbolic relationship between puppet and puppet master in a number of sketches and oil paintings based on a life-sized doll he had commissioned to represent Alma Mahler, the widow of the composer Gustav Mahler, and Kokoschka's lover between 1912 and 1914 (see Figure 6.1).[43] Designed by Kokoschka

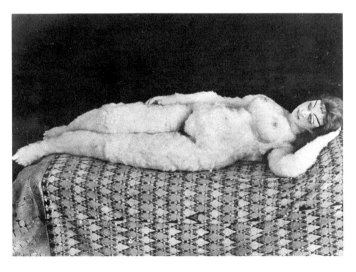

Figure 6.1 Unknown, *Oskar Kokoschka's Alma-Puppe as Venus*, circa 1918–19, photograph. Private Collection.

Source: Photo: Courtesy Richard Nagy Ltd., London.

and constructed between 1918 and 1919 by Hermine Moos, a Munich-based doll and dressmaker, the *Alma Puppe* became the subject of at least two major oil paintings and twenty drawings created by Kokoschka between 1919 and 1922. Kokoschka variously referred to the *Puppe* as "the fetish," his "beloved," and the "Silent Woman;" and given the scandalous nature of this would-be "sex surrogate," the doll understandably drew attention to the artist during the postwar period, in large part due to the fact that Kokoschka often took the *Puppe* with him in public.[44] More recently, the Alma doll has enjoyed the attention of scholars who have examined it as a metaphorical muse and object of artistic self-promotion, rather than a scandalous sex toy.[45] Peter Gorsen has argued that the doll was a clever modernization of the ancient Pygmalion myth, while Lisa Street has instead analyzed the object alongside Kokoschka's interest in turn-of-the-century puppetry and the more general interest in dolls among avant-garde Austrian writers, including Rainer Maria Rilke. She has also looked at the importance of these objects in works by Zürich and Dresden-based Dadaists that Kokoschka collaborated with.[46] Building on Street's re-evaluation of the doll as a serious work of art, Bonnie Roos has scrutinized the relationship that existed between it, Moos, and Kokoschka, as well as the manner in which this artistic collaboration was dissimilar from the proliferation of commercial mannequins in post-war Europe and the artistic interest in mannequins as lifeless objects of capitalistic desire.[47] Roos additionally suggests that Lotte Pritzel, who Kokoschka first approached with the project, apparently rejected the commission because she thought it would be too scandalous for her reputation, whereas Moos may instead have hoped to convey "a certain bravado in her character" by accepting Kokoschka's unconventional request.[48]

Two paintings in particular, *Frau in Blau* (*Woman in Blue*, circa 1920, Figure 6.2) and *Mann mit Puppe* (*Man with Doll*, circa 1922, Figure 6.3), as well as an ink drawing entitled *Sitzende "Frau" mit entblößten Brüsten* (*Seated "Woman" with Exposed Breasts*, circa 1920, Figure 6.4) all portray the Alma doll. However, the fact

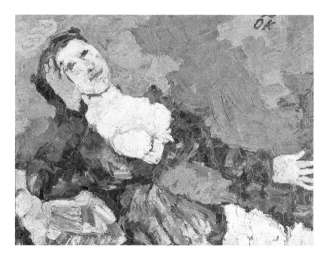

Figure 6.2 Oskar Kokoschka, *Woman in Blue*, circa 1920, oil on canvas. Staatsgalerie, Stuttgart.

that these images are representations of the puppet is not immediately clear, since it could be assumed that they contained expressionistic representations of the real (that is, the actual, living) Alma Mahler. Yet it is precisely this confusion on the part of the viewer as to whether he or she is viewing a human body or its inanimate doppelgänger that makes Kokoschka's "doll" paintings and drawings so intriguing. This conundrum returns us to the discourse surrounding the metaphorical puppet or doll, and to Kokoschka's understanding of his "fetish" as an uncanny object created around the theme of the crisis of language and vision that pervades his early work. This contention is especially relevant in relation to visual works that portray puppet-like humans, as in the double-portrait of *Hans Tietze and Erica Tietze-Conrat* (Plate 1), in prints from *The Dreaming Youths*, namely *The Awakening* (Figure 1.2), and in paintings of the actual Alma doll, such as *Woman in Blue* and *Man with Doll*.

In a letter to Moos dated 10 December 1918, Kokoschka is explicit about his belief that the Alma doll must function as something other, or more, than an inanimate thing. He states:

> I beg you again to use all your imagination, all your sensitiveness for the ghostly companion you are preparing for me and to breathe into her such life that in the end, when you have finished the body, there is no spot which does not radiate feeling, to which you have not applied yourself to overcome by the most complex devices the dead material; then will all the delicate and intimate gifts of nature displayed in the female body be recalled to me in some desperate hour by some symbolic hieroglyph, or sign with which you have secretly endowed that bundle of rags.[49]

Perhaps the best way to conceptualize Kokoschka's understanding of this doppelgänger is to see it as an uncanny, lifeless object that was supposed to be capable of articulating the "unspeakable" aspects of the now absent body of the real Alma. The Alma doll calls attention to the double vision of the doll or puppet, as previously described by Steve Tillis, insofar as it was not a mass-produced (and therefore banal or

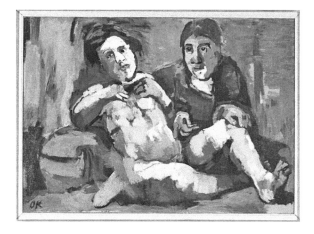

Figure 6.3 Oskar Kokoschka, *Man with Doll*, circa 1922, oil on canvas. Staatliche Museen zu Berlin, Nationalgalerie, Berlin.

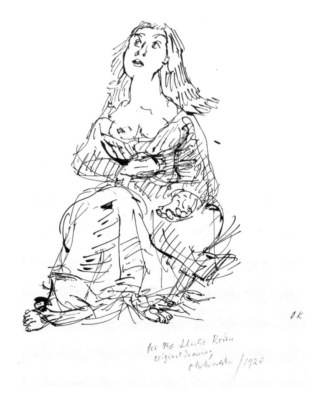

Figure 6.4 Oskar Kokoschka, *Seated "Woman" with Exposed Breasts*, circa 1920, ink on paper. Musée Jenisch, Stiftung Oskar Kokoschka, Vevey.

Source: © 2016 Fondation Oskar Kokoschka / Artists Rights Society (ARS), New York / ProLitteris, Zürich. © Oskar Kokoschka / DACS. Photo: akg-images.

characterless) mannequin, but instead a unique art object constructed on the actual measurements and corporeality of a single, living person. It seems, therefore, that the doll was deliberately created around the notion that the object *had* to be inherently uncanny, so that the "bundle of rags" would be readily familiar to Kokoschka, just as the body of the real Alma had been four years earlier.[50] But in this instance Kokoschka's artistic voyeurism reveals itself to be non-discriminating, for it desired to gaze on *any* female body, be that depictions of animate humans (including portraits of the real Alma) or inanimate *Puppen*. In this sense, the Alma doll—as the artist's fetish—joins the list of female bodies that were optically absorbed and artistically commodified by Kokoschka's modernist vision.

In *Woman in Blue*, the female doll reclines in a blue-gray dress, the bodice of which has come undone, revealing the right breast and a part of the left. When compared to the drawing entitled *Seated "Woman" with Exposed Breasts*, it is clear that the styling of the dress in both images implies that the sketch essentially served as the preparatory study for the slightly later painting. The desire to make sketches of the doll for the large-scale canvas suggests, moreover, that Kokoschka treated it as he would a living female model, albeit one whose body and gestures he could manipulate, control, and reposition with his own hands—both on the body of the actual doll, as well as in the representation of the doll in the painting. The doll's hands appear large and boneless, and her pose—which suggests that "she" is lost in dream-like revelry—gives the illusion that this body, like countless others in Kokoschka's *oeuvre*, was meant to represent a human sitter, albeit one with puppet-like features.

Kokoschka further demarcates the role of the puppet, the objectifying gaze, and the doll as a powerful doppelgänger in *Man with Doll*. The painting, which was sometimes entitled *Selbstbildnis mit liegendem Akt* (*Self-portrait with Reclining Nude*) and *Künstler und Puppe* (*Artist and Doll*) when it was shown in period exhibitions, is often regarded as an altogether unattractive self-portrait of the artist with the Alma doll. Interestingly, Kokoschka gave the painting yet another title—*Mann und Mädchen* (*Man and Girl*)—when it was shown at his 1925 retrospective exhibition in Dresden.[51] The vacillation between these slightly different titles suggests that the painter was deliberately exploiting the dual nature of the inanimate doll, which was both subject and object. In this sense, the Alma doll endures as the subject of two-dimensional paintings and drawings, but also as a three-dimensional art object whose familiarity to, and yet marked difference from, the body of the human Alma made it (and the paintings of it) all the more unsettling to the artist and the viewer.[52] In this regard, the grotesque doll—as the artist's fetish and uncanny muse—has much in common with the other manipulated, abnormal-looking female bodies that Kokoschka created during the early years of the twentieth century, including his *Portrait of Lotte Franzos* (Plate 4).

In analyzing *Man with Doll*, Roos posits that the painting introduces "Kokoschka's god-like control over the inanimate object even to the hint of ventriloquism."[53] Her suggestion that the painting may further allude to the body of the *Woman of Willendorf* (28,000–25,000 BCE)—and thus to the doll's potential function as a symbol of fertility for Kokoschka—is intriguing, particularly since the real Alma had secretly aborted their love child in 1914. As such, the Alma doll, as the uncanny body double of the real Alma, may have fulfilled Kokoschka's fantasy to successfully "procreate" with his former lover in the form of a sex doll. If this is the case, then the subject matter of the painting symbolically hints at the trauma of a love lost and then regained by means of a surrogate lover. One is left to ponder, moreover, if Kokoschka was metaphorically hoping to reinforce the notion that humans can become puppets or dolls manipulated by the hands, emotions, and whims of others—a concept that Schnitzler blatantly confronted in the *Marionettes* trilogy. As such, little distinction, if any, can be discerned visually between the inanimate features of the uncanny Alma doll, and those of Kokoschka's own "living form" in *Man with Doll*. Instead, the doll has been made flesh in the hands of the artist, or by contrast, and perhaps even more disturbingly, the living Kokoschka has been rendered lifeless in his own painting. This is a plausible reading of the image because the likeness of the real Alma was transferred to her inanimate doppelgänger, whereas Kokoschka's likeness becomes analogous to the stylistic treatment of the doll in the painting. But this artistic device operates on yet another level, since the living Kokoschka and the three-dimensional doll have both been rendered flat and lifeless within the two-dimensional picture plane. Whereas Schnitzler's marionettes could "speak" and "move" on stage, Kokoschka's doll and self-portrait exist only as muted and motionless objects in the hands of the artist-cum-puppet master. In so doing, Kokoschka reduces his own body to a flattened, doll-like form.

It is not known if Kokoschka was familiar with Freud's or Ernst Jentsch's essays on the *Unheimliche* when he was working on his own interpretation of uncanny objects, such as his painted studies of the Alma doll. This point may be inconsequential, as

Viennese artists and playwrights were all generally familiar with E. T. A. Hoffmann's "The Sandman" and Heinrich von Kleist's "On the Marionette Theater," both of which had previously addressed the role of the *Puppe* as a metaphorical entity capable of inspiring—even unsettling—its human counterparts. Within the current literature examining the *Unheimliche* and its relationship to the visual arts, it is all the more intriguing that Freud's essay remains the only pillar on which scholars have built a discourse of the uncanny body in European modern art, despite earlier analyses of this literary device having been offered by Hoffmann, Kleist, and Jentsch. The result is that few scholars have examined how painters and playwrights in turn-of-the-century Vienna, especially Kokoschka, were arguably the first to employ the puppet, doll, or marionette to convey a non-Freudian sense of the uncanny to their viewers. Kokoschka's *Man with Doll* and *Woman in Blue* are just two examples of expressionist paintings engaged in this discourse, and, more importantly, of canvases that highlight the conundrum that arises when a viewer is unsure whether or not he or she is looking at a representation of a human being or at that person's uncanny doppelgänger. More interesting still, this distinction may have been completely irrelevant to expressionists, who alternatively hoped to conflate semblances of the human body with the puppet body in order to construct the new and peculiar Viennese modern body.

Double Vision: Schiele and the Puppet Motif

Kokoschka's *oeuvre* reveals a clear interest in the metaphorical and psychologically charged puppet or doll—a fascination apparent in both his artistic and theatrical pieces, including his various puppet plays, his full-scale Alma doll, and subsequent images of the doll. Like Kokoschka, Schiele also explored the puppet motif in his visual art and actually emerges as the artist who most faithfully expressed the aesthetics of the pathological puppet body in Viennese expressionism. A number of scholars have previously suggested in passing that Schiele's artistic figures, particularly those of women, might be read as puppet-like or doll-like representations of a human sitter,[54] although to my knowledge nobody to date has seriously considered the puppet in relation to his larger *oeuvre*. Patrick Werkner, in fact, has argued that any attempt to place such a definitive reading on the artist's gestural language may be a fruitless enterprise. Werkner states that in Schiele's portraits,

> the expressive features of the face and the attitude of the hands become the trans-
> mitters of a body language, in the stylization of which a large number of recur-
> rent form motifs are to be observed. However to try to extract from this a canon
> of symbols that may be used to interpret Schiele's paintings would seem to lead
> us in the wrong direction.[55]

In contrast to this, I am asserting that the iconography of Schiele's grotesque, misshapen, and truncated figures (both male and female) are best explained alongside the *Modekrankheit* for expressive, pathological gestures, as filtered through the symbolic language of the modern puppet, doll, or marionette. As lifeless body doubles, puppets and their gestural language ostensibly demand a frank and open dialogue of otherwise unspeakable words and ideas that could more acceptably be mapped onto the bodies of these non-human doppelgängers. In other words, puppets became fitting muses—as well as deliberate targets—of socio-sexual discourses in expressionist artworks precisely because of their dialectical nature as uncanny objects.

My belief that the subjects of Schiele's various paintings and drawings share affinities with the aesthetics of the modern puppet is principally founded on the symbolic and iconographic similarities between his contorted, artistic bodies and the mechanical emulations of these inanimate objects. This connection aside, a more immediate and tangible historical anecdote reveals that the artist was interested in, and even owned, expressive puppets, particularly Javanese *wayang*. Although Schiele would certainly have known about Kokoschka's *The Speckled Egg*, and may have attended one of the performances of the show at the Fledermaus in 1907, his direct engagement with Orientalist puppetry came about through his long-time friend and promoter, Arthur Roessler. By the early twentieth century, Roessler had become a recognized essayist and critic, working for local newspapers and magazines like the daily *Wiener Arbeiterzeitung* (*Vienna Workers Newspaper*), as well as for more widely distributed art and theater journals like *Stage and World*.[56] Roessler was a supporter of Teschner's marionette theater and shared the latter's interest in the expressive qualities of *wayang*, which he discussed at length in a later book entitled *Richard Teschner* (1947).[57] Although the idea that Roessler personally introduced Schiele to Teschner is speculative, it is known that Roessler acquired a small number of Javanese puppets—presumably from Teschner—for his personal collection. A photograph of Roessler's study taken in, or around, 1920 (Figure 6.5) shows the critic's *wayang* shadow puppets hanging on the wall under Schiele's painting *Versinkende Sonne* (*Setting Sun*, 1913). The fact that Roessler juxtaposed these objects in his home highlights the importance he undoubtedly placed on Schiele's "high" art and the "low" puppets, and his curation of them represents a further challenge against such artistic distinctions.

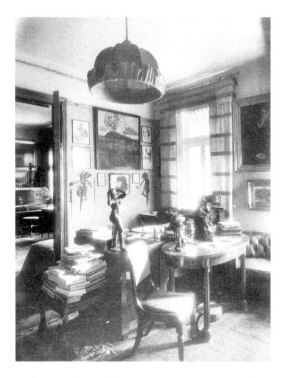

Figure 6.5 Arthur Roessler's study at Billrothstrasse 6 in Vienna, showing his Javanese puppets and Egon Schiele's *Setting Sun* on the back wall, circa 1920, photograph. Wien Museum Karlsplatz, Vienna.

Source: Photo: © Wien Museum.

In his book *Erinnerungen an Egon Schiele* (*Memories of Egon Schiele*, 1922), Roessler presents an invaluable collection of biographical essays detailing his inter-actions with the artist prior to Schiele's death in 1918. In one of these reminiscences, Roessler recalls Schiele's initial exposure to *wayang*, writing:

> For hours he could play with these figures without tiring of them and without say-ing a word. What was really astonishing from the outset was the skill with which Schiele manipulated the thin, moveable rods of the figures. When I offered him the choice of any Javanese shadow puppet to make him happy, he chose the grotesque figure of a diabolical demon with an adventurous profile. This figure greatly in-spired him. He was fascinated by the strictly stylized, expressive gestures, which were always extraordinary, and which often produced magically vivid shadow contours on the wall. "Such a figure can do more than our best female dancers. Compared to my red demon, Ruth [St. Denis] is a clodhopper," said he, as he lov-ingly admired his buffalo-hide demon. This Javanese figure remained his favorite plaything until his death, after which the artist's heirs returned it to me.[58]

Roessler's description of Schiele's interactions with the "demonic" puppet is signifi-cant for a number of reasons, as is the photograph of Roessler's study, which perhaps shows the actual puppet that Schiele had acquired from the critic. First and fore-most, Roessler's account confirms Schiele's clear interest in the expressive nature of *fin-de-siècle* puppets, as well as his more particular fascination with *wayang*. This is a significant historical point since Schiele, unlike Kokoschka, was not a playwright and therefore did not produce a body of dramatic literature centered on the *Puppenspieler* motif or the human actor in the guise of a pathological puppet. Second, Roessler's fatherly, almost endearing recollection of Schiele's childlike behavior when engaging with his "favorite plaything" reinforces the youthful sentiments latent in Schiele's manifesto for the New Art Group and in the Secession's earlier embrace of child-hood as a dominant theme in Jugendstil. It is equally helpful to note that Schiele first met Roessler in 1909, one year before he abandoned the artistic style of his student days, which had been largely derivative of Klimt's decorative approach, and instead embraced his own expressionist style. The meeting between the artist and the pro-moter in 1909 therefore chronologically verifies the theory that Schiele's personal idiom was centered on the grotesque, misshapen, and puppet-like human body, given that his unique brand of expressionism emerged only after his initial encounter with Roessler's Javanese puppets.

Moreover, Roessler's recollections reveal that Schiele believed that the gestures and outlines of his *wayang* puppet were more meaningful and aesthetically pleasing than the corporeal movements enacted by the American dancer Ruth St. Denis. This is a noteworthy claim, particularly since previous scholars have noted the presumed in-fluence of St. Denis' "Orientalist" dance movements on Schiele's lexicon of painted gestures, but not the relationship that developed between Schiele's gestural language and the bodies of the Javanese puppets that he acquired from Roessler.[59] St. Denis, who by the turn of the century had become an internationally renowned avant-garde dancer, tellingly enters the discourse surrounding Viennese expressionism because of her numerous interactions with leading Austrian figures of the period, including Hofmannsthal, and by virtue of the many modernist productions that she debuted between 1906 and 1907 in Vienna and Berlin.[60] Hofmannsthal was arguably the first

Viennese critic to celebrate St. Denis' modern gestures, doing so in his 1906 essay "The Incomparable Dancer," which I briefly discuss in Chapter 5.[61]

In the secondary literature on St. Denis, Mary Fleischer has notably examined the close rapport that developed between Hofmannsthal and the dancer, including their collaboration on a new version of *Salome* that, according to St. Denis, was to be quite unlike Oscar Wilde's, Max Reinhardt's, or Maud Allan's earlier productions, insofar as dance, rather than the spoken word, would take center stage.[62] Marjorie Warlick has further observed that the "Egyptian" figures in Klimt's *Stoclet Frieze* (1905) share a direct affinity with the corporeal gestures enacted by St. Denis during her Orientalist performances on the Viennese stage, which included productions like *Nautch*, *Cobra*, and *Yogi*.[63] Patrick Werkner has argued moreover that Schiele greatly admired St. Denis' modern dance movements and on a few occasions even cited her expressive body language with "his own exaggerated use of gesture."[64] This notwithstanding, Werkner is not quick to bring a semiotic analysis to bear on Schiele's sign language, and ultimately contends that the iconography of Schiele's painted gestures should be read alongside the vogue for modern dance at the turn of the century, as typified by St. Denis' performances and in the pantomimes staged by Schiele's friend, the mime Erwin Osen, whom he painted on a number of occasions.[65]

In terms of the *fin-de-siècle* literature, it is clear that only Roessler's work reveals the artist's fascination with the novel aesthetics offered by Javanese shadow puppets, providing a historical correlation between the artist's use of enigmatic body gestures and the semiotics of inanimate objects. This relationship manifests itself visually in a number of Schiele's works, including *Selbstportrait als heiliger Sebastian* (*Self-Portrait as Saint Sebastian*, 1914/15, Figure 6.6). In this image, which served as the promotional poster for his January 1915 exhibition at Guido Arnot's modern art gallery in Vienna, Schiele portrays his contorted body and dexterous limbs being struck by long, slender arrows, thus visually transforming himself into a representation of the Christian martyr. The placement and angularity of the arrows piercing the flesh and garments of "Saint Sebastian," which literally and theoretically invade the body of the artist, recall Roessler's description of the way that Schiele operated the rods that controlled his Javanese puppet. If Schiele intended to draw a parallel between animate and inanimate bodies, then the figure in the poster is not manipulated by the invisible strings of an unseen puppet master or artist, but is instead visibly controlled by the kinetic rods attached to the figure's awkward limbs and torso. The limp body hangs haggard in the air, supported (or suspended) by the adjoined rods, and is consequently devoid of human weight, visually mimicking the dexterity and weightlessness of a buffalo-hide puppet. The viewer might also note that the elongated features of the body and limbs—a recurring motif in Schiele's figurative works—present a striking similarity to the elongated torso of Javanese *wayang* and the disproportionate limbs that jut awkwardly from their bodies at odd angles (see Figures 5.2, 5.3 and 6.5).

The iconography of *Self-Portrait as Saint Sebastian*, which depicts a gaunt figure that is symbolically close to death, clearly references the pathological body. However, rather than arguing that Schiele drew on medical photographs as his point of reference, I want to assert that his segmented, ill-proportioned body instead alludes to the body of the pathological puppet, perhaps even one enacting hystero-theatrical gestures. The idea that Schiele was responding to the aesthetics of his own "grotesque" Javanese puppet further substantiates the assertion that *Self-Portrait as Saint Sebastian* offers the viewer a modernist interpretation of the artist/saint as a stringless,

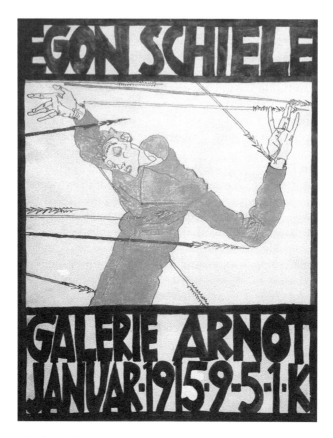

Figure 6.6 Egon Schiele, *Self-Portrait as Saint Sebastian*, 1914/15, watercolor and Indian ink
      on paper. Wien Museum Karlsplatz, Vienna.
Source: Photo: akg-images.

puppet-like martyr. The central figure—that of the self as human sacrifice—is picto-
rially rendered as if Egon/Sebastian were a marionette controlled or wounded by
the self as puppet master, rather than by outside forces. Through this visual and
theoretical paradox, the artist-as-puppet has ironically become a victim of his own
desire to control others as subjects in his art. This interpretation can also be applied
to a series of photographic images of Schiele captured by the Viennese photographer
Anton Josef Trčka. One photograph in particular shows Schiele adopting the guise of
a manipulated, stylized "puppet" whose arms and fingers communicate a language of
the inanimate or mechanized body (Figure 6.7). Given that the photograph was printed
in 1914, it also stands to reason that the unique finger gestures on Schiele's left hand
may have served as the iconographic source for the identical position of the fingers on
the right hand of the figure in *Self-Portrait as Saint Sebastian*. If this is the case, then it
is telling that Schiele was seemingly interested in portraying himself as a modern puppet
in both his personal artwork, as well as in semi-public photographs of his body. In other
words, the painted Egon and the real Egon were simultaneously being rendered lifeless
in the hands of the artist and his collaborators.

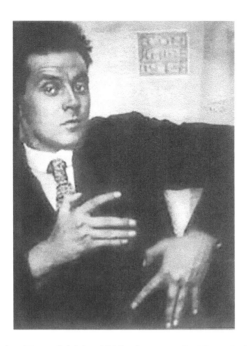

Figure 6.7 Anton J. Trčka, Egon Schiele, 1914, photograph. Neue Galerie, New York.
Source: Photo: Neue Galerie New York / Art Resource, NY.

Schiele's attempt to portray his subjects (other than himself) as lifeless puppets or dolls, and thus control them as the artist-cum-puppet master, is apparent in his drawing *Seated Female Nude with Tilted Head and Raised Arms* (1910, Plate 5). Here, the body of a woman is presented to the viewer as a contorted, twisted, and emaciated figure, whose arms and hands are seemingly being pulled or manipulated by unseen forces. Unlike *Self-Portrait as Saint Sebastian*, Schiele's female nude is not attached to physical "rods" (or arrows), and yet it is not difficult for the viewer to imagine that invisible strings or internal mechanisms are controlling her awkward, puppet-like movements. As stated in Chapter 1, Schiele's *Seated Female Nude with Tilted Head and Raised Arms* compares favorably to the androgynous figures in Kokoschka's *The Awakening* (Figure 1.2), whose strange corporeal gestures mimic the movements of adolescent "marionettes" controlled by their sexually developing bodies, and, in turn, by the libidinal forces of those who desire their bodies. In this regard, Schiele's subject could also be seen as a sexualized body, despite being pathological and unnatural. The fact that Schiele's female nude exhibits both clownish facial features and elongated arms reinforces the understanding that the figure can be read as a "living" puppet, doll, or marionette on paper. The fact that she is "missing" her lower legs altogether, likewise attests to her physiopathology.

The symbolic iconography of the rod-free or stringless puppet in Schiele's *oeuvre* is present moreover in a number of portraits of Erwin Osen executed by the artist in 1910, particularly in two gouache drawings entitled *Erwin Dominik Osen* (Figure 6.8) and *Mime van Osen* (Figure 6.9). At the turn of the century, Osen worked

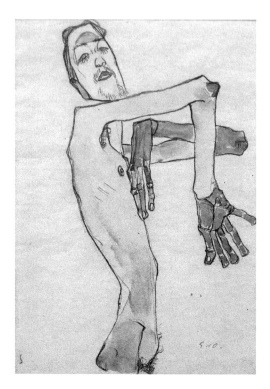

Figure 6.8 Egon Schiele, *Erwin Dominik Osen*, 1910, gouache, watercolor and black chalk on paper. Leopold Museum, Private Collection, Vienna.

Source: Photo: akg-images.

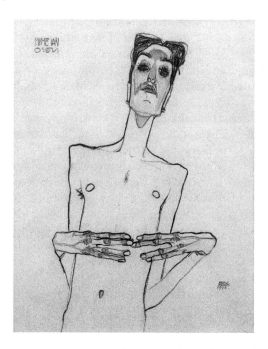

Figure 6.9 Egon Schiele, *Mime van Osen*, 1910, gouache and black chalk on paper. Leopold Museum, Private Collection, Vienna.

Source: Photo: akg-images.

as a mime, theater set designer and visual artist in Vienna, and was a member of the short-lived New Art Group alongside Schiele, Kokoschka, and Albert Paris von Gütersloh, among others. The scholarship on the Osen portraits, as well as on Schiele's and Osen's personal friendship, uniformly stresses the influence that Osen had on Schiele's understanding of theatrical gesture, and it is equally worth noting that Schiele was aware of a number of portraits that Osen had been commissioned to create in 1913 of psychiatric patients at the Steinhof Hospital in the suburbs of Vienna.[66] A photograph taken in, or around, 1910 of Osen and his paramour— the avant-garde dancer Moa Mandu—verifies that Osen had a slender build and long face, and that he was prone to striking elaborate poses and gestures with his arms and hands (Figure 6.10). This notwithstanding, Schiele's nude portraits of the mime reveal the artist's departure from reality, insofar as the emaciated and wildly elongated torso, limbs, and face of the painted Osen bear little resemblance to the physiognomy and corporeality of the actual Osen. Instead, Schiele's images present the mime as a skeletal, alien form, whose ridiculously large arms and hands recall the ill-proportioned and "weightless" arms of Schiele's *wayang* puppet or Teschner's marionettes, as well as the pathological female body in Schiele's *Seated Female Nude with Tilted Head and Raised Arms.*

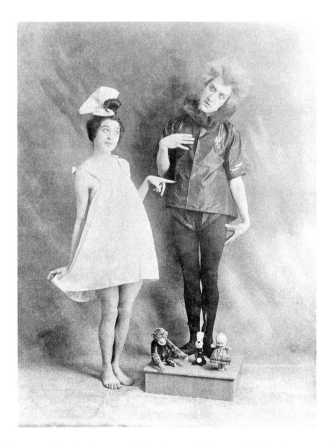

Figure 6.10 Unknown, Erwin Osen and the dancer Moa, c. 1910, photograph. Egon Schiele Archive, Albertina Museum, Vienna.

Source: Photo: akg-images / Imagno.

In *Erwin Dominik Osen*, the mime's arms extend from the body at near ninety-degree angles, with his enormous hands dangling from sticklike appendages. Similar to Klimt's *Judith I* (1901, Plate 6), Schiele's image decapitates the central figure, as Osen's head literally floats above his body. This artistic device not only reaffirms the use, and re-use, of the pathological body throughout Schiele's *oeuvre*, but in the context of this specific work also incorporates the appearance of the compartmentalized puppet body. Even the yellowish hue of Osen's face gives the impression that this "pathological puppet" may be afflicted with jaundice or some other psycho-physiological disease. Given that Osen was a mime known for his theatrics and grand gestures, it stands to reason that he was also familiar with the vogue for hystero-theatrical gestures in *fin-de-siècle* Vienna, particularly in the realm of modern theater and cabaret, and could therefore have incorporated these movements into his own avant-garde performances.

The second portrait, *Mime van Osen*, replicates the same non-naturalistic qualities of Osen's body that appear in the first portrait: the elongated face, neck, torso, arms, and hands. In *Mime van Osen*, Schiele draws the viewer's attention to Osen's fingers, which are grotesquely long, bony, and insect-like. In terms of iconography, the fingers of both hands form conspicuous and large "V" shapes—a gesture that Schiele repeated in multiple variations in other portraits, including *Nude Self-Portrait* (1910, Plate 2), *The Hermits* (1912, Figure 1.3), *Portrait of Albert Paris von Gütersloh* (1918, Plate 7), and most notably in *Selbstbildnis mit schwarzem Tongefäß und gespreizten Fingern* (*Self-Portrait with Black Vase and Spread Fingers*, 1911, Figure 6.11). Like *Mime van Osen*, Schiele's *Self-Portrait with Black Vase and Spread Fingers* depicts the sitter with an elongated hand and fingers that are spread to form the symmetrical "V." Various interpretations may explain this specific use of sign language, though I want to redirect my readers to the discourse centered on hysteria (in both males and females) as the *Modekrankheit* of the *fin de siècle*, and thus the most "modern" disorder available to visual and performing artists. When one returns to Badoureau's image of a woman afflicted with hystero-epilepcy (Figure 2.3), it is clear that the "V" shaped fingers and contorted body were initially found on the body of the pathological patient; and just as the patient was a pseudo-puppet in the hands of his or her psychiatric physician, Osen (and even Schiele himself) became pathological puppets in the hands of the young expressionist artist. Yet it is not known if Schiele actually studied Badoureau's drawing. Schiele's use of the "hysterical V" hints instead at how his images were caught in the larger European discourse centered on hystero-theatrical gestures as a particularly modern sign language of the body. It is equally apparent that Schiele subsists as the ultimate agent responsible for manipulating his pathological figures and their bodies by means of the doppelgänger motif, and in so doing, he objectifies, or even fetishizes, the unnatural body. The subjects of his non-commissioned portraits thus become objects of the artist's omnipresent gaze. This double vision, or doppelgänger vision, paradoxically renders the artist as both object and objectifier, as the ultimate manipulator but also the desired subject of his self-portraiture. This doppelgänger motif is particularly relevant to the discussion of the modern body and its relationship to the marionette if one recognizes that Schiele's figures, including images of the self, simultaneously represent living beings as well as objectified *things*, like puppets controlled by the artist's desires.

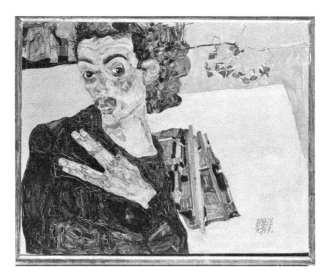

Figure 6.11 Egon Schiele, *Self-Portrait with Black Vase and Spread Fingers*, 1911, oil on
      wood panel. Wien Museum Karlsplatz, Vienna, Austria.
Source: Photo: Erich Lessing / Art Resource, NY.

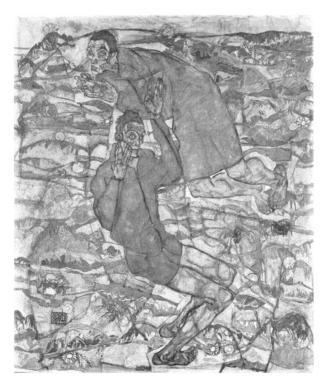

Figure 6.12 Egon Schiele, *Levitation (The Blind II)*, 1915, oil on canvas. Leopold Collection,
      Vienna.
Source: Photo: HIP / Art Resource, NY.

Schiele's *Entschwebung (Die Blinden II) (Levitation (The Blind II)*, 1915, Figure 6.12) and *Nude Self-Portrait* (Plate 2) each benefit from this reading.[67] In his self-portrait *Levitation (The Blind II)*, the doppelgänger motif—interpreted here within the context of a mirror image—is explicit. Perhaps signifying the split personality or double consciousness of the artist, the painting is somewhat ambiguous in its communication of the double vision.[68] The viewer is left to ponder a number of possibilities: is Schiele depicting two malleable, floating puppets created in his own likeness? Is he visually representing a theoretical manifestation of the split self? Or is he simply illustrating two separate people, both of whom embody aspects of the artist's personality, one aware of his puppet-like state, the other blind to this reality? The lower figure in the painting harbors a wide-eyed stare, has arms that seem to be controlled by unseen rods, and exhibits the same V-shaped finger gestures found in *Mime van Osen* and *Self-Portrait with Black Vase and Spread Fingers*. The upper figure levitates above his counterpart, seemingly asleep while he floats through the claustrophobic space of the canvas as if being dangled by invisible strings. The presence of two analogous bodies with noticeably disparate emotional states—or at least noticeably different states of consciousness—calls attention to the paradox of being the objectified *and* the objectifier in the doppelgänger complex.[69]

Nude Self-Portrait also incorporates this double vision, although in this image Schiele is more intent on exploring how it might articulate the androgynous puppet-like body—an androgyny that is made clear or, rather, is obscured by the ambiguity of the figure's sexual organs. We as viewers are left to question whether or not we are looking at a female vulva with a red interior, or a thin red phallus surrounded by enlarged testicles. Although a certain clinical "bisexuality" may be implicit in this image (recall Freud's analysis of this particular condition in the hysterical body of Dora), I propose that Schiele's dual sexuality is, in fact, a way for the artist to render himself genderless, androgynous, or even hermaphroditic. Just as a viewer cannot discern the sex of a puppet, given its lack of sexual organs, one cannot necessarily ascertain the exact gender of Schiele's self-portrait, and thus, the gender of his self. Whereas one can determine the gender of a puppet through its attributes: a dress, a bow, long hair for a female puppet; short hair, trousers, and a necktie for a male marionette, here Schiele sardonically masks his gender through the transparency of female genitalia graphed onto a male body that biologically does not belong to these parts. Within this image, the self is stripped bare, exposing what ought not to be exposed, but in the process he does not provide the viewer with what he or she expects to witness on a nude body that is otherwise codified as male. This conflict may suggest the artist's internal or psychological struggle with his own sexual identity or adolescent sexual development, though Schiele's choice to depict himself as an androgynous figure seems more closely tied to the aesthetics of the genderless puppet and its inherent symbolic assertions about the body, its construction of gender, and the viewer's preconceived notions of gender, sex, and nudity.

Like the rendering of the figure in *Self-Portrait as St. Sebastian*, the iconography of the puppet-like body in *Nude Self-Portrait* is reinforced by Schiele's vacant eye sockets and his elongated, wildly ill-proportioned limbs that jut awkwardly from his emaciated torso. If one further observes that the fingers on a Javanese *wayang* puppet are often paired three to one (an equally recurrent theme in Schiele's cryptic finger gestures), a tangible correlation is further established between the body of the puppet and the corporeal gestures in *Nude Self-Portrait*. This finger motif is also visible in numerous other self-portraits, including *Prediger (Selbstakt mit blaugrünem Hemd)* (*Preacher (Nude Self-Portrait with Blue-green Shirt)*, 1913, Figure 6.13). In this image, Schiele isolates the index finger from the other three fingers of the left hand, hiding the thumb completely. The fingers of the right hand are instead grouped together, with the thumb bent at a ninety-degree angle. Iconographically, the left hand resembles the fingers of a Javanese puppet, whereas the right hand recalls the conjoined fingers of a wooden European doll. The preacher's bent head, the doll-like eyes, the awkward protrusion of the right arm, and the relative state of undress further emphasize the semiotics of a modern marionette implicit in the artist's visual language.

Semblances of the modern puppet body are also conspicuously present in Schiele's *Selbstdarstellung mit gestreiften Ärmelschonern* (*Self-Portrait with Striped Armlets*, 1915, Figure 6.14) and *Selbstbildnis mit erhobenen Ellenbogen* (*Self-Portrait in Jerkin with Right Elbow Raised*, 1914, figure 6.15). The iconography of the expressive, though lifeless marionette is made clear through the figures' vacant, direct stares, wooden facial features, strangely cocked heads, and the elongated arms that jut awkwardly from their doll-like bodies. Once more, Schiele depicts a series of "puppets" created in his own likeness. As doppelgängers, the manifestations of the puppet-self in these drawings become stand-ins for the real, living Schiele, whose "presence" in

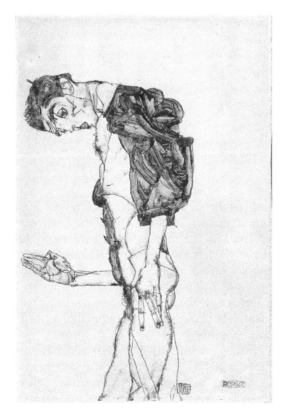

Figure 6.13 Egon Schiele, *Preacher (Nude Self-Portrait with Blue-green Shirt)*, 1913, gouache and pencil on paper. Leopold Museum, Vienna.
Source: Photo: Erich Lessing / Art Resource, NY.

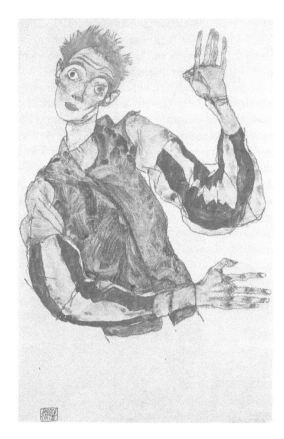

Figure 6.14 Egon Schiele, *Self-Portrait with Striped Armlets*, 1915, gouache and pencil on paper. Leopold Museum, Vienna.
Source: Photo: HIP / Art Resource, NY.

his art assumes the role of the viewer, or, alternatively, the puppet master as creator and manipulator of these images. What is more, the body gestures in *Self-Portrait with Striped Armlets* and *Self-Portrait in Jerkin with Right Elbow Raised* interestingly mirror the limbs of the left-most figure in Kokoschka's *The Awakening*, given that each figure displays a raised, puppet-like arm. Perhaps Schiele was thinking of Kokoschka's *The Dreaming Youths* when he created these two self-portraits, though the artists' common interest in the expressiveness and symbolic potency of objects whose very nature demands that they be manipulated in order to create meaning seems a more likely explanation.

Additional self-portraits created between 1910 and 1918 further emphasize the semiotics of the puppet implicit in Schiele's gestural language, though this trope can also be seen in a number of double portraits, either self-portraits with female figures, or portraits of two women, often entwined in each other's arms. Two examples of this latter type are Schiele's *Zwei Mädchen, in verschränkter Stellung liegend (Two Girls, Lying in an Entwined Position*, Plate 8) and *Frauenpaar (Two Women Embracing (Two Friends)*, Figure 6.16), both created in 1915. Each of these drawings departs from self-portraiture, and instead communicates the puppet motif through the female body, each offering the viewer a double portrait of two

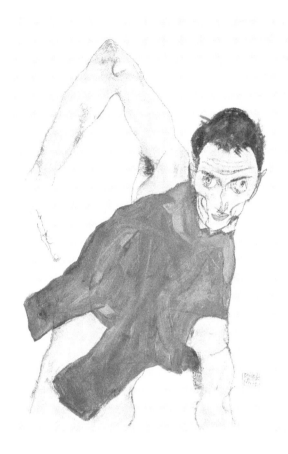

Figure 6.15 Egon Schiele, *Self-Portrait in Jerkin with Right Elbow Raised*, 1914, gouache, black chalk and pencil on paper. Private Collection.

Source: Photo: © Christie's Images/Bridgeman Images.

women: one clothed, the other naked, save for disheveled stockings or shoes. In each of these images the female figures, despite being depicted as separate entities, are intertwined, forming a cohesive mass of "femininity" that occupies and exceeds the drawings' visual planes. In *Two Girls, Lying in an Entwined Position*, the facial physiognomy of the lower figure strongly resembles the lifeless face of a doll or puppet, particularly when compared to the more naturalistically rendered facial physiognomies of the unclothed woman. More implicitly, this iconography communicates a double vision focused on a dichotomy that exists between a "living" being (the upper, naked woman) and a non-living doll (the lower, fully clothed figure). The same artistic device is at play in *Two Women Embracing*, given that the lower figure represents a living woman, whereas the clothed figure in the background resembles a stiff, lifeless doll. The impetus behind clothing the bodies of the doll-like figures may suggest that the artist once again sought to conceal the genderless, puppet-like body in order to veil its uncanniness from the viewer's stare, while simultaneously subjecting the sensuous curves of the "real" women to this same voyeuristic gaze.

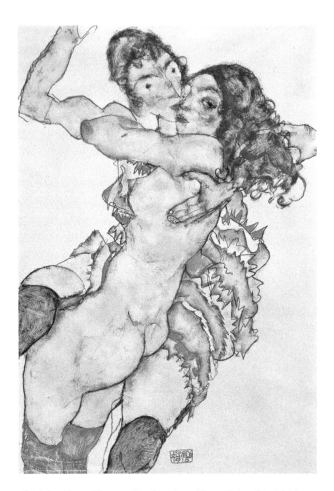

Figure 6.16 Egon Schiele, *Two Women Embracing (Two Friends)*, 1915, watercolor, gouache and pencil on paper. Museum of Fine Arts (Szépmüvészeti) Budapest, Hungary.
Source: Photo: Bridgeman Images.

Unlike other figures in Schiele's *oeuvre*, which also depict naked and contorted female bodies, the bodies that occupy *Two Girls, Lying in an Entwined Position* and *Two Women Embracing* do not confront the male gaze with a direct stare or challenge his sexualized voyeurism. Instead, the figures appear to revel in the implicit and explicit male voyeurism that transpires between object and artist, subject and viewer. These bodies ask to be looked at and, in return, they enjoy being seen. They are, in a rather misogynistic sense, bodies performing the role of objectified *things*, rather than persons. In this respect, these objects, particularly the female figures rendered as life-size dolls or stringless marionettes, also resemble pathological puppets due to their misshapen appendages and wooden facial features. If these bodies strive to articulate a double portrait of the same body, as in Schiele's double self-portrait *Levitation (The Blind II)*, then the living/sexualized, non-living/desexualized binary is clearly manifest in Schiele's visual language, particularly in these two works. When considering the use of the female body in both drawings, one might further conclude that this sexualized reduction was solely fashioned for, and consumed by, the artistic male gaze: the same gaze that reveled in the pleasure of hysterical female bodies pirouetting in the amphitheater of Charcot's Salpêtrière, and in modern theatrical performances on the Viennese stage. Expressionist renderings of the female body, especially Schiele's *Two Girls, Lying in an Entwined Position* and *Two Women Embracing*, thus bring hysteria's modernist journey full circle: from the clinics of Paris to the modern venues of Vienna. And in so doing, Schiele's images not only suggest that hystero-theatrical gestures were part-and-parcel of Viennese modernism, but that the pathological, puppet-like body had become synonymous with the Viennese modern body.

Conclusion

As a final consideration, I want to return to where this book began: Kokoschka's vision dialectic and its role in constructing semblances of the Viennese modern body. Like Schiele, Kokoschka was a young expressionist who fully embraced the dichotomy between animate and inanimate bodies, as simultaneously revealed in his emotionally charged plays and puppet-inspired paintings. The aesthetics of the agitated and compartmentalized marionette body is likewise present in Kokoschka's *Hans Tietze and Erica Tietze-Conrat* (Plate 1), a painting previously discussed in this book for its role in constructing notions of modern vision, but which also exemplifies the strangely proportioned limbs and finger gestures of its sitters. The Tietzes' extremities indeed appear to be controlled by an unseen force, perhaps by the hand of an external *Puppenspieler* who resides outside of the painting's frame. These iconographies might therefore be read as votives for the expressive body, capable of wordlessly conveying a sign language of modernity in *fin-de-siècle* Vienna. This interpretation proposes that, by the early twentieth century, what was previously (or concurrently) understood to be "pathological," could also be read, very simply, as "modern."

This realization is important to our present understanding of the genesis of Viennese expressionism, since pathological gestures in expressionist paintings can now be seen to materialize in one of two ways: either as a medical stereotype of the hysterical femme fatale, or as a language of the body that signified modernism in the Austrian capital. The latter contention is inextricably linked to the former, particularly when one recalls that modern medicine in the late nineteenth century was revealing the secrets of the mind, just as hysteria was offering the new century a fashionable disease of the body. Given the mutability of meanings that corporeal gestures enjoyed at the turn of the century, the Tietzes' doll-like movements do not, therefore, have to be read strictly as hystero-theatrical gestures conveying an appearance of hysteria. Instead, the present study has hopefully demonstrated that their gestural language might instead be contingent upon the metaphorical body of the puppet or marionette as signifiers of modern man's desire to control, or be controlled by external forces, including the hands, minds, and desires of others.

The motivation for the queries raised in this book has been the desire to understand how hystero-theatrical gestures came to inhabit Viennese paintings at the turn of the century, and to what end the expressionists utilized semblances of the modern body to articulate their vision of European modern art. By turning to disciplines outside the field of art history—namely to the realms of medicine and the performing arts—I have attempted to show that hysteria had unequivocally become the *Modekrankheit* of the *fin de siècle*, and that hystero-theatrical gestures were the progeny of this particular union between modern science, modern drama, and modern painting. This study has shown that the Viennese modern body was one that directly confronted and incorporated these gestures as a means of bringing material form to a body fashioned through the inner and outer vision of the modern artist. Expressionistic sight, in turn, was a direct result of the dialectical tension that existed between these two prevalent, though oppositional, views of artistic vision at the turn of the century. Seen to develop from the expressive body of the theatrically hysterical madwoman, as well as the metaphorical movements of the pathological puppet, the modern body thus offered expressionist artists the ultimate conflation of Kokoschka's vision dialectic: a body that was both of the material world (and thus observable through corporeal vision), as well as one that was easily refashioned, as if it were a puppet in the hands (and through the inner vision) of the modern Viennese artist. In so doing, Kokoschka, Schiele, and their interlocutors were successful in utilizing the puppet body—rather than the language of abstraction—as a metaphorical body double, or doppelgänger, for the manipulated human body, enacting through its iconography a language that was easily transplanted onto the expressionist canvas and stage. By offering their viewers a unique puppet vision of modernity, each of these individuals reinforced, in their own manner, the belief that playing with puppets in *fin-de-siècle* Vienna was far from mere child's play.

Notes

1 Arthur Roessler, *Erinnerungen an Egon Schiele* (Vienna: Verlag Carl Konegen, 1922), 38.
2 For literature on the puppet/doll/mannequin in German Dada and surrealism, see Leah Dickerman, et al., *Dada: Zürich, Berlin, Hannover, Cologne, New York, Paris* (New York: National Gallery of Art and Distributed Art Publishers, 2005), 108, 140–42; Hal Foster, *Prosthetic Gods* (Cambridge, MA: The MIT Press, 2004); Juliet Koss, "Bauhaus Theater of Human Dolls," *The Art Bulletin* 85, no. 4 (December 2003): 724–45; Susanne Lahusen, "Oskar Schlemmer: Mechanical Ballets?" *Dance Research* 4, no. 2 (Autumn 1986): 65–77; Thérèse Lichtenstein, *Behind Closed Doors: The Art of Hans Bellmer* (Los Angeles: University of California Press, 2001); and Sue Taylor, *Hans Bellmer: The Anatomy of Anxiety* (Cambridge, MA: The MIT Press, 2002).
3 In 1917 at the Cabaret Voltaire in Zurich, the Dadaist Tristan Tzara staged Kokoschka's play *Sphinx und Strohmann* (*Sphinx and Scarecrow*), which Robert Knopf calls an "Expressionist/Dada performance," in *Theater of the Avant-Garde, 1890–1950: A Critical Anthology*, ed. Robert Knopf (New Haven: Yale University Press, 2015), 240.
4 Harold Segel and Robert Tausky both discuss the puppet motif in Kokoschka's dramatic works, but they do not transfer this discourse to the artist's visual work, nor to the work of other expressionist artists. See Harold B. Segel, *Pinocchio's Progeny: Puppets, Marionettes, Automatons, and Robots in Modernist and Avant-Garde Drama* (Baltimore: Johns Hopkins University Press, 1995), 185–89; and Robert Tausky, *Hiob: Ein Mann im Lande Utz und seine Wege durch die Welt* (Würzburg: Verlag Königshausen & Neumann, 2004), 89–90.
5 See David Joravsky, "Between Science and Art: Freud versus Schnitzler, Kafka, and Musil," in *The Mind of Modernism: Medicine, Psychology, and The Cultural Arts in Europe and America, 1880–1940*, ed. Mark S. Micale (Stanford: Stanford University Press, 2004), 279; and Henri F. Ellenberger, *The Discovery of the Unconscious: The History and Evolution of Dynamic Psychiatry* (New York: Basic Books, 1970), 469–74. It is equally interesting to read the few letters exchanged between Freud and Schnitzler during the *fin de siècle*. See Sigmund Freud, "Briefe an Arthur Schnitzler," *Die Neue Rundschau* 66 (1955): 1–12; and Herbert I. Kupper and Hilda S. Rollman-Branch, "Freud und Schnitzler—(Doppelgänger)," *Journal of the American Psychoanalytic Association* 7 (January 1959): 120.

6 Lorenzo Bellettini, "Freud's Contribution to Arthur Schnitzler's Prose Style," *Rocky Mountain Review of Language and Literature* 61, no. 2 (Fall 2007): 11–27; and Ernst Jones, *The Life and Work of Sigmund Freud*, vol. 3 (New York: Basic Books, 1957), 84.

7 Sigmund Freud, *Briefe, 1879–1939*, eds. Ernst and Lucie Freud (Frankfurt: Fischer, 1960), 357. The original German reads: "Ihr Determinismus wie Ihre Skepsis, Ihr Ergriffensein von den Wahrheiten des Unbewußten, von der Triebnatur des Menschen, Ihre Zersetzung der kulturell-konventionellen Sicherheiten, das Haften Ihrer Gedanken an der Polarität von Lieben und Sterben, das alles berührt mich mit einer unheimlichen Vertrautheit." David Joravsky has instead argued that Freud was outspoken about Schnitzler's "abandonment" of science for art. See Joravsky, "Between Science and Art," 279.

8 Regarding Schnitzler's interest in Charcot's writings, see Urszula Kawalec, "Die Hypnose in der österreichischen Literatur der Jahrhundertwende. Am Beispiel der Pantomime Pierrot Hypnotiseur von Richard Beer-Hofmann," *Orbis Linguarum* 19 (2002): 161.

9 In his career as a dramatist and literary figure, Schnitzler wrote approximately sixteen plays, two novels, eleven novellas, and three works of non-fiction, which consisted of a posthumous autobiography, a diary, and collection of essays on literature and theater. He also dallied with medical studies during his early career as a physician, though to my knowledge none of these papers were ever published during his lifetime.

10 See, for example, Kawalec, "Die Hypnose in der österreichischen Literatur der Jahrhundertwende," 161–62. For the dates of Schnitzler's works, see Dagmar C. G. Lorenz, ed., *A Companion to the Works of Arthur Schnitzler* (Rochester: Camden House, 2003), vii; and Arthur Schnitzler, *Eight Plays: Performance Texts*, trans. William L. Cunningham and David Palmer (Evanston: Northwestern University Press, 2007), x. See also Arthur Schnitzler, *Paracelsus and Other One-act Plays*, trans. G. J. Weinberger (Riverside: Ariadne Press, 1995); and Heinz Politzer, "Arthur Schnitzler: The Poetry of Psychology," *MLN* 78, no. 4, German Issue (October 1963): 364.

11 Kawalec, "Die Hypnose in der österreichischen Literatur der Jahrhundertwende," 162. See also Harold B. Segel, *Turn-of-the-Century Cabaret: Paris, Barcelona, Berlin, Munich, Vienna, Cracow, Moscow, St. Petersburg, Zurich* (New York: Columbia University Press, 1987), 211.

12 The first two plays were performed in Berlin, while the third was revealed at Vienna's Lustspieltheater. See Segel, *Pinocchio's Progeny*, 173.

13 See Schnitzler, *Paracelsus and other One-act Plays*, 1–36.

14 For an analysis of this theme in Schnitzler's *Pierrot*, see G. J. Weinberger, "Marionette or 'Puppenspieler'?: Arthur Schnitzler's Pierrot," *Neophilologus* 86 (2002): 265–72.

15 See Segel, *Pinocchio's Progeny*, 174.

16 H. S. Reiss discusses Schnitzler's interest in this fate motif in the puppet plays in H. S. Reiss, "The Problems of Fate and of Religion in the Work of Arthur Schnitzler," *The Modern Language Review* 40, no. 4 (October 1945): 302–3.

17 This description of Schnitzler's play as it was initially performed on the Berlin stage with human actors in the guise of the marionettes is offered in Ralf E. Remshardt, *Staging the Savage God: The Grotesque in Performance* (Carbondale: Southern Illinois University Press, 2004), 170–71. Segel does not discuss this actor-as-puppet staging, but does argue that Schnitzler utilizes this play-within-a-play motif to mock his bourgeois real audience. See Segel, *Pinocchio's Progeny*, 178.

18 See Arthur Schnitzler, *Der tapfere Cassian: Puppenspiel in einem Akt* (Berlin: S. Fischer, 1910). For a good English translation, see Arthur Schnitzler, *Gallant Cassian: A Puppet-play in One Act*, trans. Adam L. Gowans, Third ed. (London: Gowans and Gray, Ltd., 1914).

19 The subtitles for Schnitzler's puppet plays allow us to distinguish those that involved actual marionettes or puppets—referred to as *Puppenspiel*, or puppet plays, in the case of *The Gallant Cassian*—and plays that involved human actors in the guise of marionettes—subtitled *Studie* (study), in the cases of *The Puppet Master*, and *Burleske* (burlesque), for *The Great Prater Puppet Theater*.

20 Schnitzler, *Der tapfere Cassian*, 22. The original German reads: "Die da ist von einer, die ich noch nicht einmal gesprochen habe, und die ich liebe wie ein Toller. Im Herbst war sie hier in der Stadt un hat getanzt – sie heißt Eleonora Lambriani."

21 Schnitzler, *Der tapfere Cassian*, 12. The original German reads: "Wie ich sie vor mir sehe! Gleich zuckenden Schlangen im Schnee ringelten ihr die schwarzen Locken über die Schultern. Alle, die sie sahen, waren toll vor Entzücken. Und der Erbprinz warf ihr rote Rosen hinunter auf die Bühne. O, ich weiß es noch!"

22 Schnitzler, *Der tapfere Cassian*, 13. The original German reads: "Denke, Martin, daß sie alle falsch sind, die heimatlos durch die Welt ziehen."

23 For the original dialogue, which is too lengthy to reproduce here, see Schnitzler, *Der tapfere Cassian*, 22–23.

24 Segel, *Pinocchio's Progeny*, 185. See also Michael Buhrs, Barbara Lesák, and Thomas Trabitsch, eds., *Fledermaus Kabarett 1907 bis 1913, ein Gesamtkunstwerk der Wiener Werkstätte: Literatur, Musik, Tanz* (Vienna: Christian Brandstätter und Österreichisches Theatermuseum, 2007).

25 Henry I. Schvey, *Oskar Kokoschka: The Painter as Playwright* (Detroit: Wayne State University Press, 1982), 67–88.

26 See the cover page for *Der Sturm: Wochenschrift für Kultur und die Künste* 1, no. 54, March 11, 1911.

27 Segel, *Pinocchio's Progeny*, 187.

28 Oskar Kokoschka, "Sphinx und Strohmann: Komödie für Automaten," *Wort in der Zeit: Österreichische Literaturzeitschrift* 2, no. 3 (March 1956): 145–48.

29 Concerning the social morality of *fin-de-siècle* Vienna, see Stefan Zweig, *The World of Yesterday* (Lincoln, NE: University of Nebraska Press, 1964), 74–76.

30 Helen Borowitz discusses the primacy of the "youth theme," as it pertains to adolescent sexuality in both dramatic literature and expressionist painting, in Helen O. Borowitz, "Youth as Metaphor and Image in Wedekind, Kokoschka, and Schiele," *Art Journal* 33, no. 3 (Spring 1974): 219–25. See also Henry I. Schvey, "Oskar Kokoschka's 'The Dreaming Youths'," *Books Abroad* 49, no. 3 (Summer 1975): 484–85.

31 See, for example, reviews reproduced in Ludwig Hevesi, *Altkunst—Neukunst: Wien 1894–1908*, ed. Otto Breicha, Reprint ed. (1909; Klagenfurt: Ritter Verlag, 1984).

32 Oskar Kokoschka, *Die Träumenden Knaben* (Vienna: Wiener Werkstätte mit Berger und Chwala, 1908). The original German, written in lowercase, reads: "ich will das kindliche zittern deiner schultern erwarten und sehen / wie dein mund / ohne worte zu suchen / für mich spricht."

33 Segel, *Pinocchio's Progeny*, 72; and Robert Weldon Whalen, *Sacred Spring: God and the Birth of Modernism in Fin de Siècle Vienna* (Cambridge: Eerdmans Publishing Co., 2007), 223.

34 Oskar Kokoschka and Ernst Reinhold, *Kokoschka-Matinee Einladung*, March 29, 1909, 1–2. See also Oskar Kokoschka, *Der Weisse Tiertöter* (Vienna: Genossenschaftsverlag, 1920).

35 Segel, *Pinocchio's Progeny*, 72.

36 Segel, *Pinocchio's Progeny*, 38.

37 Peter Jelavich, *Berlin Cabaret*, vol. 11, *Studies in Cultural History* (Cambridge, MA: Harvard University Press, 1996), 26. One could obviously debate what constitutes a modern puppet play, as European puppet theater has enjoyed a long history, developing early in the Medieval period in Italy. Puppetry in general, however, can be traced back to ancient Egypt and Greece, and may, in fact, have its origins in prehistoric cultures.

38 Armond Fields, *Le Chat Noir: A Montmartre Cabaret and Its Artists in Turn-of-the-Century Paris* (Santa Barbara: Santa Barbara Museum of Art, 1993), 31.

39 Jelavich, *Berlin Cabaret*, 26–27.

40 Jelavich, *Berlin Cabaret*, 27, 34–35.

41 Günter Böhmer, *Puppets*, trans. Gerald Morice (Munich: Verlag F. Bruckmann KG, 1969), 49–50.

42 Segel, *Turn-of-the-Century Cabaret*, 197.

43 After the death of Gustav Mahler in 1911, Alma and Kokoschka began a turbulent love affair in 1912, which lasted until 1914, when Alma chose to secretly abort the child they conceived. See Françoise Giroud, "Alma Oskar Kokoschka," trans. R. M. Stock, in *Alma Mahler, or, The Art of Being Loved* (Oxford: Oxford University Press, 1991), 96–117,

204–5; Susanne Keegan, *The Eye of God: A Life of Oskar Kokoschka* (London: Blooms-bury, 1999), 177–201; Alfred Weidinger, *Kokoschka and Alma Mahler: Testimony to a Passionate Relationship* (Munich: Prestel, 1996), 79–88; Oskar Kokoschka, *My Life*, trans. David Britt (New York: Macmillan Publishing Co., 1974); and Frank Whitford, *Oskar Kokoschka: A Life* (New York: Atheneum, 1986), 91.

44 Oskar Kokoschka, "Der Fetisch," in *Oskar Kokoschka: Die frühen Jahre, Aquarelle und Zeichnungen (1906–1924)* (Hannover: Kestner-Gesellschaft, 1983), 67–79; and Kokoschka, *My Life*, 118.

45 See Richard Calvocoressi, *Kokoschka: Paintings* (New York: Rizzoli, 1992), 14.

46 See Peter Gorsen, "Pygmalions stille Frau. Oskar Kokoschka und die Puppe," in *Sex-ualästhetik. Grenzformen der Sinnlichkeit im 20. Jahrhundert* (Reinbek bei Hamburg: Rowohlt-Taschenbuch-Verlag, 1987), 248–58; and Lisa J. Street, "Oskar Kokoschka's Doll: Symbol of Culture" (PhD diss., Emory University, 1993), 81–83, 249–52, 57–70.

47 Bonnie Roos, "Oskar Kokoschka's Sex Toy: The Women and the Doll Who Conceived the Artist," *Modernism/Modernity* 12, no. 2 (2005): 291–309.

48 Roos, "Oskar Kokoschka's Sex Toy," 307.

49 Oskar Kokoschka quoted and translated in Edith Hoffmann, *Kokoschka: Life and Work* (London: Faber and Faber, 1947), 147. The original German version of this letter was later published in Kokoschka, "Der Fetisch," 73.

50 When Kokoschka received the doll, he ironically despised it, and expressed deep disap-pointment, stating that the skin of the doll felt like a "polar bear pelt." See Kokoschka, "Der Fetisch," 78–79.

51 See Chelius-Zitzewitz, *Oskar Kokoschka: Gemälde, Handzeichnungen, Aquarelle, Drucke* (Dresden: Galerie Ernst Arnold, 1925), cat. no. 44.

52 Kokoschka, "Der Fetisch," 78–79.

53 Roos, "Oskar Kokoschka's Sex Toy," 303–4.

54 Kirk Varnedoe, *Vienna 1900: Art, Architecture & Design* (New York: The Museum of Modern Art, 1986), 176; Renée Price, ed., *Egon Schiele: The Ronald S. Lauder and Serge Sabarsky Collections* (New York: Prestel, 2005), 85; Reinhard Steiner, *Egon Schiele, 1890–1918: The Midnight Soul of the Artist*, trans. Michael Hulse (Cologne: Taschen, 2000), 74; Frank Whitford, *Egon Schiele* (London: Thames and Hudson, 1981), 111, 158.

55 Patrick Werkner, *Austrian Expressionism: The Formative Years*, trans. Nicholas T. Parsons (New York: The Society for the Promotion of Science and Scholarship, 1993), 126.

56 For a comprehensive bibliography of Roessler's work, see Tobias G. Natter and Ursula Storch, ed., *Egon Schiele & Arthur Roessler: Der Kunstler und sein Forderer. Kunst und Networking im fruhen 20. Jahrhundert* (Ostfildern-Ruit: Hatje Cantz, 2004), 199–206. Unlike his contemporaries, whose theater reviews often appeared in the non-liberal *Wiener Abendpost*, Roessler was a staff writer for *Wiener Arbeiterzeitung*, a liberal newspaper politically affiliated with the Social Democratic Workers' Party of Austria at the turn of the century.

57 See Arthur Roessler, *Richard Teschner* (Vienna: Gerlach & Wiedling, 1947).

58 Roessler, *Erinnerungen an Egon Schiele*, 38. The original German reads:

> Stundenlang konnte er mit diesen Figuren spielen, ohne zu ermüden und ohne dabei auch nur ein Wort zu sprechen. Das eigentlich Erstaunliche hierbei war die Geschicklichkeit, mit der Schiele die dünnen Bewegungsstäbchen der Figuren gleich von Anbeginn handhabte. Als ich, ihn zu erfreuen, ihm die Wahl einer solchen javanischen Schattenspielfigur freistellte, wählte er die groteske Gestalt eines teuflischen Dämons mit abenteuerlichem Profil. Ihr hatte er manche Anregung zu danken. Es faszinierten ihn die streng stilisierten, ausdrucksstarken Gebärden, die immer ungewöhnlichen, oft zauberhaft eindringlichen Umrißlinien der Schattenrisse an der Wand, die das Spiel ergab. 'Solch eine Figur kann mehr als unsere besten Tänzerinnen. Gegen meinen roten Dämon ist die Ruth...' er nannte eine berühmte Tänzerin, 'eine schwerfällige Kanone,' sagte er, seinen büffelledernen Dämon liebevoll bewundernd. Diese javanische Figur blieb sein Lieblingsspielzeug bis zu seinem Tode, nach dem sie mir von des Künstlers Erben wieder zurückgegeben wurde.

59 Kimberly A. Smith, *Between Ruin and Renewal: Egon Schiele's Landscapes* (New Haven: Yale University Press, 2004), 141; Steiner, *Egon Schiele*, 42; and Patrick Werkner, "The Child-Woman and Hysteria," in *Egon Schiele: Art, Sexuality, and Viennese Modernism*, ed. Patrick Werkner (Palo Alto: The Society for the Promotion of Science and Scholarship, 1994), 72.

60 Mary Fleischer provides a succinct account of the history of St. Denis' performances in Vienna. See Mary Fleischer, *Embodied Texts: Symbolist Playwright-Dancer Collaborations* (Amsterdam: Editions Rodopi, 2007), 93–148.

61 Hugo von Hofmannsthal, "Die unvergleichliche Tänzerin," in *Reden und Aufsätze I: 1891–1913*, vol. 8, Gesammelte *Werke*, ed. Bernd Schöler (Frankfurt: Bernd Schöler, 1979), 496–501. A good English translation can be found in David Berger, "Her Extraordinary Immediacy," *Dance Magazine* XLII (September 1968): 36–38.

62 Fleischer, *Embodied Texts*, 109, 11.

63 M. E. Warlick, "Mythic Rebirth in Gustav Klimt's Stoclet Frieze: New Considerations of Its Egyptianizing Form and Content," *The Art Bulletin* 74, no. 1 (March 1992): 127.

64 Werkner, *Austrian Expressionism*, 126.

65 Werkner, *Austrian Expressionism*, 126.

66 For a review of this literature, see Peter Vergo and Barnaby Wright, eds, *Egon Schiele: The Radical Nude* (London: The Courtauld Gallery and Paul Holberton Publishing, 2014), 98–99. For literature on Osen's clinical portraits, see Alessandra Comini, *Egon Schiele's Portraits* (Berkeley: University of California Press, 1974), 203–4n66; and Gemma Blackshaw and Leslie Topp, eds., *Madness and Modernity: Mental Illness and the Visual Arts in Vienna 1900* (Farnham: Lund Humphries, 2009), 35.

67 When approaching the subject of "self" in his self-portraits, scholars have noted a connection between Schiele's and Nietzsche's writings. Reinhard Steiner notes the affinity between Schiele's preoccupation with his naked form and Nietzsche's treatment of the body in *Thus Spoke Zarathustra*. See Steiner, *Egon Schiele*, 11.

68 Double consciousness was a term first coined by Ralph Waldo Emerson and later expounded upon by W. E. B. Du Bois, who concluded that it is the act of always seeing one's self through the eyes of another. In Schiele's image, he sees himself through the eyes of his double, which, ironically, are still his own eyes. For a theoretical examination of double consciousness, see Doris Sommer, "A Vindication of Double Consciousness," in *A Companion to Postcolonial Studies*, eds. Henry Schwarz and Sangeeta Ray (Malden: Blackwell Publishers, Inc., 2000), 165.

69 In keeping with the doppelgänger theme, Lori Felton alternatively reads a religious connotation into the painting, which she translates as *Transfiguration (The Blind II)*. See Lori A. Felton, "Beyond the *Self-Seers*: The Creative Strategies within Egon Schiele's Double Self-Portraiture," in *The Doppelgänger*, ed. Deborah Ascher Barnstone, vol. 3 of *German Visual Culture*, eds. Deborah Ascher Barnstone and Thomas O. Haakenson (Bern: Peter Lang, 2016), 39–42.

Bibliography

Adair, Mark J. "Plato's View of the 'Wandering Uterus'." *The Classical Journal* 91, no. 2 (December 1995–January 1996): 153–63.

Allan, Maud. *My Life and Dancing*. London: Everett & Co., 1908.

Altenberg, Peter. "Authentisch." *Simplicissimus* 16, no. 36 (1911): 621.

Armstrong, Carol. "Probing Pictures." *Artforum International* 42, no. 1 (September 2003): 55–56.

Armstrong, Richard H. "Oedipus as Evidence: The Theatrical Background to Freud's Oedipus Complex." *PsyArt: An Online Journal for the Psychological Study of the Arts* 2, no. 6a (January 1999): n.p.

Bahr, Hermann. *Dialog vom Tragischen*. Berlin: S. Fischer, 1904.

———. "Marionetten." In *Das Hermann-Bahr-Buch*, edited by S. Fischer, 214–24. Berlin: S. Fischer, 1913.

———. *Expressionismus*. Third edn. Munich: Delphin-Verlag, 1919.

———. "Expressionism." In *Art in Theory, 1900–1990: An Anthology of Changing Ideas*, edited by Charles Harrison and Paul Wood, 116–21. Oxford: Blackwell Publishers, 1992.

Bahr, Hermann, ed. *Gegen Klimt: Historisches, Philosophie, Medizin, Goldfische, Fries*. Vienna: Eisenstein & Co., 1903.

Baker, Oswald Georg. "… 'Daß Der Ausdruck Eindruck Werde.' Gustav Mahler Und Alfred Roller: Die Reform Der Wiener Wagner-Szene." *Bayerische Akademie der Schönen Künste Jahrbuch* 11 (1996–97): 55–95.

Baragwanath, Nicholas. "Anna Bahr-Mildenburg, Gesture, and the Bayreuth Style." *Musical Times* 148, no. 1901 (Winter 2007): 63–74.

Behrendt, Klaus. "Austria: Puppet Theatre." In *The World Encyclopedia of Contemporary Theatre*, edited by Don Rubin, Péter Nagy, and Philippe Rouyer, 72–73. Vol. 1: Europe. London and New York: Routledge, 1994.

Beizer, Janet L. *Ventriloquized Bodies: Narratives of Hysteria in Nineteenth-Century France*. Ithaca: Cornell University Press, 1994.

Bell, John, ed. *Puppets, Masks, and Performing Objects*. Cambridge, MA: The MIT Press, 2001.

Beller, Steven, ed. *Rethinking Vienna 1900*. Vol. 3 of *Austrian Studies*. New York: Berghahn Books, 2001.

Bellettini, Lorenzo. "Freud's Contribution to Arthur Schnitzler's Prose Style." *Rocky Mountain Review of Language and Literature* 61, no. 2 (Fall 2007): 11–27.

Beniston, Judith. *Welttheater: Hofmannsthal, Richard von Kralik, and the Revival of Catholic Drama in Austria, 1800–1934*. Vol. 46 of *MHRA Texts and Dissertations*. London: W. S. Maney & Son Ltd, 1998.

Benjamin, Walter. "What Is Epic Theater?" In *Illuminations*, 147–54. Edited by Hannah Arendt. New York: Schocken Books, 1977.

Bentley, Toni. *Sisters of Salome*. Lincoln: Bison Books, 2005.

Bergel, Kurt. "Rilke's *Fourth Duino Elegy* and Kleist's Essay *Über das Marionettentheater*." *Modern Language Notes* 60, no. 2 (February 1945): 73–78.

Berger, David. "Her Extraordinary Immediacy." *Dance Magazine* XLII (September 1968): 36–38.

Berland, Rosa J. H. "The Exploration of Dreams: Kokoschka's *Die Träumenden Knaben* and Freud." *Source: Notes in the History of Art* 27, no. 2/3, Special Issue on Art and Psycho-analysis (Winter/Spring 2008): 25–31.

Blackshaw, Gemma. *Facing the Modern: The Portrait in Vienna 1900*. London: National Gallery Company and Yale University Press, 2013.

———. "The Pathological Body: Modernist Strategising in Egon Schiele's Self-Portraiture." *Oxford Art Journal* 30, no. 3 (2007): 377–401.

Blackshaw, Gemma, and Leslie Topp. *Madness and Modernity: Mental Illness and the Visual Arts in Vienna 1900*. Farnham: Lund Humphries, 2009.

Blum, Harold. "Setting Freud and Hysteria in Historical Context." In *The Psychoanalytic Century: Freud's Legacy for the Future*, edited by David E. Scharff, 159–63. New York: Other Press, 2001.

Bogatyrëv, Peter. "A Contribution to the Study of Theatrical Signs." Translated by John Burbank, Olga Hasty, Manfred Jacobson, Bruce Kochis, and Wendy Steiner. In *The Prague School: Selected Writings, 1929–1946*, edited by Peter Steiner, 55–64. Austin: University of Texas Press, 1982.

Böhmer, Günter. *Puppets*. Translated by Gerald Morice. Munich: Verlag F. Bruckmann KG, 1969.

Borowitz, Helen O. "Youth as Metaphor and Image in Wedekind, Kokoschka, and Schiele." *Art Journal* 33, no. 3 (Spring 1974): 219–25.

Brandes, Friedrich. "Dresdener Uraufführung Der Salome Von Wilde-Strauss." *Deutsche Tageszeitung*, December 11, 1905, n.p.

Breuer, Josef, and Sigmund Freud. *Studies on Hysteria*. Translated and edited by James Strachey. New York: Basic Books, 2000.

Bronner, Stephen Eric, and F. Peter Wagner, eds. *Vienna: The World of Yesterday, 1889–1914*. Atlantic Highlands: Humanities Press International, Inc., 1997.

Brooks, Peter. *Body Work: Objects of Desire in Modern Narrative*. Cambridge, MA: Harvard University Press, 1993.

Buhrs, Michael, Barbara Lesák, and Thomas Trabitsch, eds. *Fledermaus Kabarett 1907 bis 1913, Ein Gesamtkunstwerk der Wiener Werkstätte: Literatur, Musik, Tanz*. Vienna: Christian Brandstätter und Österreichisches Theatermuseum, 2007.

Butler, E. M. "Hoffmannsthal's [sic] 'Elektra'. A Graeco-Freudian Myth." *Journal of the Warburg Institute* 2, no. 2 (October 1938): 164–75.

Calico, Joy H. "Staging Scandal with *Salome* and *Elektra*." In *The Arts of the Prima Dona in the Long Nineteenth Century*, edited by Rachel Cowgill and Hilary Poriss, 61–82. New York: Oxford University Press, 2012.

Calvocoressi, Richard. *Kokoschka: Paintings*. New York: Rizzoli, 1992.

Caradec, François. *Jane Avril: Au Moulin Rouge avec Toulouse-Lautrec*. Paris: Fayard, 2001.

Carr, G. J. "'Organic' Contradictions in Alfred Kerr's Theatre Criticism." *Oxford German Studies* 14 (1983): 111–24.

Carus, Paul. "Indonesian Legend of Nabi Isa." *The Open Court* 22 (1908): 499–502.

Cernuschi, Claude. *Re/Casting Kokoschka: Ethics and Aesthetics, Epistemology and Politics in Fin-de-Siècle Vienna*. Madison: Fairleigh Dickinson University Press, 2002.

Charcot, Jean-Martin. *Oeuvres complètes*. Vol. 3. Paris: Progrès médical/Lecrosnier & Babé, 1886–1893.

———. *Leçons sur les maladies du système nerveux*. Vol. 3. Paris: Delahaye & Lecrosnier, 1887.

———. "Sur un Cas d'Amnésie Rétro–Antérograde: Probablement d'Origine Hysterique." *Revue de médecine* 12 (1892): 81–96.

———. *Leçons sur l'hystérie virile*. Edited by Michèle Ouerd. Paris: Le Sycomore, 1984.

Charcot, Jean-Martin, D. M. Bourneville, and Paul Régnard. *Iconographie photographique de la Salpêtrière*. 3 Vols. Paris: Progrès médical/Adrien Delahaye, 1876–1880.

Chelius-Zitzewitz. *Oskar Kokoschka: Gemälde, Handzeichnungen, Aquarelle, Drucke*. Dresden: Galerie Ernst Arnold, 1925.

Claretie, Jules. *Les amours d'un interne*. Paris: Dentu, 1881.

Cohen, Matthew Isaac. "Contemporary Wayang in Global Contexts." *Asian Theatre Journal* 24, no. 2 (Fall 2007): 338–69.

Comini, Alessandra. *Egon Schiele's Portraits*. Berkeley: University of California Press, 1974.

———. *Gustav Klimt*. New York: George Braziller, 1975.

Crabtree, Adam. *From Mesmer to Freud: Magnetic Sleep and the Roots of Psychological Healing*. New Haven: Yale University Press, 1994.

Craig, Edward Gordon. "The Actor and the Über-Marionette." *The Mask: A Monthly Journal of the Art of the Theatre* 1, no. 2 (April 1908): 3–8.

David-Ménard, Monique. *Hysteria from Freud to Lacan: Body and Language in Psychoanalysis*. Translated by Catherine Porter. Ithaca: Cornell University Press, 1989.

Davis, W. Eugene. "Oscar Wilde, Salome, and the German Press 1902–1905." *English Literature in Transition, 1880–1920* 44, no. 2 (2001): 149–80.

Der Sturm: Wochenschrift für Kultur und die Künste 1, no. 54, March 11, 1911.

Dickerman, Leah, et al. *Dada: Zürich, Berlin, Hannover, Cologne, New York, Paris*. New York: National Gallery of Art and Distributed Art Publishers, 2005.

Didi-Huberman, Georges. *Invention of Hysteria: Charcot and the Photographic Iconography of the Salpêtrière*. Translated by Alisa Hartz. Cambridge, MA: The MIT Press, 2003.

Die Bühnen des Richard Teschner. Wien: Österreichisches Theater Museum, 2013.

Dobai, Johannes, and Fritz Novotny. *Gustav Klimt*. Edited by Friedrich Welz. Salzburg: Galerie Welz, 1967.

Effenberger, Hans. "Richard Teschners Indisches Theater." *Deutsche Kunst und Dekoration* 32 (April–September 1913): 217–22.

Ellenberger, Henri F. *The Discovery of the Unconscious: The History and Evolution of Dynamic Psychiatry*. New York: Basic Books, 1970.

Erdheim, Mario. "Psychoanalyse Jenseits von Ornament und Askese: Zur Entdeckungsgeschichte des Unbewußten." In *Ornament und Askese: Im Zeitgeist des Wien der Jahrhundertwende*, edited by Alfred Pfabigan, 230–41. Vienna: C. Brandstätter, 1985.

Eulenburg, Albert. "Schauspieler-Krankheiten." *Bühne und Welt: Zeitschrift für Theaterwesen, Litteratur und Musik* 4, no. 9 (February 1902): 388–91.

Eysoldt, Gertrud. *Der Sturm Elektra: Gertrud Eysoldt, Hugo von Hofmannsthal Briefe*. Salzburg: Residenz Verlag, 1996.

Falret, Jules, and Brierre de Boismont. *Über gefährliche Geisteskranke und die Special-Asyle für die sogenannten verbrecherischen Irren. Zwei psychiatrische Abhandlungen*. Translated by Carl Stark. Stuttgart: H. Lindemann, 1871.

Farrar, F. W. "The Bible on the Stage." *The New Review* 8 (January–June 1893): 185.

Fechter, Paul. *Der Expressionismus*. Munich: R. Piper & Co., 1914.

Federn, Ernst, and Herman Nunberg, eds. *The Minutes of the Vienna Psychoanalytic Society*. Vol. 2. New York: International Universities Press, 1967.

Felton, Lori A. "Beyond the *Self-Seers*: The Creative Strategies within Egon Schiele's Double Self-Portraiture." In *The Doppelgänger*, edited by Deborah Ascher Barnstone, 13–44. Vol. 3 of *German Visual Culture*, edited by Deborah Ascher Barnstone and Thomas O. Haakenson. Bern: Peter Lang, 2016.

Fields, Armond. *Le Chat Noir: A Montmartre Cabaret and its Artists in Turn-of-the-Century Paris*. Santa Barbara: Santa Barbara Museum of Art, 1993.

Fischer, Wolfgang Georg. *Egon Schiele 1890–1918: Desire and Decay.* Translated by Michael Hulse. Cologne: Taschen, 2004.

Fischer-Lichte, Erika. *The Semiotics of Theater.* Translated by Jeremy Gaines and Doris L. Jones. Bloomington: Indiana University Press, 1992.

Fisher-Dieskau, Dietrich. *Wagner and Nietzsche.* Translated by Joachim Neugroschel. New York: The Seabury Press, 1976.

Fleischer, Mary. *Embodied Texts: Symbolist Playwright-Dancer Collaborations.* Amsterdam: Editions Rodopi, 2007.

Foster, Hal. *Prosthetic Gods.* Cambridge, MA: The MIT Press, 2004.

Foucault, Michel. *The History of Sexuality: An Introduction.* Vol. 1, translated by Robert Hurley. New York: Vintage Books, 1978.

———. *Madness and Civilization: A History of Insanity in the Age of Reason.* Translated by Richard Howard. Second edn. Oxford: Routledge, 2001.

Freud, Sigmund. *The Etiology of Hysteria.* Vol. 3 of *The Standard Edition of the Complete Psychological Works of Sigmund Freud.* Translated and edited by James Strachey. London: The Hogarth Press and the Institute of Psycho-Analysis, 1953–74.

———. *The Uncanny.* Vol. 17 of *The Standard Edition of the Complete Psychological Works of Sigmund Freud.* Translated and edited by James Strachey. London: The Hogarth Press and the Institute of Psycho-Analysis, 1953–74.

———. "Briefe an Arthur Schnitzler." *Die Neue Rundschau* 66 (1955): 1–12.

———. *Briefe, 1879–1939.* Edited by Ernst and Lucie Freud. Frankfurt: Fischer, 1960.

———. *Letters of Sigmund Freud.* Translated by Tania and James Stern. Edited by Ernst L. Freud. New York: Basic Books, 1960.

———. *Dora: An Analysis of a Case of Hysteria.* Translated by Philip Rieff. Edited by Philip Rieff. New York: Collier Books, 1963.

———. "General Remarks on Hysterical Attacks." In *Dora: An Analysis of a Case of Hysteria,* edited by Philip Rieff, 120–24. New York: Collier Books, 1963.

———. "Hysterical Fantasies and Their Relation to Bisexuality." In *Dora: An Analysis of a Case of Hysteria,* edited by Philip Rieff, translated by Douglas Bryan, 113–19. New York: Collier Books, 1963.

———. *The Interpretation of Dreams.* Translated and edited by James Strachey. Third revised English edn. New York: Avon, 1965.

———. *Three Essays on the Theory of Sexuality.* Translated and edited by James Strachey. Revised edn. New York: Basic Books, 2000.

Friedmann, Armin. "Feuilleton: Bildende Kunst. Salon Miethke: Beardsley." *Wiener Abendpost: Beilage zur Wiener Zeitung,* no. 1, January 2, 1905.

Fürst, L. "Das Pathologische auf der Bühne." *Bühne und Welt: Zeitschrift für Theaterwesen, Litteratur und Musik* 5, no. 9 (February 1903): 375–79.

Gallagher, Catherine, and Thomas Walter Laqueur, eds. *The Making of the Modern Body: Sexuality and Society in the Nineteenth Century.* Berkeley: University of California Press, 1987.

Gilliam, Bryan. *Richard Strauss's Elektra.* Oxford: Oxford University Press, 1996.

Gilman, Sander L. "Strauss, the Pervert, and Avant Garde Opera of the Fin De Siècle." *New German Critique,* no. 43, Special Issue on Austria (Winter 1988): 35–68.

———. "The Image of the Hysteric." In *Hysteria Beyond Freud,* edited by Sander L. Gilman, 345–452. Berkeley: University of California Press, 1993.

———. "Salome, Syphilis, Sarah Bernhardt and the 'Modern Jewess'." *The German Quarterly* 66, no. 2 (Spring 1993): 195–211.

Gilman, Sander L., ed. *Hysteria Beyond Freud.* Berkeley: University of California Press, 1993.

Giroud, Françoise. "Alma Oskar Kokoschka." Translated by R. M. Stock. In *Alma Mahler, or, the Art of Being Loved,* 96–117, 204–05. Oxford: Oxford University Press, 1991.

Goetz, Christopher G., Michel Bonduelle, and Toby Gelfand. *Charcot: Constructing Neurology*. New York: Oxford University Press, 1995.

Goldberg, Itzhak. "Talking Hands." In *Vienna 1900: Klimt, Schiele, Moser, Kokoschka*, edited by Marie-Amélie zu Salm-Salm, 75–84. London: Ashgate, 2005.

Goldstein, Jan. "The Uses of Male Hysteria: Medical and Literary Discourse in Nineteenth-Century France." *Representations* 34 (Spring 1991): 134–65.

Gordon, Rae Beth. *Why the French Love Jerry Lewis: From Cabaret to Early Cinema*. Stanford: Stanford University Press, 2001.

———. "From Charcot to Charlot: Unconscious Imitation and Spectatorship in French Cabaret and Early Cinema." In *The Mind of Modernism: Medicine, Psychology, and the Cultural Arts in Europe and America, 1880–1940*, edited by Mark S. Micale, 93–124. Stanford: Stanford University Press, 2004.

Gorsen, Peter. "Pygmalions stille Frau. Oskar Kokoschka und die Puppe." In *Sexualästhetik. Grenzformen der Sinnlichkeit im 20. Jahrhundert*, 248–58. Reinbek bei Hamburg: Rowohlt-Taschenbuch-Verlag, 1987.

Greiner, Leo. "Münchener Theater." *Revue franco-allemande/Deutsch-französische Rundschau* 2, no. 21 (November 1899): 294–95.

Groddeck, Wolfram. "Nachwort." In *Duineser Elegien, Die Sonette an Orpheus*, 137–55. Stuttgart: Philipp Reclam, 1997.

Grüner, Franz. "Oskar Kokoschka." *Die Fackel* 12, no. 317/318 (February 28, 1911): 18–23.

Gütersloh, Albert Paris von. *Egon Schiele: Versuch Einer Vorrede*. Vienna: Brüder Rosenbaum, 1911.

Gyökér, Sarolta Katalin. "Egon Schiele's Self-Portraiture." MA thesis, Queen's University, 1994.

Haberfeld, Hugo. *Aubrey Beardsley: Galerie Miethke Ausstellung von Werken alter und moderner Kunst*. Vienna: Galerie Miethke, 1905.

Hadamowsky, Franz, ed. *Richard Teschner und Sein Figurenspiegel*. Vienna: Eduard Wancura, 1956.

Hamburger, Michael. "Hofmannsthals Bibliothek." *Euphorion* 55 (1955): 27.

Harrington, Anne. "Hysteria, Hypnosis, and the Lure of the Invisible: The Rise of Neo-Mesmerism in *fin-de-siècle* French Psychiatry." In *The Anatomy of Madness: Essays in the History of Psychiatry*, vol. 3, edited by Roy Porter, W. F. Bynum, and Michael Shepherd, 226–46. London: Routledge, 1988.

Harrison, Charles. "Abstraction." In *Primitivism, Cubism, Abstraction: The Early Twentieth Century*, edited by Francis Frascina, Charles Harrison, and Gill Perry, 184–250. New Haven: Yale University Press, 1993.

Harrison, Thomas. *1910: The Emancipation of Dissonance*. Berkeley: University of California Press, 1996.

Haxell, Nichola A. ""Ces Dames du Cirque": A Taxonomy of Male Desire in Nineteenth-Century French Literature and Art." *MLN* 115, no. 4 (2000): 783–800.

Hevesi, Ludwig. *Altkunst—Neukunst: Wien 1894–1908*. Edited by Otto Breicha. Reprint edn. Klagenfurt: Ritter Verlag, 1984.

———. "Das Kind als Künstler." In *Altkunst-Neukunst: Wien 1894–1908*, edited by Otto Breicha, 449–54. Reprint edn. Klagenfurt: Ritter Verlag, 1984.

Hibberd, J. L. "The Spirit of the Flesh: Wedekind's Lulu." *The Modern Language Review* 79, no. 2 (April 1984): 336–55.

Hirschfeld, Georg. "Neue Puppen von Lotte Pritzel–München." *Deutsche Kunst und Dekoration* 31 (October 1912–March 1913): 254–60.

Hofen, Franz. "Sarah Bernhardt in Deutschland." *Bühne und Welt: Zeitschrift für Theaterwesen, Litteratur und Musik* 5, no. 3 (November 1902): 89–93.

Hoffmann, E. T. A. *The Best Tales of Hoffmann*. Edited by E. F. Bleiler. New York: Dover Publications, Inc., 1967.

Hoffmann, Edith. *Kokoschka: Life and Work.* London: Faber and Faber Limited, 1947.

Hofmann, Paul. *The Viennese: Splendor, Twilight, and Exile.* New York: Anchor Press, 1988.

Hofmannsthal, Hugo von. "Über die Pantomime." *Süddeutsche Monatshefte* 9, no. 1 (October 1911): 100–3.

———. *Briefe 1900–1909.* Vienna: Bermann-Fischer Verlag, 1937.

———. *Prosa.* Vol. 1. Frankfurt: S. Fischer, 1956.

———. "Die Unvergleichliche Tanzerin." In *Reden und Aufsätze I: 1891–1913*, edited by Bernd Schoeller. Vol. 8 of *Gesammelte Werke*, edited by Bernd Schoeller, 496–501. Frankfurt: S. Fischer Taschenbuch Verlag, 1979.

———. *The Lord Chandos Letter.* Translated by Russell Stockman. Marlboro: The Marlboro Press, 1986.

———. *Elektra.* Stuttgart: Schauspiel Staatstheater, 2003.

Holland, Norman N. "Freud and the Poet's Eye: His Ambivalence toward the Artist." *PsyArt: An Online Journal for the Psychological Study of the Arts* 2 (1998): n.p.

Hustvedt, Asti. *Medical Muses: Hysteria in Nineteenth-Century Paris.* New York: W. W. Norton & Company, 2011.

Huter, Michael. "Body as Metaphor: Aspects of the Critique and Crisis of Language at the Turn of the Century with Reference to Egon Schiele." In *Egon Schiele: Art, Sexuality, and Viennese Modernism*, edited by Patrick Werkner, 119–29. Palo Alto: The Society for the Promotion of Science and Scholarship, 1994.

Huysmans, Joris-Karl. *Against Nature (À Rebours).* Translated by Robert Baldick and Patrick McGuinness. London: Penguin Books, 2003.

Huyssen, Andreas. "The Disturbance of Vision in Vienna Modernism." *Modernism/Modernity* 5, no. 3 (1998): 33–47.

Innes, Christopher. *Edward Gordon Craig: A Vision of the Theatre.* Second edn. Amsterdam: Hardwood Academic Publishers, 1998.

Jelavich, Peter. *Munich and Theatrical Modernism: Politics, Playwriting, and Performance, 1890–1914.* Cambridge, MA: Harvard University Press, 1985.

———. *Berlin Cabaret.* Cambridge, MA: Harvard University Press, 1993.

Jensen, Robert. "A Matter of Professionalism: Marketing Identity in *Fin-de-Siècle* Vienna." In *Rethinking Vienna 1900*, edited by Steven Beller, 195–219. New York: Berghahn Books, 2001.

Jentsch, Ernst. "Zur Psychologie des Unheimlichen." *Psychiatrisch-Neurologische Wochenschrift* 8, no. 22 (August 25, 1906): 195–98.

———. "Zur Psychologie des Unheimlichen." *Psychiatrisch-Neurologische Wochenschrift* 8, no. 23 (September 1, 1906): 203–05.

———. "On the Psychology of the Uncanny (1906)." *Angelaki: A New Journal in Philosophy, Literature, and the Social Sciences* 2, no. 1, translated by Roy Sellars (1996): 7–16.

Jones, Ernst. *The Life and Work of Sigmund Freud.* Vol. 3. New York: Basic Books, 1957.

Joravsky, David. "Between Science and Art: Freud Versus Schnitzler, Kafka, and Musil." In *The Mind of Modernism: Medicine, Psychology, and the Cultural Arts in Europe and America, 1880–1940*, edited by Mark S. Micale, 277–97. Stanford: Stanford University Press, 2004.

Kaes, Anton. "The Debate about Cinema: Charting a Controversy (1909–1929)." *New German Critique*, no. 40, Special Issue on Weimar Film Theory (Winter 1987): 7–33.

Kallir, Jane. *Gustav Klimt: 25 Masterworks.* New York: Harry N. Abrams, 1995.

———. *Egon Schiele: Life and Work.* New York: Harry N. Abrams, 1996.

Kandel, Eric R. *The Age of Insight: The Quest to Understand the Unconscious in Art, Mind, and Brain, from Vienna 1900 to the Present.* New York: Random House, 2012.

Kandinsky, Wassily. *Über das Geistige in der Kunst: Insbesondere in der Malerei.* München: R. Piper & Co., 1912.

Kaplan, Ellen W., and Sarah J. Rudolph, eds. *Images of Mental Illness Through Text and Performance.* Vol. 33 of *Studies in Theatre Arts.* Lewiston: The Edwin Mellen Press, 2005.

Karnes, Kevin C. *A Kingdom Not of This World: Wagner, the Arts, and Utopian Visions in Fin-de-Siècle Vienna.* New York: Oxford University Press, 2013.

Karpfen, Fritz, ed. *Das Egon Schiele Buch.* Vienna: Verlag der Wiener Graphischen Werkstätte, 1921.

Katalog der Kunstschau Wien 1908. Vienna: Holzhausen, 1908.

Kawalec, Urszula. "Die Hypnose in der Österreichischen Literatur der Jahrhundertwende. Am Beispiel der Pantomime Pierrot Hypnotiseur von Richard Beer-Hofmann." *Orbis Linguarum* 19 (2002): 161–69.

Keegan, Susanne. *The Eye of God: A Life of Oskar Kokoschka.* London: Bloomsbury, 1999.

Kelley, Susanne. "Perceptions of Jewish Female Bodies Through Gustav Klimt and Peter Altenberg." *Imaginations* 3, no. 1 (May 2012): 109–22.

Kerr, Alfred. "Rose Bernd und Elektra." *Neue Deutsche Rundschau* 14 (1903): 1311–17.

———. *Die Welt im Drama.* Vol. 2. Berlin: S. Fischer, 1917.

Klaar, Alfred. ["Elektra,"] *Vossische Zeitung,* no. 511, (October 31, 1903).

Kleist, Heinrich von. "On the Marionette Theatre." *The Drama Review* 16, no. 3, The "Puppet" Issue. Translated by Thomas G. Neumiller (September 1972): 22–26.

———. "Über das Marionettentheater." *Berliner Abendblätter,* nos. 63–66, (December 12–15, 1810), 247–61.

Kleist, Heinrich von. *Über das Marionettentheater: Aufsätze und Anekdoten.* Zweite edn. Frankfurt: Insel, 1982.

Knafo, Danielle. "Egon Schiele's Self-Portraits: A Psychoanalytic Study in the Creation of a Self." In *The Annual of Psychoanalysis,* edited by Chicago Institute for Psychoanalysis, 59–90. Chicago: Chicago Institute for Psychoanalysis, 1991.

Knopf, Robert, ed. *Theater of the Avant-Garde, 1890–1950: A Critical Anthology.* New Haven: Yale University Press, 2015.

Kohn, Hannah. "Richard Teschners Figurenspiegel als Spiegel des Zeitgeistes einer Epoche." M.Phil. thesis, Universität Wien, 2012.

Kokoschka, Oskar. *Die Träumenden Knaben.* Vienna: Wiener Werkstätte mit Berger und Chwala, 1908.

———. *Der Weisse Tiertöter.* Vienna: Genossenschaftsverlag, 1920.

———. "On the Nature of Visions." Translated by Heidi Medlinger and John Thwaites. In *Kokoschka, Life and Work,* edited by Edith Hoffmann, 285–87. London: Faber and Faber, 1947.

———. "Sphinx und Strohmann: Komödie für Automaten." *Wort in der Zeit: Österreichische Literaturzeitschrift* 2, no. 3 (March 1956): 145–48.

———. "Von der Natur der Gesichte." In *Oskar Kokoschka: Schriften 1907–1955,* edited by Hans Maria Wingler, 337–41. Munich: Langen Müller, 1956.

———. *My Life.* Translated by David Britt. New York: Macmillan Publishing Co., Inc., 1974.

———. "Der Fetisch." In *Oskar Kokoschka: Die Frühen Jahre, Aquarelle und Zeichnungen (1906–1924),* edited by Carl Albrecht Haenlein, 67–79. Hannover: Kestner-Gesellschaft, 1983.

Kokoschka, Oskar, and Ernst Reinhold. *Kokoschka-Matinee Einladung.* (March 29, 1909).

Koss, Juliet. "Bauhaus Theater of Human Dolls." *The Art Bulletin* 85, no. 4 (December 2003): 724–45.

Krafft-Ebing, Richard von. *Psychopathia Sexualis: Eine Klinisch-Forensische Studie.* Stuttgart: Ferdinand Enke, 1886.

———. *Hypnotische Experimente.* Second extended edn. Stuttgart: Ferdinand Enke, 1893.

———. *Über Gesunde und Kranke Nerven.* Fifth revised edn. Tübingen: H. Laupp'sche Buchhandlung, 1903.

Kramer, Lawrence. "Culture and Musical Hermeneutics: The Salome Complex." *Cambridge Opera Journal* 2, no. 3 (November 1990): 269–94.

———. "*Fin-de-Siècle* Fantasies: *Elektra*, Degeneration and Sexual Science." *Cambridge Opera Journal* 5, no. 2 (July 1993): 141–65.

Kultermann, Udo. "The 'Dance of the Seven Veils': Salome and Erotic Culture around 1900." *Artibus et Historiae* 27, no. 53 (2006): 187–215.

Kumar, Ann. *Java and Modern Europe: Ambiguous Encounters*. Richmond: Curzon Press, 1997.

Kupper, Herbert I., and Hilda S. Rollman-Branch. "Freud und Schnitzler—(Doppelgänger)." *Journal of the American Psychoanalytic Association* 7 (January 1959): 109–26.

Lahusen, Susanne. "Oskar Schlemmer: Mechanical Ballets?" *Dance Research* 4, no. 2 (Autumn 1986): 65–77.

Lankheit, Klaus. "A History of the Almanac." In *The Blaue Reiter Almanac*, edited by Klaus Lankheit, 11–48. New York: Da Capo Press, 1974.

Lenman, Robin. *Artists and Society in Germany, 1850–1914*. Manchester: Manchester University Press, 1997.

Leopold, Elisabeth, et al. *Egon Schiele: Letters and Poems 1910–1912 from the Leopold Collection*. Munich: Prestel, 2008.

Lerner, Paul. *Hysterical Men: War, Psychiatry, and the Politics of Trauma in Germany, 1890–1930*. Ithaca: Cornell University Press, 2003.

Lichtenstein, Thérèse. *Behind Closed Doors: The Art of Hans Bellmer*. Los Angeles: University of California Press, 2001.

Lomas, David. *The Haunted Self: Surrealism, Psychoanalysis, Subjectivity*. New Haven: Yale University Press, 1999.

Lorenz, Dagmar C. G., ed. *A Companion to the Works of Arthur Schnitzler*. Rochester: Camden House, 2003.

Man, Paul de. *The Rhetoric of Romanticism*. New York: Columbia University Press, 1984.

Marinis, Marco de. *The Semiotics of Performance*. Translated by Áine O'Healy. Bloomington: Indiana University Press, 1993.

Martens, Lorna. "The Theme of the Repressed Memory in Hofmannsthal's *Elektra*." *The German Quarterly* 60, no. 1 (Winter 1987): 38–51.

———. *Shadow Lines: Austrian Literature from Freud to Kafka*. Lincoln: University of Nebraska Press, 1996.

Martensen, Karin. "Anna Bahr-Mildenburg." In *MUGI. Musikvermittlung und Genderforschung: Lexikon und Multimediale Präsentationen*, edited by Beatrix Borchard und Nina Noeske. Hamburg: Hochschule für Musik und Theater Hamburg, 2003.

McCarren, Felicia. "The 'Symptomatic Act' circa 1900: Hysteria, Hypnosis, Electricity, Dance." *Critical Inquiry* 21, no. 4 (Summer 1995): 748–74.

McGuire, William, ed. *The Freud/Jung Letters: The Correspondence between Sigmund Freud and C. G. Jung*. Translated by Ralph Manheim and R. F. C. Hull. Vol. 94 of *Bollingen Series*. Princeton: Princeton University Press, 1974.

McMullen, Sally. "From the Armchair to the Stage: Hofmannsthal's 'Elektra' in its Theatrical Context." *The Modern Language Review* 80, no. 3 (July 1985): 637–51.

Medicus, Thomas. "Das Theater der Nervosität. Freud, Charcot, Sarah Bernhardt und die Salpêtrière." *Freibeuter* 41 (1989): 93–103.

Meyden, H. van der. "Belle Epoque: Klimt and Schiele." *Apollo* CXXVI (December 1987).

Micale, Mark. *Hysterical Men: The Hidden History of Male Nervous Illness*. Cambridge, MA: Harvard University Press, 2008.

Micale, Mark S. "Charcot and the Idea of Hysteria in the Male: Gender, Mental Science, and Medical Diagnosis in Late Nineteenth-Century France." *Medical History* 34, no. 4 (October 1990): 363–411.

———. "Discourses of Hysteria in Fin-De-Siècle France." In *The Mind of Modernism: Medicine, Psychology, and the Cultural Arts in Europe and America, 1880–1940*, edited by Mark S. Micale, 71–92. Stanford: Stanford University Press, 2004.

Michel, Wilhelm. "Puppen von Lotte Pritzel." *Deutsche Kunst und Dekoration* 27 (October 1910–March 1911): 329–38.

Mrázek, Jan. "Javanese Wayang Kulit in the Times of Comedy: Clown Scenes, Innovation, and the Performance's Being in the Present World: Part One." *Indonesia* 68 (October 1999): 38–128.

Myslobodsky, Michael S. *The Fallacy of Mother's Wisdom: A Critical Perspective on Health Psychology.* Hackensack: World Scientific Publishing Co., 2004.

Natter, Tobias G., and Max Hollein, eds. *The Naked Truth: Klimt, Schiele, Kokoschka and Other Scandals.* Translated by Elizabeth Clegg. Munich: Prestel, 2005.

Natter, Tobias G., and Ursula Storch, eds. *Egon Schiele & Arthur Roessler: Der Kunstler und Sein Forderer. Kunst und Networking im Fruhen 20. Jahrhundert.* Ostfildern-Ruit: Hatje Cantz, 2004.

Nebehay, Christian M. *Egon Schiele, 1890–1918: Leben, Briefe, Gedichte.* Salzburg: Residenz Verlag, 1979.

Nelson, Claudia. "The 'Child-Woman' and the Victorian Novel." *Nineteenth Century Studies* 20 (2007): 1–12.

Nietzsche, Friedrich. *Thus Spoke Zarathustra: A Book for Everyone and No One.* Translated by R. J. Hollingdale. New York: Penguin, 1969.

Nunberg, Herman, and Ernst Federn, eds. *The Minutes of the Vienna Psychoanalytic Society.* Vol. 2. New York: International Universities Press, 1967.

Ostini, Fritz von. "Die VIII. Internationale Kunstausstellung im KGL Glaspalast zu München." *Die Kunst für Alle: Malerei, Plastik, Graphik, Architektur* 16, no. 23 (September 1, 1901): 538–48.

Paupié, Kurt. *Handbuch der Osterreichischen Pressegeschichte, 1848–1959.* Vol. 1. Vienna: Wilhelm Braumüller, 1960.

Pelizzon, V. Penelope. "Memoire on the Heliographe." *Fourth Genre: Explorations in Nonfiction* 6, no. 2 (2004): 35–48.

Perkins, Geoffrey. *Contemporary Theory of Expressionism.* Bern: Peter Lang, 1974.

Pfabigan, Alfred, ed. *Ornament und Askese: Im Zeitgeist des Wien der Jahrhundertwende.* Vienna: C. Brandstätter, 1985.

Pierce, Jennifer L. "The Relation between Emotion Work and Hysteria: A Feminist Reinterpretation of Freud's *Studies on Hysteria.*" *Women's Studies* 16 (1989): 255–70.

Politzer, Heinz. "Arthur Schnitzler: The Poetry of Psychology." *MLN* 78, no. 4, German Issue (October 1963): 353–72.

———. "Hugo von Hofmannsthal's 'Elektra': Geburt der Tragödie aus dem Geiste der Psychopathologie." *Deutsche Vierteljahrschrift* 47 (1973): 95–119.

Price, Renée, ed. *Egon Schiele: The Ronald S. Lauder and Serge Sabarsky Collections.* New York: Prestel, 2005.

Price, Steven, and William Tydeman. *Wilde: Salome.* Cambridge: Cambridge University Press, 1996.

Reiss, H. S. "The Problems of Fate and of Religion in the Work of Arthur Schnitzler." *The Modern Language Review* 40, no. 4 (Oct. 1945): 300–8.

Remshardt, Ralf E. *Staging the Savage God: The Grotesque in Performance.* Carbondale: Southern Illinois University Press, 2004.

"Richard Teschner's Figure Theatre." *Theatre Arts Monthly* 23, no. 7 (1928): 490–95.

Richet, Charles. "Le Somnambulisme Provoqué." *Journal d'Anatomie et de Physiologie Normale et Pathologique* 11 (1875): 348–78.

Rilke, Rainer Maria. *Auguste Rodin.* Vol. 10 of *Die Kunst.* Berlin: Bard, 1903.

———. *Puppen.* München: Hyperionverlag, 1921.

———. *Briefe an Auguste Rodin.* Leipzig: Insel-Verlag, 1928.

———. *Duineser Elegien, Die Sonette an Orpheus.* Stuttgart: Philipp Reclam, 1997.

———. *The Duino Elegies.* Translated by John Waterfield. Lewiston: Edwin Mellen Press, 1999.

Roessler, Arthur. "Neukunstgruppe. Ausstellung im Kunstsalon Pisko." *Arbeiter Zeitung*, no. 336, December 7, 1909, 21.

———. *Erinnerungen an Egon Schiele.* Vienna: Verlag Carl Konegen, 1922.

———. *Richard Teschner.* Vienna: Gerlach & Wiedling, 1947.

Roessler, Arthur, ed. *Briefe und Prosa von Egon Schiele.* Vienna: Buchhandlung Richard Lányi, 1921.

Roos, Bonnie. "Oskar Kokoschka's Sex Toy: The Women and the Doll Who Conceived the Artist." *Modernism/Modernity* 12, no. 2 (2005): 291–309.

Roth, Michael. "Falling into History: Freud's Case of Frau Emmy von N." In *The Psycho-analytic Century: Freud's Legacy for the Future*, edited by David E. Scharff, 5–20. New York: Other Press, 2001.

Ryan, Judith. *Rilke, Modernism and Poetic Tradition.* Cambridge: Cambridge University Press, 2004.

Schaumberg, Georg. "Münchener Brief." *Bühne und Welt: Zeitschrift für Theaterwesen, Litteratur und Musik* 3, no. 16 (May 1901): 696–700.

Schechner, Richard. "Wayang Kulit in the Colonial Margin." *TDR* 34, no. 2 (Summer 1990): 25–61.

Schiele, Egon. "Skizzen." *Die Aktion* 4, no. 9 (February 1914): 234.

———. "Gedichte." *Die Aktion* 4, no. 15 (April 1914): 323.

———. "Die Kunst der Neukünstler." *Die Aktion* 4, no. 20 (May 1914): 428.

———. "Zwei Gedichte." *Die Aktion* 5, no. 3/4 (January 1915): 37–38.

———. "Ährenfeld." *Die Aktion* 5, no. 31/32 (August 1915): 398.

———. "Abendland." *Die Aktion* 6, no. 35/36 (September 1916): 493.

Schjeldahl, Peter. "Golden Girl: The Neue Galerie's new Klimt." *The New Yorker*, July 24, 2006, n.p.

Schneider, Manfred. *Der Expressionismus im Drama.* Stuttgart: Julius Hoffmann, 1920.

———. "Hysterie als Gesamtkunstwerk." In *Ornament und Askese: Im Zeitgeist des Wien der Jahrhundertwende*, edited by Alfred Pfabigan, 212–29. Vienna: C. Brandstätter, 1985.

Schnitzler, Arthur. *Der Tapfere Cassian: Puppenspiel in einem Akt.* Berlin: S. Fischer, 1910.

———. *Gallant Cassian: A Puppet-Play in One Act.* Translated by Adam L. Gowans. Third edn. London: Gowans and Gray Ltd, 1914.

———. *Paracelsus and Other One-Act Plays.* Translated by G. J. Weinberger. Riverside: Ariadne Press, 1995.

———. *Eight Plays: Performance Texts.* Translated by William L. Cunningham and David Palmer. Evanston: Northwestern University Press, 2007.

Schorske, Carl E. *Fin-de-Siècle Vienna: Politics and Culture.* New York: Vintage Books, 1981.

Schreder, Karl. "Kunstuntergang im 'Hagenbund'." *Deutsches Volksblatt* 23, no. 7941, February 9, 1911, 1–2.

Schröder, Klaus Albrecht. *Egon Schiele: Eros and Passion.* Translated by David Britt. Munich: Prestel, 1989.

Schuler-Will, Jeannine. "Wedekind's Lulu: Pandora and Pierrot, the Visual Experience of Myth." *German Studies Review* 7, no. 1 (February 1984): 27–38.

Schvey, Henry I. "Oskar Kokoschka's 'The Dreaming Youths'." *Books Abroad* 49, no. 3 (Summer 1975): 484–85.

———. *Oskar Kokoschka: The Painter as Playwright.* Detroit: Wayne State University Press, 1982.

Schweiger, Werner J. *Der Junge Kokoschka: Leben und Werk, 1904–1914.* Vienna: Christian Brandstätter, 1983.

Scott, Jill. *Electra After Freud: Myth and Culture.* Ithaca: Cornell University Press, 2005.

Segel, Harold B. *Turn-of-the-Century Cabaret: Paris, Barcelona, Berlin, Munich, Vienna, Cracow, Moscow, St. Petersburg, Zurich.* New York: Columbia University Press, 1987.

————. *Pinocchio's Progeny: Puppets, Marionettes, Automatons, and Robots in Modernist and Avant-Garde Drama*. Baltimore: The Johns Hopkins University Press, 1995.

Sekula, Allan. "The Body and the Archive." *October* 39 (Winter 1986): 3–64.

Selz, Peter. *German Expressionist Painting*. Berkeley: University of California Press, 1957.

Servaes, Franz. "Neue Theaterpuppen von Richard Teschner." *Deutsche Kunst und Dekoration* 33 (October 1912–March 1913): 169–73.

Seshadri, Anne L. "The Taste of Love: Salome's Transfiguration." *Women & Music: A Journal of Gender and Culture* 10 (2006): 24–44.

Shershow, Scott Cutler. *Puppets and "Popular" Culture*. Ithaca: Cornell University Press, 1995.

Sine, Nadine. "Cases of Mistaken Identity: Salome and Judith at the Turn of the Century." *German Studies Review* 11, no. 1 (February 1988): 9–29.

Smith, Kimberly A. "The Tactics of Fashion: Jewish Women in Fin-De-Siècle Vienna." *Aurora: The Journal of the History of Art* 4 (2003): 135–54.

————. *Between Ruin and Renewal: Egon Schiele's Landscapes*. New Haven: Yale University Press, 2004.

Sommer, Doris. "A Vindication of Double Consciousness." In *A Companion to Postcolonial Studies*, edited by Henry Schwarz and Sangeeta Ray, 165–79. Malden: Blackwell Publishers, Inc., 2000.

Sonne, Otto. "Strauss–Hofmannsthal *Elektra*." *Illustrirte Zeitung*, January 28, 1909, n.p.

Stefan, Paul. *Anna Bahr-Mildenburg*. Vienna: Wiener Literar. Anst., 1922.

Stein, Erwin. "Mahler and the Vienna Opera." In *The Opera Bedside Book*, edited by Harold Rosenthal, 296–317. London: V. Gollancz, 1965.

Stein, Philipp. "Ibsen auf den Berliner Bühnen 1876/1900." *Bühne und Welt: Zeitschrift für Theaterwesen, Litteratur und Musik* 3, no. 12 (March 1901): 489–504.

Steiner, Reinhard. *Egon Schiele, 1890–1918*. Translated by Michael Hulse. Cologne: Taschen Verlag, 2000.

Street, Lisa J. "Oskar Kokoschka's Doll: Symbol of Culture." PhD diss., Emory University, 1993.

Strzygowski, Josef. "Junge Künstler im Hagenbund." *Die Zeit* 10, no. 3010, February 9, 1911, 1–2.

Stümcke, Heinrich. "Von Den Berliner Theatern 1902/03." *Bühne und Welt: Zeitschrift für Theaterwesen, Litteratur und Musik* 5, no. 3 (November 1902): 167–70.

————. "Von Den Berliner Theatern 1902/03." *Bühne und Welt: Zeitschrift für Theaterwesen, Litteratur und Musik* 5, no. 4 (November 1902): 167–70.

————. "Von Den Berliner Theatern 1902/03." *Bühne und Welt: Zeitschrift für Theaterwesen, Litteratur und Musik* 5, no. 5 (December 1902): 211–15.

————. "Von Den Berliner Theatern 1902/03." *Bühne und Welt: Zeitschrift für Theaterwesen, Litteratur und Musik* 5, no. 6 (December 1902): 254–56.

————. "Von Den Berliner Theatern 1902/03." *Bühne und Welt: Zeitschrift für Theaterwesen, Litteratur und Musik* 5, no. 7 (January 1903): 298–300.

Suleiman, Susan Rubin. *Subversive Intent: Gender, Politics, and the Avant-Garde*. Cambridge, MA: Harvard University Press, 1990.

Symons, Arthur. "Aubrey Beardsley." *Ver Sacrum: Organ der Vereinigung bildender Kuenstler Österreichs* 6, no. 6. Translated by Anna Muthesius (March 15, 1903): 117–38.

Szecsödy, Imre. "Dora: Freud's Pygmalion?" In *The Psychoanalytic Century: Freud's Legacy for the Future*, edited by David E. Scharff, 125–38. New York: Other Press, 2001.

Tausky, Robert. *Hiob: Ein Mann im Lande Utz und seine Wege durch die Welt*. Würzburg: Verlag Königshausen & Neumann, 2004.

Taylor, Sue. *Hans Bellmer: The Anatomy of Anxiety*. Cambridge, MA: The MIT Press, 2002.

Tillis, Steve. *Toward an Aesthetics of the Puppet: Puppetry as a Theatrical Art*. Westport: Greenwood Press, 1992.

Topp, Leslie. *Architecture and Truth in Fin-de-Siècle Vienna*. Cambridge: Cambridge University Press, 2004.

Toro, Fernando de. *Theatre Semiotics: Text and Staging in Modern Theatre*. Translated by John Lewis. Edited by Carole Hubbard. Toronto: University of Toronto Press, 1995.

———. "L'attitude et la Marche dans L'Hémiplégie Hystérique." In *Nouvelle Iconographie de la Salpêtrière: Clinique des Maladies du Système Nerveux*, plates I and II. Paris: Lescronier et Babbé, 1888.

Tourette, Gilles de la. *L'hypnotisme et les états analogues au point de vue médico-légal*. Paris: Plon, Nourrit et Cie, Imprimeurs-Éditeurs, 1887.

Uhr, Horst. *Lovis Corinth*. Berkeley: University of California Press, 1990.

Urban, Bernd. *Hofmannsthal, Freud und die Psychoanalyse*. Frankfurt: Peter Lang, 1978.

Valiani, Leo. *The End of Austria-Hungary*. New York: Alfred A. Knopf, 1973.

Varnedoe, Kirk. *Vienna 1900: Art, Architecture & Design*. New York: The Museum of Modern Art, 1986.

Vergo, Peter. "Gustav Klimts 'Philosophie' und das Programm der Universitätsgemälde." *Mitteilungen der Österreichischen Galerie* 22/23, no. 66/67, Klimt-Studien (1978/79): 69–100.

———. *Art in Vienna, 1898–1918: Klimt, Kokoschka, Schiele and their Contemporaries*. Third edn. London: Phaidon Press Limited, 1993.

Vergo, Peter, and Barnaby Wright, eds. *Egon Schiele: The Radical Nude*. London: The Courtauld Gallery and Paul Holberton Publishing, 2014.

Veyrac, S. "Nos Interviews: Une Heure Chez Sarah Bernhardt." *La Chronique Médicale: Revue Bi-mensuelle de Médecine, Historique, Littéraire et Anecdotique* 4, no. 19 (October 1, 1897): 609–18.

Wagner, Manfred. *Alfred Roller in Seiner Zeit*. Salzburg: Residenz Verlag, 1996.

Ward, Philip Marshall. "Hofmannsthal, *Elektra* and the Representation of Women's Behaviour Through Myth." *German Life and Letters* 53, no. 1 (2003): 37–55.

Warlick, M. E. "Mythic Rebirth in Gustav Klimt's Stoclet Frieze: New Considerations of Its Egyptianizing Form and Content." *The Art Bulletin* 74, no. 1 (March 1992): 115–34.

Wedekind, Frank. *Erdgeist (Earth-Spirit)*. Translated by Jr. Samuel A. Eliot. New York: Albert and Charles Boni, 1914.

Weidinger, Alfred. *Kokoschka and Alma Mahler: Testimony to a Passionate Relationship*. Munich: Prestel, 1996.

Weinberger, G. J. "Marionette or 'Puppenspieler'?: Arthur Schnitzler's Pierrot." *Neophilologus* 86 (2002): 265–72.

Weininger, Otto. *Geschlecht und Charakter: Eine Prinzipielle Untersuchung*. Vienn: Wilhelm Braumüller, 1904.

Weißenböck, Jarmila. *Der Figurenspiegel Richard Teschner*. Vienna: Böhlau, 1991.

Werkner, Patrick. *Austrian Expressionism: The Formative Years*. Translated by Nicholas T. Parsons. New York: The Society for the Promotion of Science and Scholarship, 1993.

———. "The Child-Woman and Hysteria: Images of the Female Body in the Art of Schiele, in Viennese Modernism, and Today." In *Egon Schiele: Art, Sexuality, and Viennese Modernism*, edited by Patrick Werkner, 51–78. Palo Alto: The Society for the Promotion of Science and Scholarship, 1994.

Werkner, Patrick, ed. *Egon Schiele: Art, Sexuality, and Viennese Modernism*. Palo Alto: The Society for the Promotion of Science and Scholarship, 1994.

Whalen, Robert Weldon. *Sacred Spring: God and the Birth of Modernism in Fin de Siècle Vienna*. Cambridge: Eerdmans Publishing Co., 2007.

Wheeler, Graham. "Gender and Transgression in Sophocles' 'Electra'." *The Classical Quarterly* 53, no. 2 (Nov. 2003): 377–88.

Whitford, Frank. *Egon Schiele*. London: Thames and Hudson Ltd, 1981.

———. *Oskar Kokoschka: A Life*. New York: Atheneum, 1986.

Wittels, Fritz. *Freud and the Child Woman: The Memoirs of Fritz Wittels*. Edited by Edward Timms. New Haven: Yale University Press, 1996.

Wölfflin, Heinrich. *Principles of Art History: The Problem of the Development of Style in Later Art*. Translated by M. D. Hottinger. New York: Dover Publications, 1950.

Worps, Michael. *Nervenkunst*. Frankfurt: Europäische Verlagsanstalt, 1983.

Worringer, Wilhelm. *Abstraktion und Einfühlung: Ein Beitrag zur Stilpsychologie*. Third edn. Munich: R. Piper & Co., 1911.

Wright, Alastair. *Matisse and the Subject of Modernism*. Princeton: Princeton University Press, 2005.

Wright, John P. "Hysteria and Mechanical Man." *Journal of the History of Ideas* 40, no. 2 (April–June 1980): 233–47.

Yates, W. E. *Theatre in Vienna: A Critical History, 1776–1995*. Cambridge: Cambridge University Press, 1996.

Zuckerkandl, Berta. "The Klimt Affair." In *Gustav Klimt: The Ronald S. Lauder and Serge Sabarsky Collections*, edited by Renée Price, 459–61. Munich: Prestel, 2007.

Zuelsdorf, Dean. "Implications of Creativity, Artistic Expression, and Psychological Cohesion: The Self-Portrait as a Reparative Self-Object of Egon Schiele." PhD diss., The Chicago School of Professional Psychology, 1995.

Zweig, Stefan. *The World of Yesterday*. Lincoln, NE: University of Nebraska Press, 1964.

Index

Adrienne Lecouvreur (play) 69–70
Akademie der bildenden Künste Wien
  (Academy of Fine Arts, Vienna) 30, 32, 35
Akademischen Verband für Literatur
  und Musik (Academic Association for
  Literature and Music, Vienna) 19
Aktion, Die (*The Action*, magazine) 32–33
Allan, Maud 91, 108, 110–11, 120 n50; *see
  also* Salome
Alma doll: *see* Alma Mahler
Altenberg, Peter 27–28
anti-Semitism 9, 54, 92, 103
Arnot, Guido 171
art nouveau 30, 108; *see also* Jugendstil;
  Secession
Asian puppetry 135, 138, 162, 169–71,
  178–79
Augustine 10, 51–55, 58–59
Austrian Theater Museum 81, 94, 136
Avril, Jane 68–71, 77; *Jane Avril
  Dancing* (painting) by Henri de
  Toulouse-Lautrec 71

Badoureau, Jean-François: *Hystero-epileptic
  attack: period of contortions* (drawing)
  59–60, 71, 176
Bahr, Hermann 13, 19, 23–25, 27, 33,
  37, 78–79, 81, 91, 93–94, 121–22,
  125, 127–28, 130, 133, 141–42;
  Expressionismus (*Expressionism*, book)
  23–24, 142; *Marionetten* (*Marionettes*,
  essay) 127, 142
Bahr-Mildenburg, Anna 14, 81, 91, 93–96,
  98–101, 103–04, 158
Baragwanath, Nicholas 81
Bauer, Ida: *see* Dora
Beardsley, Aubrey 108, 123, 133
Beer-Hofmann, Richard 155
Beizer, Janet 103
Beller, Steven 8
Bellmer, Hans 153
Benjamin, Walter 144
Bernhardt, Sarah 60, 68–73, 93

Blackshaw, Gemma 9, 11, 44, 60, 122–23
Blaue Reiter 25, 40 n32
Blum, Harold 50, 54–55
body/bodies: *see* Viennese modern body
Böhmer, Günter 163
Bourneville, D. M. 49
Brandes, Friedrich 66, 80–81, 101
Breuer, Josef 13, 43, 46–50, 54–56, 78–79, 86
  n71, 103
Brooks, Peter 124, 131
Brouillet, Pierre Aristide André: *A Clinical
  Lesson at the Salpêtrière* (painting)
  53–54, 59
Bühne und Welt (*Stage and World*, journal)
  72, 74, 77, 169
Burgtheater, Vienna 141

catalepsy 59, 107–08, 118 n21 & n22
Cernuschi, Claude 9, 16 n16, 30–31
Charcot, Jean-Martin 9–10, 13, 44–53, 55–60,
  62 n19 & n20, 66–71, 79, 99, 103, 110–11,
  118 n21, 121, 123, 153–54, 183; *Nouvelle
  Iconographie de la Salpêtrière* (*New
  Iconography of the Salpêtrière*, medical
  journal) 9, 55; *Iconographie photographique
  de la Salpêtrière* (*Photographic Iconography
  of the Salpêtrière*, medical journal) 9, 49–55,
  55, 57, 59, 67
Chat Noir, Le (The Black Cat, cabaret) 163
Claretie, Jules 69, 71, 83 n21
Comini, Alessandra 9, 31, 112
Craig, Edward Gordon 130–31

Dada 146, 153, 164, 184 n3
David-Ménard, Monique 56
Deutsche Kunst und Dekoration (*German
  Art and Decoration*, magazine) 132–34,
  138–40, 150 n48
Deutsches Theater 102
Deutsches Volksblatt (*German People's Paper*,
  newspaper) 18, 114
dialectics of vision: *see* Vision dialectic
Didi-Huberman, Georges 45, 51–52

Divéky, Josef von: *Poster for the Cabaret Fledermaus* (lithograph) 112–13
doll 6, 11, 14, 35, 116, 123–25, 127, 129–35, 140–42, 144, 146, 153–54, 158, 160, 162–68, 173, 179, 181–83
doppelgänger 14, 121, 125, 127, 129–30, 138, 141, 154, 156, 158, 165, 167–68, 176, 178–79, 184
Dora (pseudonym for Ida Bauer) 48, 51, 54–55, 58, 78, 93, 116, 124, 131, 178
Durieux, Tilla 14, 74, 91
Duse, Eleonora 131

Effenberger, Hans 138–39
Elektra 14, 75, 78–81, 91–99, 102–03, 117 n11, 131; *Elektra* (play) by Hugo von Hofmannsthal and Max Reinhardt 14, 75, 78–80, 92–93, 102–03, 131; *Elektra* (opera) by Richard Strauss and Hugo von Hofmannsthal 78, 81, 91–99, 117 n11; Anna Bahr-Mildenburg in *Elektra* (photographs) 94–95; Annie Krull in *Elektra* (photograph) 96; Maria Gärtner in *Elektra* (photograph) 97
Ernst, Max 153
Eulenburg, Albert 77
expressionism, Viennese 2, 9, 12–13, 17, 19–26, 29–32, 36–38, 45, 50, 60, 66, 116, 142, 153, 160, 168, 170, 183; expressionism, German 21–25, 37; *see also* Hermann Bahr; Paul Fechter; Oskar Kokoschka; Egon Schiele; Wilhelm Worringer
Eysoldt, Gertrud 14, 74–76, 78–79, 81, 84 n45, 91, 93, 97

Fackel, Die (*The Torch*, newspaper) 18
Falret, Jules 66–68
Fechter, Paul: *Der Expressionismus* (*Expressionism*, book) 13, 19, 22–23, 37
femme fatale 13, 38, 43, 47, 51–52, 56–60, 67, 75–79, 84 n45, 92–95, 99, 102, 104–08, 110–15, 119 n34, 124, 127, 133, 138, 156–61, 183
Ferdinand, Franz (Archduke of Austria-Hungary) 12, 17–18, 26, 36, 74
Fledermaus, Cabaret 14, 78, 91–92, 112–13, 123, 154–55, 158–59, 162, 169; *Poster for the Cabaret Fledermaus* by Josef von Divéky 113
Fleischer, Mary 171
Foucault, Michel 50, 52, 63 n33
Franzos, Lotte 17–18, 26; *Portrait of Lotte Franzos* (painting) by Oskar Kokoschka 17, 44, 59–60, 88, 167
Freud, Sigmund 4, 9, 12–13, 38, 43–51, 53–58, 60–61, 66, 68, 78–79, 91, 93, 99, 102–03, 110, 115–16, 123–25, 127,
131, 153–55, 167–68, 178; *Allgemeines über den hysterischen Anfall* (*General Remarks on Hysterical Attacks*, essay) 54–55; *Dora* (case study) 48, 54, 116; *Drei Abhandlungen zur Sexualtheorie* (*Three Essays on the Theory of Sexuality*, essays) 38, 54; *Hysterische Phantasien und ihre Beziehung zur Bisexualität* (*Hysterical Fantasies and Their Relation to Bisexuality*, essay) 54, 56; *Die Traumdeutung* (*Interpretation of Dreams*, book) 65 n63, 79; *Studien über Hysterie* (*Studies on Hysteria* (book, with Josef Breuer) 13, 46–48, 50, 54–56, 99; *Das Unheimliche* (*The Uncanny*, essay) 124–25, 127, 167–68; *Zur Ätiologie der Hysterie* (*The Etiology of Hysteria*, book) 46
Fuller, Loïe 110–11

Gärtner, Maria 97–99, 103; Maria Gärtner in *Elektra* (photograph) 97
Gallagher, Catherine 4
Gesamtkunstwerk 91–92, 98, 141, 159
Gesicht(e) 13, 19–20, 22–23, 26, 33, 122; *see also* Vision
Gilman, Sander 92–93
Goethe, Johann Wolfgang von 25
Goldberg, Itzhak 123
Gordon, Rae Beth 67, 69
Gorsen, Peter 164
Greiner, Leo 73
Grüner, Franz 18, 38, 59
Gütersloh, Albert Paris von 4, 14, 144–45, 147, 175; *Egon Schiele* (book) 144–45; *Portrait of Albert Paris von Gütersloh* (painting) by Egon Schiele 90, 144, 146, 176

Hagenbund, Vienna (exhibitions) 17–19, 27, 160
Harrison, Charles Townsend 21, 31
Hartel, Johannes Wilhelm Rittér von (Austrian Minister of Education) 26
Hauptmann, Gerhart 73, 75, 77; *Der arme Heinrich* (*Poor Heinrich*, play) 75; *Kollege Crampton* (play) 73
Henry, Marc (pseudonym for Achille Georges d'Ailly-Vaucheret) 72–73
Hibberd, J. L. 76
historicism, Viennese 30, 45
Höch, Hannah 153
Hodler, Ferdinand 6
Hofen, Franz 72
Hoffmann, E. T. A. 123–25, 127, 139, 168
Hoffmann, Josef 28
Hofmannsthal, Hugo von 12, 14, 74–75, 78–80, 85 n70, 91–95, 97–98, 102–03,

121–22, 130–31, 142–46, 153, 155, 162, 170–71; *Der Brief des Lord Chandos* (*The Letter of Lord Chandos*, essay) 122, 142–43; *Elektra* (play) 14, 75, 78–80, 93–94, 97–98, 102–03, 131, 147 n3; *Das Gerettete Venedig* (*Venice Preserved*, play) 130; *Oedipus Rex* (play) 91, 102–04, 153; *Über die Pantomime* (*On the Pantomime*, essay) 143; *Die unvergleichliche Tänzerin* (*The Incomparable Dancer*, essay) 143, 171

Holland, Norman 116

Huter, Michael 123

Huysmans, Joris-Karl: *À rebours* (*Against Nature*) 106–08

Huyssen, Andreas 122–24, 126–27

hypnotism 48–49, 53, 56, 58, 62 n19, 83 n21, 99, 118 n21, 154–55

hysteria/hysterical bodies 3–4, 9, 10–15, 38, 43–61, 62 n20, 63 n33 & n35, 66–75, 77–81, 91–92, 94–99, 101–08, 110–11, 114–16, 121, 123–24, 127, 129, 131, 146, 153–55, 176, 178, 183–84; *L'arche de pont* (print) by the French School 53; *A Clinical Lesson at the Salpêtrière* (painting) by Pierre Aristide André Brouillet 54; *Hystero-epileptic attack* (drawing) by Jean-François Badoureau 60; *Tétanisme* (photograph) by Paul Régnard 10

hystero-theatrical gestures 4, 11–15, 44, 46–47, 58–61, 66, 71–72, 77, 80–81, 91–92, 95, 99, 103–04, 108, 121–23, 153–54, 158, 171, 176, 183

Ibsen, Henrik 73, 75, 77, 84 n46

Iconographie photographique de la Salpêtrière (*Photographic Iconography of the Salpêtrière*, medical journal) 9, 49–55, 55, 57, 59, 67; *see also* Jean-Martin Charcot

Illustrirte Zeitung (*Illustrated Newspaper*) 96

Isolde 6–7, 14, 37, 88, 91–92, 98–105, 108, 115; *Der Liebestrank–Tristan und Isolde* (*The Love Potion–Tristan and Isolde*, painting) by Koloman Moser 6–7, 37, 88, 98–99, 102, 104–05; *Tristan and Isolde* (opera) by Richard Wagner 6, 91, 98–101, 103–05; Anna Bahr-Mildenburg in *Tristan and Isolde* (photograph) 100; Costume design for *Tristan and Isolde* by Alfred Roller (drawing) 101

Japanese woodblock prints 160

Javanese puppet theater 135–36, 138–39, 150 n59, 153, 169–71, 178–79; *see also* shadow puppet theater

Jelavich, Peter 162–63

Jensen, Robert 24, 39 n15

Jentsch, Ernst 124–25, 129, 167–68; *see also* uncanny

Jews/Jewish 54–55, 92–93, 103, 111, 113–14, 117 n5, 154; *see also* anti-Semitism

Jugendstil 30, 33, 36, 170; *see also* art nouveau

Jung, Carl 102

Jung Wien (Young Vienna) 27–28, 33, 44, 78, 158

Kallir, Jane 9, 111–12

Kandel, Eric 12

Kandinsky, Wassily 2–4, 13, 19, 22, 25, 37, 40 n32; *Untitled* (drawing) 2–3; *Über die Formfrage* (*On the Question of Form*, essay) 25; *Über das Geistige in der Kunst* (*Concerning the Spiritual in Art*, essay) 25

Kasperletheater 138

Kawalec, Urszula 154

Kelley, Susanne 111–12

Kerr, Alfred 79–80

Kleines Theater (Little Theater) 73–75, 78, 92, 94, 108, 158

Kleist, Heinrich von 14, 125–28, 130, 133, 139, 168

Klimt, Gustav 1–2, 6–9, 13, 24, 26–32, 35–36, 38, 43–45, 59, 89, 92, 108, 111–15, 123, 129, 136, 144, 159–60, 170–71, 176; *Adele Bloch-Bauer I* (painting) 1–2; *Fakultätsbilder* (*Faculty Paintings*) 6–9, 26–28, 114, 123, 129; *Judith I* (painting) 89, 111–15, 160, 176; *Judith II (Salome)* (painting) 28–29, 43, 59, 114–15; *Medicine* (painting) 6, 8–9, 26, 43, 59, 114; *Philosophy* (painting) 6, 7, 9, 26, 43, 114; *Stoclet Frieze* (painting) 171

Klimtgruppe (Klimt Group) 28, 31–32, 44

Klinger, Max 108

Klosterneuburg 32

Kokoschka, Oskar 4–7, 9, 11–15, 16 n16, 17–33, 35, 37–38, 40 n32, 43–44, 59, 74, 87–88, 116, 121–23, 129, 131, 142, 144, 146–47, 153–55, 158–70, 173, 175, 180, 183–84; *Die Erwachenden* (*The Awakening*) from *Die Träumenden Knaben* (*The Dreaming Youths*, lithograph) 29–31, 35, 159–62, 165, 173, 180; *Das getupfte Ei* (*The Speckled Egg*, puppet play) 159, 162, 169; *Frau in Blau* (*Woman in Blue*, painting) 164–66, 168; *Mann mit Puppe* (*Man with Doll*, painting) 164–65, 167–68; *Mörder, Hoffnung der Frauen* (*Murderer, Hope of Women*, play) 159; *Portrait of Lotte Franzos* (painting) 17, 44, 59, 88, 167; *Sitzende "Frau" mit entblößten*

Brüsten (*Seated "Woman" with Exposed Breasts*, drawing) 164, 166; *Sphinx und Strohmann* (*Sphinx and Scarecrow*, play) 159–61, 184 n3; *Von der Natur der Gesichte* (*On the Nature of Visions*, essay) 13, 19–26, 32; *Der Weisse Tiertöter* (*The White Animal Slayer*, puppet play) 162

Krafft-Ebing, Richard von 57–58, 65 n74; *Hypnotische Experimente* (*Hypnotic Experiments*, book) 58; *Über gesunde und kranke Nerven* (*On Healthy and Diseased Nerves*, book) 57; Purkersdorf Sanatorium 58

Kramer, Lawrence 92–93

Kraus, Karl 18

Krull, Annie 96–99, 103; Annie Krull in *Elektra* (photograph) 96

Kunst, Die (*Art*, journal) 111

Kunstschau, Vienna (exhibitions) 28–29, 33, 35, 114, 135, 159

Laqueur, Thomas 4

Lenman, Robin 112

Lichtenstein, Thérèse 67

Loos, Adolf 16 n16, 31, 35

Mahler, Alma 163, 165, 186 n43; Alma doll 164–68; *Oskar Kokoschka's Alma-Puppe as Venus* (photograph) 163

Mahler, Gustav 91, 99, 163, 186 n43

Makart, Hans 5

Mallarmé, Stéphane 111

Man, Paul de 126–28

Mandu, Moa 175; Erwin Osen and the dancer Moa (photograph) 175

Marc, Franz 25

Marinis, Marco de 68

marionette/marionette theater 6, 11, 14–15, 29, 35, 116–17, 121–23, 125–32, 134–36, 138–42, 144, 147, 153–56, 158–60, 162–63, 167–69, 172–73, 175–76, 178–79, 182–83; *Marionetten* (*Marionettes*, essay) by Hermann Bahr 127, 142; *Über das Marionettentheater* (*On the Marionette Theater* (essay) by Heinrich von Kleist 125–28, 168; *see also* Oskar Kokoschka; Rainer Maria Rilke; Arthur Schnitzler; Richard Teschner

Matisse, Henri 45

McCarren, Felicia 110–11

mesmerism: *see* hypnotism

Micale, Mark 51, 67

Michel, Wilhelm 132–33

Mirliton, Le (The Reed Pipe, cabaret) 163

Modekrankheit 13, 43, 60, 61 n3, 77, 80–81, 93, 98, 101, 108, 111, 114, 118 n27, 131, 146, 168, 176, 183

Moissi, Alexander 102–04; Alexander Moissi in *Oedipus Rex* (photograph) 102

Moos, Hermine 164–65

Moreau, Gustave: *L'Apparition* (*The Apparition*, painting) 106–08

Moser, Koloman 4, 6–7, 11, 28, 32, 37–38, 88, 92, 98–105, 131; *Der Liebestrank– Tristan und Isolde* (*The Love Potion— Tristan and Isolde*, painting) 6–7, 37–38, 88, 98–105

Munch, Edvard 108

Munich Secession 108

Neue Deutsche Rundschau (*New German Review*, journal) 79–80

Neue Preußische Zeitung (*New Prussian Newspaper*) 80

Neues Wiener Journal (*New Vienna Journal*) 93

Neukunstgruppe (New Art Group) 32, 144, 170, 175

Nietzsche, Friedrich 98, 127, 148 n27, 188 n67

Oedipus Rex (play) 91, 102–04, 153

opera 6–7, 11, 80–81, 91–100, 104–05, 108, 114–15, 117, 125, 153; Vienna Opera 81, 93–94, 96–99

Oppenheimer, Max 108, 122

Osen, Erwin 11, 171, 173–76, 178; *Erwin Dominik Osen* (drawing) by Egon Schiele 173–76; *Mime van Osen* (drawing) by Egon Schiele 173–76, 178; Erwin Osen and the dancer Moa (photograph) by unknown artist 175

Ostini, Fritz von 111

Pelizzon, V. Penelope 52

Picasso, Pablo 1–2, 4; *Les Demoiselles d'Avignon* (painting) 1–2

Piegl, Fräulein Cl. 58

Pisko, Kunstsalon 32

Politzer, Heinz 79, 95

Prange, Ernst: *Kain* (play) 73, 75

Prater (amusement park) 138

Pre-Raphaelite Brotherhood 30, 98

Pritzel, Lotte 131–34, 141, 144, 164; *Puppen für die Vitrine* (*Puppets for the Cabinet*, photograph) 134

psychoanalysis: *see* Sigmund Freud

psychology 9, 14, 31, 44, 48, 73, 116, 124, 133, 155, 158

Puppe: see doll; marionette/marionette theater; puppet/puppet theater

Puppenspieler motif: *see* Arthur Schnitzler

puppet/puppet theater 3, 5–6, 11–12, 14–15, 29, 35, 37, 108, 116–17, 121–42, 144–47, 153–65, 167–73, 175–76, 178–84, 185 n19, 186 n37; Asian puppetry 135, 138, 162; Javanese/Indonesian puppets 135–36, 138–39, 150 n59, 153, 169–71, 178–79; *Puppen* (*Puppets*, essay) by Rainer Maria Rilke 127, 131–32; *Puppen für die Vitrine* (*Puppets for the Cabinet*) by Lotte Pritzel; 134; *see also* Oskar Kokoschka; Egon Schiele; Arthur Schnitzler; Richard Teschner

Purkersdorf Sanatorium 58

Régnard, Paul 49, 53, 55; *Tétanisme* (photograph) 10
Reichel, Dr. Oskar 36
Reinhardt, Max 14, 74–78, 80–81, 91–94, 102–03, 108, 130–31, 171; *Elektra* (play) 75, 78–81, 92–94, 102–03, 131; *Erdgeist* (*Earth Spirit*, play) 75–77, 81; *Oedipus Rex* (play) 91, 102–03; *Salome* (play) 74–75, 92, 108, 131, 171
Revue franco-allemande/Deutsch-französische Rundschau (*French-German Review/ German-French Review*, journal) 72–73
Richet, Charles 118 n21
Rilke, Rainer Maria 14, 73, 122, 125–34, 143, 148 n20, 149 n29, 164; *Duineser Elegien* (*The Duino Elegies*, poems) 125, 127–30; *Puppen* (*Puppets*, essay) 127, 131–32
Rivière, Henri 163
Roessler, Arthur 33, 140, 153, 169–71; *Erinnerungen an Egon Schiele* (*Memories of Egon Schiele*, book) 170; *Richard Teschner* (book) 169; Arthur Roessler's study (photograph) 169
Roller, Alfred 91, 97, 99–101, 136; Costume design for *Tristan and Isolde* by Alfred Roller (drawing) 101
Roos, Bonnie 164, 167

Salis, Rodolphe 163
Salome 14, 28–29, 43, 59, 73–81, 83 n36 & n37, 91–93, 103–15, 117 n5, 119 n34 & n41, 131, 171; *L'Apparition* (*The Apparition*, painting) by Gustave Moreau 106–08; *Dancing Salome* (painting) by Franz von Stuck 108–09, 111, 119 n41, 120 n50; *Judith II* (*Salome*) (painting) by Gustav Klimt 28–29, 43, 59, 114–15; *Salome* (painting) by Franz von Stuck 108–09, 111, 119 n41, 120 n50; *Salome* (opera) by Richard Strauss 80, 92–93; *Salomé* (play) by Oscar Wilde 14, 73–74, 83 n36 & n37, 107, 171; *Salome* (production) by Max Reinhardt 74–78, 81, 103, 131, 171; *The Vision of Salomé* (play) by Maud Allan 91,

108, 110–11, 171; Maud Allan as Salome (photograph) 110
Salpêtrière Hospital: *see* Jean-Martin Charcot; *L'arche de pont* (print) by the French School 53; *A Clinical Lesson at the Salpêtrière* (painting) by Pierre Aristide André Brouillet 54; *Hystero-epileptic attack* (drawing) by Jean-François Badoureau 60; *Tétanisme* (photograph) by Paul Régnard 10
Sandmann, Der (*The Sandman*, short story): *see* E. T. A. Hoffmann
Schaumberg, Georg 73
Schiele, Egon 4, 6–7, 9–15, 19, 24, 28, 31–38, 43–45, 59, 87, 89–90, 92, 103–05, 123, 129, 131, 144–47, 153–54, 163, 168–84; *Aktselbstbildnis* (*Nude Self-Portrait*, drawing) 6, 37, 45, 59, 87, 176, 178; *Empfindung* (*Sensation*, poem) 36–37; *Entschwebung* (*Die Blinden II*) (*Levitation* (*The Blind II*), painting) 177–78, 182; *Die Eremiten* (*The Hermits*, painting) 35–36, 59, 176; *Erwin Dominik Osen* (drawing) 173–76; *Frau mit blauem Haar* (*Woman with Blue Hair*, drawing) 103–05; *Frauenpaar* (*Two Women Embracing* (*Two Friends*), drawing) 180–83; *Mime van Osen* (drawing) 173–76, 178; *Nude Pregnant Woman Reclining* (drawing) 10, 59; *Das Porträt des Stillbleichen Mädchens* (*Portrait of a Silent Pale Girl*, poem) 34; *Portrait of Albert Paris von Gütersloh* (painting) 90, 144–46, 176; *Prediger* (*Selbstakt mit blaugrünem Hemd*) (*Preacher* (*Nude Self-Portrait with Blue-green Shirt*), drawing) 179; *Sitzender Frauenakt mit geneigtem Kopf und erhobenen Armen* (*Seated Female Nude with Tilted Head and Raised Arms*, drawing) 34–35, 44, 89, 173, 175; *Selbstbildnis mit schwarzem Tongefäß und gespreizten Fingern* (*Self-Portrait with Black Vase and Spread Fingers*, painting) 176–78; *Selbstbildnis mit erhobenen Ellenbogen* (*Self-Portrait in Jerkin with Right Elbow Raised*, drawing) 179–81; *Selbstportrait als heiliger Sebastian* (*Self-Portrait as Saint Sebastian*, drawing) 171–73; *Selbstdarstellung mit gestreiften Ärmelschonern* (*Self-Portrait with Striped Armlets*, drawing) 179–80; *Versinkende Sonne* (*Setting Sun*, painting) 169; *Visionen* (*Visions*, poem) 33–34, 36; *Zwei Mädchen, in verschränkter Stellung liegend* (*Two Girls, Lying in an Entwined Position*, drawing) 90, 180–83

Schlemmer, Oskar 153
Schnitzler, Arthur 12, 15, 78, 122,
    147, 154–60, 163, 167, 185 n9 &
    n19; *Anatol* (play) 155; *Marionetten*
    (*Marionettes* trilogy) 155, 158, 167;
    Der Puppenspieler (*The Puppet Master*,
    puppet play) 155; *Paracelsus* (play) 155;
    Reigen (*Roundelay*, play) 154; *Der tapfere*
    Cassian (*The Gallant Cassian*, puppet
    play) 155–58; *Traumnovelle* (*Dream*
    Story, novella) 154; *Die Verwandlungen*
    des Pierrot (*The Metamorphoses of*
    Pierrot, play) 155; *Zum großen Wurstel*
    (*The Great Prater Puppet Theater*, puppet
    play) 155–56, 159
Schorske, Carl 8, 11, 25, 44
Schreder, Karl 18, 27, 38, 59
Schröder, Klaus Albrecht 9, 63 n42, 67
Schwabinger Schattenspiele (Schwabing
    Shadow Theater) 163
Scott, Jill 78, 86 n71, 93, 147 n3
Secession, Vienna 4, 6, 13, 24, 26, 28, 30–33,
    36, 38, 44, 46, 91–92, 97–99, 105, 123,
    153, 158, 170
Secessionstil/Secessionists: *see* Secession
Segel, Harold 73, 131, 155, 162–63,
    184 n4
Selz, Peter 39 n3 & n14
Sembach, Johannes 96–97; Johannes
    Sembach in *Elektra* (photograph) 96
Semperoper, Dresden (Dresden State
    Opera) 93
Servaes, Franz 139
Seshadri, Anne 93
shadow puppet theater 136, 153, 159,
    162–63, 169–71
Shershow, Scott 129, 162
Sine, Nadine 111
sleepwalking/sleepwalker 6, 98–100, 103,
    107–08
Smith, Kimberly 32, 118 n27, 147 n3
somnambulism/somnambulist 6–7, 69,
    99–100, 102–03, 118 n21 & n22; *see also*
    sleepwalking
Sonne, Otto 96
Sophocles 78–79, 102
St. Denis, Ruth 91, 143, 170–71
Stein, Erwin 93, 96
Steiner, Reinhard 9, 61 n7, 67, 188 n67
Steinhof Hospital 11, 175
Strauss, Richard 74, 78, 80–81, 91–98, 108,
    114; *Elektra* (opera) 78, 81, 91–98, 114;
    Salome (opera) 80, 92–93, 108, 114
Street, Lisa 164
Strzygowski, Josef 17–18, 38
Stuck, Franz von: *Dancing Salome* (painting)
    108–09, 111, 119 n41, 120 n50 & n56;

Salome (painting) 108–09, 111, 119 n41,
    120 n50 & n56
Stümcke, Heinrich 74–77, 83 n25
Sturm, Der (*The Storm*, journal) 159
surrealism 146, 153

Teschner, Richard 134–42, 144, 150 n59
    & n61, 153, 155, 158–59, 162–63, 169,
    175; Figurenspiegel (Figure Mirror, puppet
    stage) 136–37, 141; Der goldener Schrein
    (Golden Shrine, puppet stage) 136–37,
    140, 162; *Kusomos Opfertod* (*Kusomo's*
    Sacrifice, puppet play) 138; *Nabi Isa*
    (*The Prophet Jesus*, puppet play) 138;
    Nachstück (*Night Play*, puppet play) 139;
    Nawang Wulan (puppet play) 138–140;
    Prinzessin und Wassermann (*Princess and*
    Water Elf, puppet play) 139–41; Richard
    Teschner's *Figure Mirror* (photograph)
    137; Richard Teschner's *Golden Shrine*
    (photograph) 137; Scene from Richard
    Teschner's *Nawang Wulan* (photograph)
    138; Scenes from Richard Teschner's
    Princess and Water Elf (photographs)
    140–41
theater/dramatic arts 3, 5, 8–9, 11–15, 22–23,
    43–44, 46, 51, 58–61, 66–81, 82 n8,
    91–92, 94, 98–99, 101–03, 105, 107–08,
    115–16, 121–31, 133–36, 138–42, 147,
    153–56, 158–63, 168–70, 175–76, 184; *see*
    also marionette/marionette theater; puppet/
    puppet theater
Theater an der Wien 72
Tietze, Hans, and Erica Tietze-Conrat: *Hans*
    Tietze and Erica Tietze-Conrat (painting)
    by Oskar Kokoschka 5–7, 37, 87, 146–47,
    165, 183
Tillis, Steve 129–30, 165
Topp, Leslie 9, 44, 57, 60
Toulouse-Lautrec, Henri de: *Jane Avril*
    Dancing (painting) 71
Tourette, Gilles de la 99, 118 n22
Trčka, Anton Josef: Photograph of Egon
    Schiele (photograph) 172–73
Tristan and Isolde (opera) 91, 98–101,
    103–04; *Der Liebestrank–Tristan und*
    Isolde (*The Love Potion—Tristan and*
    Isolde, painting) by Koloman Moser 6–7,
    37–38, 88, 98–105
Tzara, Tristan 153

Über das Marionettentheater (*On the*
    Marionette Theater, essay): *see* Heinrich
    von Kleist
uncanny (concept of) 13, 14, 53, 80, 124–25,
    127, 129, 132, 141–42, 153–54, 158, 161,
    165–68; *Das Unheimliche* (*The Uncanny*,

essay) by Sigmund Freud 124–25, 127, 167–68; *Zur Psychologie des Unheimlichen* (*On the Psychology of the Uncanny*, essay) by Ernst Jentsch 124–25, 167–68
University of Vienna 6, 11, 26, 44, 59, 154

Viennese modern body 1, 3–6, 8, 11–12, 19, 25, 29, 31, 37, 98–99, 104, 111, 114–15, 123, 168, 183–84
vision(s) 4, 12–13, 15, 17–38, 43–44, 46–48, 55, 57–58, 61, 72, 77, 92, 99, 116, 122–24, 130, 142–44, 146, 154, 165–66, 168, 176, 178, 181, 183–84
vision dialectic 13, 19–20, 23–27, 31, 33, 36–37, 43, 116, 122, 130, 142, 146, 183–84; *see also* Oskar Kokoschka

Wagner, Richard: *Tristan and Isolde* (opera) 6, 91, 98–101, 104–05, 118 n18 & n20
Warlick, Marjorie 171
wayang puppets 135–36, 138–40, 169–71, 175, 178; wayang golek puppets (photograph) 135; wayang kulit shadow puppets (photograph) 136
Wedekind, Frank 14, 75–77, 110, 160; *Erdgeist* (*Earth Spirit*, play) 14, 75–77; *Lulu* plays 75; *Spring Awakening* (play) 160
Weininger, Otto 114, 133

Weissen Blätter, Die (*The White Pages*, journal) 131
Werkner, Patrick 9, 168, 171
Whalen, Robert 162
Wiener Arbeiterzeitung (*Vienna Workers Newspaper*) 169
Wiener Hofoper (Vienna Court Opera): *see* opera
Wiener Kunstgewerbeschule (Vienna School of Arts and Crafts) 32, 158
Wiener Werkstätte (Viennese Workshops) 6, 32, 91–92, 98–99, 135, 159
Wiesenthal, Grete 143
Wilde, Oscar: *Salomé* (play) 14, 73–74, 83 n36 & n37, 107, 171; *see also* Salome
Wölfflin, Heinrich 24, 40 n23
Worringer, Wilhelm 13, 19–25, 33, 37, 116–17, 138; *Abstraktion und Einfühlung* (*Abstraction and Empathy*, book) 21–25, 139
Wright, Alastair 45
Wursteltheater: *see* Prater

Yates, W. E. 72, 92

Zeit, Die (*The Times*, newspaper) 17
Zirkus Busch 102
Zirkus Schumann 102
Zweig, Stefan 78

T - #0522 - 071024 - C4 - 246/174/10 - PB - 9780367736187 - Gloss Lamination